The Heart and Science of Yoga

A Blueprint for Peace, Happiness and Freedom from Fear

"A true work of art that explains the transformational power of classical yoga science in clear and practical terms. A manual for creatively meeting the challenges of everyday life."
LILIAS FOLAN
Author and host of the groundbreaking PBS yoga series, *Lilias!*

"A comprehensive and practical guide to the yogic practices as tools for transformation."
DEAN ORNISH, MD
Founder, president, and director of the Preventive Medicine Research Institute and author of *Dr. Dean Ornish's Program for Reversing Heart Disease*

"Comprehensively outlines the holistic benefits of yoga and brought joy to this heart surgeon's heart."
MEHMET OZ, MD
Vice-chairman, Department of Surgery, Professor of Surgery, Columbia University

"An all-inclusive manual of safe, effective practices for achieving optimal wellness and longevity. An encyclopedic resource for experiencing the healing connection between mind, body and spirit."
DR. ABBAS QUTAB, Ayurvedic physician
Author and founder of Élan Vital Medical Center and Spa, Worcester, Massachusetts

"An admirable guide to one of the world's greatest wisdom traditions. This excellent book presents not only yoga techniques but also the philosophy behind them."
LARRY DOSSEY, MD
Author of *Healing Beyond the Body, Reinventing Medicine* and *Healing Words*

"This important teaching faithfully interprets the wisdom of the ancient yoga masters and is a great service to humanity. A powerful tool for spiritual growth."
ACHARYA SIVAGURU: K.S. DIXITAR
Sivaguru Ashram, Paulsboro, NJ and Hindu Temple Society, Albany, NY

"A very basic yet truly profound offering—a feast for the soul."
LINDA JOHNSEN, author of *A Thousand Suns*

"The Heart and Science of Yoga introduces us to yoga as an essential part of daily life. Leonard inspires us to be passionate about yoga…and he practices what he preaches! Read it yourself and see!"
RADU TEODORESCU
Owner of Radu Physical Culture, author of *Kid Fitness* and *Radu's Simply Fit*

"A magnificent interpretation of the science of yoga through the heart. Only selfless, daily practitioners of the art and science can deliver writing with this clarity. A must for every seeker as a daily reference and aid to practice."
HORST M. RECHELBACHER
Founder of Aveda and Intelligent Nutrients

"An in-depth and stimulating examination of yoga in its many dimensions of body, mind and consciousness, The Heart and Science of Yoga is bound to take your yoga practice into new realms of life transformation."
DR. DAVID FRAWLEY
Author of *Yoga* and *Ayurveda* and *Yoga and the Sacred Fire*

The Heart
and Science
of Yoga

*A Blueprint for Peace, Happiness
and Freedom from Fear*

LEONARD PERLMUTTER
with Jenness Cortez Perlmutter

Foreword by
Linda Johnsen

AMI Publishers
Averill Park, New York 12018

AMI Publishers

PO Box 430, Averill Park, New York 12018, Tel. (518) 674-8714 or (800) 234-5115

www.amipublishers.org   info@amipublishers.org

The American Meditation Institute, Inc.

Averill Park, New York, Tel. (518) 674-8714 or (800) 234-5115

www.americanmeditation.org

The paper used in this book meets the minimum requirements of the American National Standard for Information Sciences—Permanence of Paper for Printed Library Materials, ANSI Z39.48-1984.

Printed in the United States of America

Cover Designs by Foster and Foster

LIMIT OF LIABILITY/DISCLAIMER OF WARRANTY:

This is not a medical text, but a compendium of remarks concerning how yoga science and philosophy can correlate to physical, mental and emotional well-being. Any medical questions regarding whether or not to proceed with particular practices or postures should be referred to a health professional. The accuracy and completeness of the information provided and the opinions stated herein are not guaranteed or warranted to produce any particular results, and the advice and practices contained herein may not be suitable for every individual. The publisher and the author disclaim any specific or implied warranties of fitness for a particular purpose. There are no warranties that extend beyond the descriptions contained in this paragraph. Neither the publisher nor author shall be liable for any loss of profit or any other personal or commercial damages, including but not limited to special, incidental, consequential, or other damages.

Acknowledgements on the last page constitute an extension of the copyright page.

Library of Congress Cataloging-in-Publication Data

Perlmutter, Leonard T.
    The heart and science of yoga : a blueprint for peace, happiness and freedom from fear / Leonard Perlmutter with Jenness Cortez Perlmutter ; foreword by Linda Johnsen.
        p. cm.
    Includes bibliographical references and index.
    ISBN 0-9753752-8-8 (alk. paper)
    1. Yoga. I. Perlmutter, Jenness Cortez. II. Title.

B132.Y6P395 2005
181'.45--dc22

                                                                                2005004130

10 9 8 7 6 5 4 2 1 First Edition, 2005

Dedication

With humility, love and respect, we dedicate this book to the One Creative Spirit of every tradition and to our most revered teacher, Shri Swami Rama of the Himalayas, the blessed emissary whose teachings continue to reflect the Light of intuitive wisdom.

Table of Contents

Part II—YOGA SCIENCE

Part III—MANTRA SCIENCE

Part IV—MEDITATION

CHAPTER 15

CHAPTER 16

Part VI—DEEPENING YOUR PRACTICE

Part VII—POWER OF BREATH

Part VIII—POWER OF THE MIND

Part IX—AYURVEDA

Acknowledgements

We gratefully acknowledge the love and teachings of our families: Clara and Julius Perlmutter, Frances and Jesse Northerner, Charles Caplan, Carol Hershkowitz, Lee Ellen Slabach and Jed Northerner.

We humbly thank the following teachers who have inspired and clarified our understanding: Jesus the Christ, Shri Eknath Easwaran, Adi Shankara, Patanjali, Moses, Arjuna, Shri Krishna, Compassionate Buddha, Swami Dhyananda Saraswati, Paramahansa Yogananda, Shri Yukteswar, Lahiri Mahasaya, Babaji, Nisargadatta Maharaj, Ramana Maharshi, Ramesh Balsekar, Jean Klein, Mohandas K. Gandhi, Swami Rama Tirtha, Swami Pranananda, Ashtavakra, King Janaka, Bengali Baba, Swami Veda Bharati, Swami Hariharananda, Swami Nijananda, Swami Ajaya, Pandit Rajmani Tigunait, Ramakrishna, Sarada Devi, Swami Shivananda, Swami Vivekananda, Swami Abhedananda, Swami Prabdhavananda, Meher Baba, Alan Watts, Teilhard de Chardin, Dr. David Frawley, Dr. Deepak Chopra, Maharishi Mahesh Yogi, Nachiketa, Lord Yama, St. Francis of Assisi, St. Paul, Abraham, David the Shepherd, Isaac, Solomon, the Talmudists, Muhammad, Teresa of Avila, Mother Teresa, Thomas Jefferson, James Madison, Abraham Lincoln, Martin Luther King, Black Elk, Meister Eckhart, William Shakespeare, Ralph Waldo Emerson, Henry David Thoreau, Antonius Raemaekers,

Mangala Sugandhi, Hanumappa Visweswaraiah, M.D., Pandit Shiva Guru Dixitar and Elvis Aron Presley.

We thank our generous patrons John and Sandy Smith, Nataraja and Arul Balasubramanian, M.D.s and Kathleen and George McNamee.

We express our deep appreciation to our beloved secretary Elaine Peterson, AMI retreat coordinator Robert J. Washington and our entire Board of Directors (past and present) for their tireless service.

Completing this manuscript has required a great deal of professional assistance. We respectfully thank Linda Johnsen for her meticulous editing and gracious foreword, Dr. Abbas Qutab for his thorough review of the Ayurveda material, Dr. David Coulter for his technical expertise in book publishing and George Foster for his keen eye in assisting with our cover designs.

To Dr. K. Scott Christianson, Dr. Sanjay Kumar, Jan Wohl, Laurie Rosin, Kim Smithgall, Mike Swertinski, Mike Cassidy and the entire staff of Tech Valley Printing Company in Watervliet, New York, we extend our gratitude for their contributions to this book.

We also thank Mary Balsam, Donna Bunker-Panzl, Anita Burock, M.D., Kathie Carroll, Leslie Fallon, Kimberly Funck, Jeanne Laiacona, Anita Patka, Carl Patka, Jim Whiting, Mari Selby and Nancy Kahan for their dedication and creativity in bringing this book to publication.

Last, but not least, we are eternally grateful for the profound lessons taught to us by the courageous seekers we have been privileged to teach and to serve.

Special Notes

ॐ

Whenever you encounter the OM symbol in the text, please pause. Take a few moments for quiet contemplation and to assimilate the meaning of what has been presented before continuing your reading.

Italic Usage

Please note that Sanskrit words and names of practices are printed in italic to enhance your familiarity with them.

Capitalizations

Certain words are capitalized to denote that they refer to the Divine Reality.

Foreword

It wasn't what I'd expected. I'd spoken at many yoga centers before; they were often large, empty rooms where students could unroll their hatha mats and launch into a series of stretches and twists imported from India. When I'd show up to lecture, folding chairs would materialize from hidden closets and an audience would listlessly filter in from the dirty city streets.

The American Meditation Institute, it turned out, was more like a beautiful estate than a yoga business. The grounds were magnificent, colored with an astonishing array of flowers and flowering shrubs. A sparkling pond brimming with minnows and a small, man-made waterfall interrupted the rolling green lawn. This oasis twenty minutes outside Albany, New York was a paradise of tranquility and fragrant blossoms.

The *AMI* building was friendly and clean, scented with the inviting aroma of vegetarian cooking and filled with co-founder Jenness Cortez Perlmutter's paintings of country landscapes, scenes from Indian mythology and especially— everywhere—horses. Jenness herself was tall and lean, exuding both warmth and intelligence. Her husband and fellow *AMI* founder Leonard Perlmutter had a thick beard that made him look like an Indian *baba* who'd just come down out of the Himalayas after years of meditation. He appeared very serious but the moment he began to speak, not only his vast knowledge of the world's mystical traditions but also his totally disarming sense of humor were immediately evident.

I didn't for a moment feel I was visiting a yoga "institute." Len and Jen made all of us at the seminar feel like family. Their emphasis on yoga as a preeminently practical form of spiritual discipline kept their teaching very real, grounded and relevant to their students' everyday lives.

The Perlmutters are students of Swami Rama of the Himalayas, the yogi who revolutionized our understanding of human physiology back in the 1970s. Before Swami Rama allowed researchers at the Menninger Institute in Topeka, Kansas to hook him up to their EEGs, EKGs and temperature monitors, Western scientists had never believed India's yogis could do what the Indians always claimed they could, controlling every component of their physical bodies to the extent that they could appear virtually lifeless according to the electronic printouts, yet remain fully conscious. The swami repeatedly demonstrated full mastery of his autonomic nervous system, which until then most Western doctors had assumed was impossible.

I studied with Swami Rama for some years when he founded a graduate program in Eastern Studies here in the United States in the 1980s. Swamiji complained that the experiments the researchers conducted at Menninger were comparatively trivial. The real value of yoga lay not so much in stopping one's heartbeat or regulating the temperature in individual cells in his body (skills he actually demonstrated there) but in its deep and transforming effect on human consciousness. That, unfortunately, the scientists didn't know how to measure.

Swami Rama left his body permanently in November, 1996. He died like a yogi, having announced the exact moment of his departure earlier that day. He sat up in a yoga posture and, in full consciousness, vacated the body we'd come to love so well. He taught us how to live and, in his final moments, showed us how to die.

Swami Rama's work lives on through the efforts of his

students. Swamiji strongly encouraged the Perlmutters to teach. His blessings have transformed their originally modest home into one of the finest yoga centers in North America. *The Heart and Science of Yoga* is the story of yoga as they live it, in the vibrant tradition of Swami Rama of the Himalayas.

Linda Johnsen
Sonoma, California

Part I
YOGA PHILOSOPHY

Introduction

There is no path to peace. The path is peace.

THICH NHAT HAHN

The realization of peace, happiness and freedom from fear begins with the recognition that you are a citizen of two worlds. Clearly, you are a citizen of the ever-changing material world of animal, vegetable and mineral matter. In this familiar environment, the body is your vehicle for action and your mind is your most powerful instrument for evaluating circumstances and motivating your body into action. For every action your body-mind-sense complex takes, a consequence results.

You are also a citizen of the distinctly non-material, yet profoundly real world of consciousness. Within this subtle world exists an intuitive library of knowledge that unerringly identifies which of your possible actions will lead you to realize peace, happiness and freedom from fear and which will lead to physical, mental, emotional and spiritual dis-ease.

When, as a citizen of the material world, your outer actions reflect the perfection of your inner, subtle wisdom, you will be led for your highest and greatest good. The choice to base your outer action on your own inner wisdom is the essence of all forms of yoga. Yoga means union, and the heart and science of yoga provides a reliable blueprint for building a trustworthy, ever-accessible bridge to your own inner wisdom.

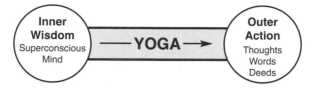

Yoga means union. It represents a bridge between inner wisdom and outer actions. When your outer actions are based on your inner wisdom, you are always led for your highest and greatest good and there is no cause for worry.

Yoga science is a very practical tool that can be applied easily in every circumstance and relationship. By employing this blueprint you will learn to deal confidently and skillfully with common, everyday situations. Take worrying for example.

To one extent or another, we all worry. If the truth were known, most of us squander a tremendous amount of creative energy attending to notions of what the future might or might not hold. Just as Gulliver was hopelessly bound by the Lilliputians' slender threads, many of us are held captive by habitual thoughts generated from our own fertile imaginations.

How alluring that unending train of hypothetical "what if" situations can be! "What if this should happen? Oh, dear, what if that should happen? And what if neither happens?" So much of life is spent imagining things that never were and never will be. Because of all our concerns, we often can't even get a good night's sleep. And the more attention we give our worries, the worse we feel—physically, mentally, emotionally and spiritually.

But this need not be the case.

When you have done all that you can do in a situation, but still find yourself plagued by worries, use this checklist to transform the power of those worrisome thoughts into reserves of energy, will power and creativity. But remember, perennial Happiness is never realized by simply dismissing your concerns for the future, nor by repressing them. Rather, when you become a yoga scientist, you can face thoughts that tempt you to worry as they arise by experimenting with a gentle and loving time-tested procedure.

First-Aid Kit for Worries

1. Before you address your anxiety, ask yourself the question, "Who am I?" Through this form of quiet contemplation, your attention becomes centered in the peace and fullness of the Eternal Witness who is the thinker of the thought.

2. Attend to the inhalation and exhalation of your breath at the bridge between the two nostrils.

3. As you remain centered in the equanimity of the Eternal Witness, practice detachment and dispassionately welcome, witness and honor your concerns—allowing yourself to be present with these thoughts, desires and emotions without being controlled by them.

4. Listening to the inner wisdom of your conscience, willingly surrender the worrisome thought back to its Origin—the Origin of every person, every thing and every thought (the Divine Reality).

5. Lovingly direct your attention to your *mantra* (the name of the Divine Reality).

6. If it's possible, go for a *mantra* walk. Take a brisk fifteen to twenty minute walk just listening to the silent repetition of your *mantra*.

7. Try to recognize an opportunity (it's probably in front of you right now) to engage in some selfless service. This transforms the energy of worry into the energy of love, fearlessness and strength.

Throughout history, the profound insights of yoga science and philosophy (such as this *First-Aid Kit for Worries*) have been taught and re-experienced within the culture and idioms of changing times, so that their healing and nurturing effects can be embraced anew by each successive generation. Whenever their inner wisdom has been realized and relied upon, individuals have experienced the greatest freedom of all: the freedom from worry and fear. When you learn to embrace this freedom, your life will become a great and meaningful adventure—in which you naturally blossom to your fullest potential.

Because this ageless truth is intrinsically universal and democratic, many people in every age have realized the freedom of enlightenment without ever having heard the word "yoga" or knowing anything about Eastern philosophy. Yet, the science and philosophy of yoga have always provided quiet, reliable encouragement and concrete guidance to seekers in every culture, tradition and religion.

The American experiment that aspires to this wisdom began in 1776 with rebellion against the tyranny of rule by a distant, sovereign monarch. True freedom, the founding fathers insisted, rests on the bedrock of the self-evident truth that all people are "created equal . . . endowed by the Creator with (the) unalienable rights of Life, Liberty and the Pursuit of Happiness." This noble truth is not only the ideal upon which our republic was founded, but is also the heart of yoga science. According to the ancient sages, realizing those precious, inherent and unalienable rights in our daily lives is the surest evidence of union with the Divine. That union is the singular goal of all yoga.

Now, from within the cultural milieu of twenty-first century America, *The Heart and Science of Yoga* presents a practical, modern interpretation of the perennial yogic wisdom.

Our promise to you is simple. If you are willing to follow the blueprint this book offers, you will live your life joyfully, free from worry and supported by an imperishable wellspring of loving and creative energy.

CHAPTER 1

How Meditation Benefits You

Man has three ways of acting wisely:
First, on meditation, this is the noblest;
Second, on imitation, this is the easiest;
Third, on experience, this is the bitterest.

CONFUCIUS

In March, 1775, a group of patriots convened at St. John's Church in Richmond, Virginia. At that convention, a thirty-nine-year-old man rose to his feet to deliver one of the most inspiring speeches in world history. Although he spoke about the desire to be free from the tyranny and oppression of the British Crown, Patrick Henry's words could very well apply to the stressful, complicated and uncertain nature of modern American life and our own personal desire for unbounded Life, Liberty and the pursuit of Happiness. "They tell us that we are weak, unable to cope. But when shall we be stronger? Will it be the next week or the next year? Shall we gather strength by irresolution and inaction—by lying supinely on our backs hugging the delusive phantom of hope—until our enemies shall have bound us hand and foot? Sir, we are not weak—if we make a proper use of those means which the God of Nature has placed in our power."

In some ways things have changed dramatically since

Patrick Henry's "Give me liberty or give me death" speech, but most human beings are no less plagued today by the painful stress of daily life, the desire for freedom from worry and the endless search for happiness. In addition to our own personal duties and responsibilities, the world around us presents many formidable challenges. With apologies to Thomas Paine, "These (too) are the times that try men's souls."

With history as our guide, it's easy to conclude that the desire to end pain, misery and bondage is both universal and timeless. How to fulfill that desire to be truly free—in the midst of every circumstance and relationship—is the essence of our teaching and the heart and science of yoga.

Concerning such perplexing issues, Henry David Thoreau offered some helpful insight. "I went to the woods," Thoreau explained, "because I wished to live life deliberately, to front only the essential facts of life, and see if I could not learn what it had to teach, and not, when I came to die, discover that I had not lived." Unlike Thoreau, yoga science and philosophy does not require that we "go to the woods" to learn the essential facts of life. In fact, true freedom and unbounded Happiness can only be experienced from within the constellation of our own relationships. Toward that goal, life itself is the greatest of all teachers—if we can develop an ear to hear and an eye to see.

This teaching provides a practical framework to experience the peace of mind and fulfillment we seek. Just as the physical sciences investigate the laws of the external universe, the spiritual practice of *sadhana* is a tool for knowing our internal landscape, the nature of our consciousness. We are citizens of two worlds—the outer world of names and forms and the inner world of thoughts, desires and emotions. To be free, we must learn to act skillfully according to our objective knowledge of both worlds.

This book offers step-by-step instruction on how to create a bridge between these two realities. By employing precise scientific techniques, you will learn how to access an intuitive library of wisdom and how to employ that knowledge skillfully in all your relationships through mind, action and speech. Through sincere effort you will discover how to employ your greatest human resource—the energy of the mind—to attain your most deeply held desires.

As you learn to master your internal states by harmonizing the body and mind with the Divine wisdom of the spirit, the vast, hidden power of the unconscious mind will become manifest in healthy, creative, loving and rewarding relationships and experiences.

Like the American melting pot of multi-ethnic, cultural and political influences, the material contained in this book represents a mosaic of Eastern and Western spiritual truth which has been reconfirmed in the crucible of our thirty years of study and practice. Though much of this teaching has its origins in the ancient Himalayan tradition of India, its truth is echoed in every major religion and indigenous tradition including Hebrew, Christian, Hindu, Buddhist, Muslim and Native American. But yoga science is not a religion. It is a body of knowledge that does not interfere with any religious or cultural belief. In fact, a spiritual practice based on the philosophy and science of yoga enhances the understanding of, and appreciation for, every religion and culture.

Yoga science began as an oral tradition—transmitted anew in each generation directly from teacher to student. Around 200 A.D., the teaching was codified into modern yoga science by the Indian sage Patanjali in the text known as the *Yoga Sutras*. This knowledge was originally referred to as *ashtanga*, a yoga path composed of eight identifiable limbs. In the last quarter of the nineteenth century, the Indian sage Swami Vivekananda taught these same disciplines as *raja yoga*, or the royal path.

The practice of meditation has never been difficult to learn. It can be taught in a very short time, but the skill can just as easily be forgotten without proper preparation and supporting practices. In Patanjali's original *Yoga Sutras*, meditation appears as the seventh in a series of eight steps of knowledge. Historically, the teaching of meditation itself always presupposed a certain level of understanding and preparation by the student. A house must have a structurally sound roof to keep the elements out of the living quarters, but without a solid foundation and good sturdy walls, the roof is going to be of little value. The same is true of meditation.

Meditation is most useful if you understand how it is practiced in relation to the entire philosophy and science of yoga. Traditionally, before spiritual seekers were instructed in the art of meditation (*dhyana*), they were required to prepare their body, breath, senses and mind for many years.

Eight Steps of Yoga Science

The eight steps of yoga science are generally described in reverse order since the ladder being used by the spiritual seeker starts at ground level and ascends to the culmination of union. The *yamas*, *niyamas*, *pranayama* and *asana* together are known as *hatha yoga*. These preliminary practices prepare the student for the demands of *pratyahara*, *dharana* and *dhyana* and are intended to lead the seeker sequentially toward *samadhi*.

8. Samadhi – absorption into the superconscious state or Godhead; also known as Self-realization
7. Dhyana – meditation
6. Dharana – concentration (one-pointed attention)
5. Pratyahara – control of the senses
4. Pranayama – control of breath and *prana* (vital energy)
3. Asana – physical postures
2. Niyamas – constructive observances designed to organize our personal daily lives. These are:
    saucha (purity)
    santosha (contentment)
    tapas (self-discipline)
    svadhyaya (self-study)
    Ishvara pranidhana (self-surrender)
1. Yamas – disciplines and restraints regulating external relationships with other people as well as with one's own body, energy and senses. These are:

ahimsa (non-harming)
satya (truthfulness)
asteya (non-stealing)
bramacharya (conservation and moderation of energy)
aparigraha (non-possessiveness)

According to yoga philosophy, our deepest driving desire for unbounded Life, Liberty and Happiness can be fulfilled only in the realization of our Essential Nature. This ultimate state of enlightenment comes to us in *samadhi*—absorption in the Divine. In preparation for experiencing this truth, eight progressive spiritual practices, or *sadhana*, were designed to purify the body and mind through a process of experiments in self-discipline.

As you willingly practice these various steps, you will gain increasing access to the intuitive wisdom of the superconscious mind—the perfect, all-encompassing intelligence that surpasses the capabilities of the rational mind. It is this Divine knowledge—beyond that of the conscious and unconscious portions of the mind—that allows you to know the state of liberation known as *moksha*.

While incorporating the fundamental eight-fold path of traditional yoga science, this teaching also provides modern technologies for creating new mental software that empowers you to make conscious, discriminating choices—choices that will unerringly lead you for your highest and greatest good. The basic instruction for every meditation tradition is found in *Psalms*: "Be still and know that I am God." In yoga science this stillness is learned through the practice of seated meditation.

The origin of the word meditation is similar to that of the word medical. It means to heal by seeing—by consciously directing one's attention. In seated meditation, you dispassionately observe your innermost thoughts, desires and emotions in a calm and concentrated manner. There is nothing dangerous nor difficult associated with this inner attention.

During the practice of seated meditation, you ask your mind to let go of its many attachments, distractions and the passing thoughts and associations of your normal waking experience. You do this not by attempting to stop or repress your thoughts, but by encouraging the mind to focus continuously on one subtle element or object in the present moment. This internal focus of attention helps rest the mind by allowing it to cease its habitual and often stressful mental processes.

As when listening to a beautiful concert, in meditation you are fully alert, but you are not aware of yourself. As your capacity to witness your thoughts is developed, meditation encourages the mind to slow down its customary chatter by surrendering its persistent tendencies to solve problems, analyze and entertain memories of the past or concerns for hypothetical situations in the future. The practice of meditation does not encourage the mind to meander aimlessly, nor to engage in some fascinating internal dialogue. Seated meditation is simply a silent, effortless, one-pointed focus of attention and awareness.

The skills you gain in seated meditation—to witness and transform the power of your thoughts, desires and emotions— can then be employed in all your relationships through the practice of *meditation in action*. Instead of always reacting impulsively to your emotional attachments to fears (worry), anger and desires, you learn to observe and transform their inherent power into thoughts, words and deeds that enable you to experience greater happiness, creativity and contentment.

For individuals recovering from surgery or an emotional ordeal, meditation is profoundly therapeutic. Meditation helps relax muscle tension and the autonomic nervous system, and it facilitates freedom from mental stress. Individuals who meditate attain a tranquility of mind that enhances the immune system by limiting the mind's reaction to worry and anxiety.

After just a few days of sincere efforts, meditation will begin to establish new, healthy habit patterns. These skills increase individual will power and help you make constructive choices in life. Sound decisions concerning a beneficial diet, daily exercise, diaphragmatic breathing and lifestyle selection all become possible when the mind is no longer controlled by habit.

In life, everything is constantly changing, and yet the habits of the mind resist that change. To facilitate positive change, all of yoga science serves one simple goal: to know the true Self in every circumstance and relationship. Knowing this true Self introduces you to the wisdom of consciousness beyond the mind—that prepares you to make reliably beneficial choices.

Sigmund Freud admitted that the ideal of psychoanalysis is to bring an individual from painful neurosis to "ordinary unhappiness." In order to end stress and dis-ease we must begin the earnest exploration of the vast frontier that lies beyond the limitations of the ordinary mind. To find true joy and contentment, we must acknowledge and serve the wisdom of our spiritual center by learning to steward the power of our thoughts, desires and emotions. *The Heart and Science of Yoga* is a road map for this inward journey. It is a program of holistic practices and time-honored techniques to improve physical, mental and emotional well-being. The only two requirements for benefitting from its use are your own determination and earnestness.

Ten Meditation Benefits
Reduce stress, anxiety and worry
Enhance your immune system
Achieve and maintain a healthy weight
End unnecessary health care costs
Lower blood pressure and reduce pain
Increase energy, focus and creativity
Learn how to love yourself
Resolve marriage and family issues
Cultivate loving, nurturing relationships
Realize your Divine Self and life purpose

CHAPTER 2

What is the Purpose of Life?

It is your body, your mind and your thoughts. They should listen to you. When you become lazy and negligent, they begin to boss you. Remember, you are the master of yourself. Your body, mind, thoughts and everything else around you are gifts of nature. By using these gifts you can accomplish your highest purpose—to recognize that the infinite library of knowledge lies within you. And when you start studying the book of life, you start gaining that knowledge which dispels the darkness of ignorance and fear.

SWAMI RAMA OF THE HIMALAYAS

To begin the study of yoga science, it is essential to know the purpose of your life. Some might say that the purpose of life is to know God. But that is not true. Those who claim that knowing God is the purpose of life have usually heard someone else make that assertion, and have accepted it as their own belief.

The sages of all traditions claim that the true purpose of life is to be free of the pains, miseries and bondages of human existence. "If you think you know God and have a relationship with the Divine," Swami Rama taught, "but are still ravaged by pain, miseries and bondages, of what use is God?" If, however, you are free from the sorrow of human existence, the sages would conclude that you have already found God.

The great value of this human life is that it provides both the capacity and the means to end our suffering. We now have a human body, mind and discriminative faculty—all the requisites for making the transition from the animal to the Divine. The sages promise that we can be free in this very lifetime. Further, they urge us not to postpone the endeavor. "Enlightenment," Swami Rama said, "is our birth state—a state free from pains, miseries and bondages. It is not something to be acquired or something new. It is already within us." Each of us, therefore, can realize this state by transforming our habits and purifying our personalities. We have been granted this rare opportunity by Providence to make ourselves fit to receive our full inheritance. This is our challenge as human beings.

No doubt you have chosen to read this book, in whole or in part, because you've been experiencing some form of dis-ease that you'd prefer to live without. Or, you may be searching for spiritual fulfillment. In order to be free from all limitations and to fulfill the purpose of your life, you must be your true Self and rely on the wisdom within to guide your actions in the world.

If, however, you remain ignorant of the Absolute Reality within, your thoughts, words and actions will remain enslaved to the power of the fear, anger and self-willed desires stored in the unconscious mind, and you will continue to feel pain and discontentment. The choice is yours.

Contemplate the Question "Who am I?"

Every desire that motivated you to read this book and investigate the science and philosophy of yoga can be fulfilled if you earnestly contemplate the question "Who am I?" This inquiry, called *vichara* in ancient yogic texts, has been esteemed for thousands of years as a reliable method of knowing the true Self. If you are sincere and persistent in posing this question to yourself, the answer will come. And, as the truth of that answer motivates you to steward the energy of your innumerable desires, large and small, you will begin to experience freedom from your fear, anger, anxiety and dis-ease.

This process occurs differently for each human being. Guided by the philosophy of yoga science, you will begin to follow your own distinct path to Self-realization and freedom. Each of us has been born with a unique body-mind-sense complex, and through this vehicle each of us experiences a different reality. Yet, from that transitory individuality, each human being has the capacity to know union with the Divine.

Absolute peace and contentment is the fruit of earnestly seeking the answer to the profound question "Who am I?" The contemplation of this question begins the systematic, step-by-step procedure to focus your mind. With this focus, you can transcend the indiscriminate call of the senses and the ego's fascination with the past or future. Then, as your mind becomes ever more focused, you will enter a timeless state as you become present to the joyful and creative oneness of your own true nature.

Begin this practice by repeatedly asking yourself the question: Who am I? During the contemplation, remember this:

I have a body. I am aware of the body, but I am not the body.
I have a mind. I am aware of the mind, but I am not the mind.
I have thoughts. I am aware of thoughts, but I am not the thoughts.
I have desires. I am aware of desires, but I am not the desires.
I have emotions. I am aware of emotions, but I am not the emotions.

Who, then, is aware of the body?
Who is aware of the mind?
Who is aware of the thoughts, desires and emotions?
Who is the thinker of every thought?
Who is the experiencer of every experience?
Who am I?

Beginning today, and for the rest of your life, contemplate

the question "Who am I?" If you are earnest in your effort—allowing consciousness to observe consciousness—the answer will appear, because the question and the answer are two sides of the same coin.

Whenever there is consternation in your mind, you are reacting from the limited perspective of the personality. It's a clear indication that the ego—not the real You—has its hands on the wheel of the bus. When thoughts, desires and emotions arise in your awareness, do not automatically pursue them with your attention, but rather, inquire: "To whom did this thought arise?" It doesn't matter how many thoughts arise. As each thought arises, inquire with diligence: "To whom has this thought arisen?" The answer that will emerge is: "To me." If you earnestly inquire "Who am I?" at this point, the mind will go deeper to consider its Source, and the thought that arose will become less seductive. Seeking the answer to the question "Who am I?" will eventually give rise to the realization that within you dwells an Eternal Witness which *is* the Divine Reality.

This dialogue requires attentive introspection. Be sensitive and patient as you consider your feelings and thoughts. Be gentle with yourself, as you would with any good friend. Don't condemn yourself or be judgmental, and you will begin to trust your inner Self and realize that a constantly faithful companion and guide resides within.

Enlightenment is Your Birthright

You may use the personal pronoun "I" hundreds or even thousands of times a day, but who is it that you are actually referring to? When you think or speak of "me," which me are you referring to? The physical body? Your thoughts, desires, emotions? Who exactly is this "me"? Who am I?

As the profound truth begins to unfold, you will find that everything you need in order to fulfill your life's purpose will spontaneously appear, and the objects and relationships that do not serve your highest good will begin to fall away. This means that your life will gradually become uncluttered, unstressed, vibrant, productive and creative. As old habits drop away, you will find yourself increasingly free to explore new possibilities.

CHAPTER 3

Who Am I?

You create your own disharmony and then complain! When you desire and fear, and identify yourself with your feelings, you create sorrow and bondage. When you create with love and wisdom, and remain unattached to your creations, the result is harmony and peace. But whatever be the condition of your mind, in what way does it really reflect on you? It is only your self-identification with the thoughts and suggestions of your mind that makes you happy or unhappy. Rebel against your slavery to your mind, see your bonds as self-created and break the chains of attachment and revulsion. Keep in mind your goal of freedom, until it dawns on you that you are already free; that freedom is not something in the distant future to be earned with painful efforts, but perennially one's own, to be used! Liberation from fear is not an acquisition but a matter of courage, the courage to believe that you are free already and to act on it.

NISARGADATTA MAHARAJ

We define ourselves physically, mentally and emotionally every day. We might define ourselves as tall or short, heavy or thin, flexible or inflexible, happy or sad, focused or unfocused, calm or stressed, angry or forgiving, bored or interested, fearful or fearless. The list could go on and on.

When we review the ways we define ourselves, one thing becomes clear. Each potential definition of "I" implies the existence of its polar opposite. The reason for this is obvious, yet profound. We live in a world of relativity replete with pairs of opposites. We cannot know *up* without knowing *down*. We cannot know *in* without knowing *out*. We cannot know *black* without knowing *white*.

If you look up from where you're presently sitting, the ceiling will appear high to you—and so it is. However, if you were on the roof, that same ceiling would seem low. While that observation would also be true, it would only be relatively true. On this plane of existence, the human being is subject to the laws of relativity. The height of the ceiling, for example, is subject to the laws of time, space and causation. The ceiling height is only relatively true, and relative truths are always subject to change.

The very same can be said about any definition we attribute to the personal pronoun "I." Any information derived through the senses is always only relatively true. Right now I am tall, but when I was five years old I was short. Today I am thin. When I was a child I was heavy. Today I am a teacher. Yesterday I was a student. Last week I was calm. This week I am anxious. When I fly in an airplane twenty thousand feet in the air I am fearful. When the plane lands safely I become fearless.

I | AM

Tall / Short
Rich / Poor
Teacher / Student
Happy / Unhappy
Focused / Unfocused
Stressed / Calm
Bored / Interested
Fearful / Fearless

} Any words defining the subject "**I**" in the phrase "**I am**" are transitory— subject to change, death and decay.

Based on our memory, the only truth about ourselves that we can declare with one hundred percent certainty is "I AM." When we try to define ourselves, we invariably settle on a meaning that reflects a relative truth that is ever-changing. Everyday definitions of the "I" are never absolutely true.

Contemplate this point for a moment. Based on your personal memory, was there ever a time in your life when the statement "I am" was not absolutely true?

ॐ

Certainly the size and shape of your body have changed over a lifetime, as has your mental and emotional landscape. You might have been heavy as a child, but now you are thin. Yesterday you might have been fearful, but now you're fearless. This morning you were angry, but now you're forgiving.

The *I-amness* that has continued as the only constant in your life is the most persuasive indication that consciousness exists beyond time and space, the body and mind. This inherent capacity to be present every moment—to witness—is what allows you to perceive the words on this page and to comprehend them. The same facility to witness and direct attention also enabled the authors to order their thoughts and craft their words into the form of this book.

Consciousness, referred to as awareness or attention, exists both within and beyond time, with and without an object to observe. As a meditator begins to observe his thoughts, the consciousness that is the Eternal Witness can be known in the stillness between and surrounding two thoughts. Consciousness is the background of all reality—a cosmic soup of awareness from which and into which all gross and subtle objects appear for limited periods of time in space.

What are these gross and subtle objects that continuously appear in your awareness? The book you are holding in your hands is a gross object. The chair you are sitting in is a gross object. Anything that can be perceived through the five senses is a gross object—including the body. The sages conclude, therefore, that we have a body, that we are aware of the body, and yet, that we are *not* the body.

Two hours ago, the gross object in the form of this book might not have been in your awareness. Now, the book has appeared. Gross objects appear in your awareness for a limited period of time, and then they depart. This phenomenon is not very different from the weather. Yesterday it was sunny. Today it's raining, and tomorrow it may snow.

Subtle objects, such as thoughts, desires and emotions also appear in your awareness. Like gross objects, subtle objects also have a form, but they vibrate at a frequency too high to be perceived through the rudimentary instrumentation of the five senses. You can't see them, taste them, or touch them. Yet, through your most powerful instrument, the mind, you are made aware of these subtle objects. Seemingly out of nowhere, a thought comes into your awareness. It could be a thought that provokes a desire, fear or anger. It might not have been in your awareness a few seconds ago, yet you're aware of it *now*—in the present moment. In an hour you may hardly remember the thought.

By this teaching, the sages encourage you to dis-identify with anything that is transitory. It is clear you have a body, but you are not the body. You have a mind with thoughts, desires and emotions, but you are not the mind, nor are you the thoughts, desires or emotions appearing in your awareness through the instrument of the mind. Essentially, you are awareness itself—pure consciousness without any object—consciousness that, by its very nature, is able to perceive all the gross and subtle objects appearing for limited periods of time in space.

Our Three Characteristics

While the sages insist that we can never define who we are through the limitations of language, they do claim that we can experience the truth. Encouraging us to remain on the spiritual path, the sages provide some helpful clues. They describe our Essential Nature as being a composition of three fundamental qualities.

Sat – Eternal Existence

The first characteristic of your Essential Nature is described by the Sanskrit word *Sat*, meaning eternal existence. That internal witnessing capacity that allows you to perceive all gross and subtle objects is eternal. The ultimate "I" was never born and will never die, the sages teach. It is self-existent. Unlike every gross and subtle object, awareness is not dependent on anything else for its existence.

No object can claim to be eternal. The book in your hands is neither eternal nor self-existent. It is dependent on many different things for its existence: trees, a lumberjack, trucker, paper mill, printer, bindery, author, editor, publisher, salesperson and bookstore. Objects like the book you are reading, or even the desire for the knowledge presented in the book, may be impermanent, but your own awareness—which empowers perception—is eternal.

Jesus the Christ taught us that, "Before Abraham was, I am." What was He speaking of, if not the eternal capacity to witness? When Moses was in the desert, he stood before a bush that was burning yet not consumed by the flame. Acknowledging the sacredness of the experience, Moses asked the bush, "Who are you?" Whereupon the bush replied to Moses, "I am that I am." Moses grasped the import of the Divine pronouncement, but still was doubtful that others would. He asked the bush, "What shall I tell the Hebrew people? Who shall I tell them has sent me?" To this the Lord responded by saying, "Tell the Hebrew people that 'I am' has sent you."

Chit – Consciousness and Wisdom

The second characteristic of your Essential Nature is *Chit*, meaning consciousness, your capacity for awareness, attention and wisdom.

Every day, thousands of gross objects come into your awareness. You have countless relationships with human beings, animals, plants and inanimate objects. You also witness thousands of subtle objects: those thoughts, desires and emotions that come into your awareness for a limited length of time. The sages teach us that the nature of the "I" you are seeking to know is Eternal Awareness (*Sat* and *Chit*)—capable of providing all the wisdom necessary for you to skillfully fulfill your life's purpose.

Ananda – Bliss or Fullness

The last of the three characteristics of your Essential Nature is *Ananda*, which means bliss or complete fullness. There is no gross or subtle object you can know, experience or obtain that can make you any fuller or more content than you already are. On the highest level of consciousness, you are the Eternal Witness—the attentive background—eternally content in the bliss and fullness of your own transcendent perfection.

You have already glimpsed the unspeakable joy, bliss, fullness and contentment that the sages refer to as *Ananda*, and yet, may not have recognized it. You might have experienced this *Ananda* when you fell in love, or at the sight of your own newborn child. Or, the rapture of *Ananda* might have briefly come to you as you jogged, gardened or read; as you lost yourself in a beautiful painting or musical composition; or as you stood in awe before the majesty of a glorious sunset on a secluded lake in the Adirondacks. When your attention is completely captured, there is no room for thinking. You neither entertain memories of the past nor imaginations of the future. Instead, at that singular point in space and time, when all your attention becomes fixed on a particular object, the perceiver and the object of perception both disappear, and what reflects into the awareness of the Inner Witness is *Ananda*—an indescribable contentment.

After some time, of course, new, compelling thoughts stream into your awareness. New, subtle objects appear, diverting you from the bliss of one-pointed attention, and you once again begin to think and question. You may have been momentarily absorbed in the absolute beauty of a rose, but the mind eventually intervenes by entertaining a thought. "Is this rose as magnificent as the one I grew last summer?" The intellect diffuses your focus and the bliss of *Ananda* fades from conscious awareness. Once more you are swept away into the unending procession of memories of the past and hypotheticals for the future that effectively dissipate your mental energy.

Those fleeting, bliss-filled moments might be termed peek experiences. Through them, you have been granted a tiny glimpse of the bliss that is your very own Divine Nature. When your attention is thoroughly one-pointed, the individual self, the little ego, that limited sense of "I" disappears, leaving only *Sat-Chit-Ananda*, the eternal, bliss-filled consciousness and wisdom of the Eternal Witness.

In that twilight moment on an Adirondack lake, the habitual procession of mental distractions temporarily abates. In that stillness you feel wonderful. This contentment, the sages remind us, is nothing other than the bliss of *Ananda* reflecting into your own consciousness (*Chit*). It is your eternal Self. It is fullness. It is perfection. No object or relationship could make you feel any more content than you already are in that stillness.

These experiences are a taste of what yoga science contends is your birthright. The sages explain that there is nothing you have to get from outside yourself to be free of fear, anxiety, stress, phobias, sorrow, spiritual longing, or any kind of physical, mental or emotional suffering. You merely have to recognize That which you are. When a sculptor stands before a raw block of marble, she might have a vision of an elephant. As she takes hammer and chisel in hand, she proceeds to remove everything from the block that is not elephant—until all that remains is the elephant.

There are really no physical or mental requirements you need to place on yourself to be happy. The truth is that you are already attained. It is your misidentification with your limited body, mind, thoughts, desires and emotions that motivates you habitually to choose options that give rise to dis-ease.

As twentieth century Indian mystic Ramana Maharshi said, "The mind is consciousness which has put on limitations. You are originally unlimited and perfect. Later, you put on limitations and identify with the mind."

If you acknowledge that you are essentially spirit (*Sat-Chit-Ananda*) having a human experience, your practice of yoga science can help you tap into your own Divine wisdom to remove all the ignorance that is not you. Then, centered in the fullness and bliss of your true Essential Nature, your thoughts, words and actions will lead you for your highest and greatest good.

CHAPTER 4
Unbounded Life, Liberty and Happiness

The poor long for riches.
The rich long for heaven.
But the wise long for a state of tranquility.
SWAMI RAMA OF THE HIMALAYAS

Because every aspect of creation is a microcosm or a macrocosm of everything else, we can view the three most powerful human desires as expressions of the limitless and perfect Absolute Reality within us.

Sat—The Desire for Unbounded Life
The *Sat* (eternal) characteristic of our Essential Nature is expressed in the human longing for unbounded Life. The human being is consciously or unconsciously motivated by the thoughts, "I want to live. I don't want to be sick. I don't want to die." Why? Because in the depth of our consciousness we know intuitively that we are eternal. When we mistakenly identify with the body, the desire for immortality instantaneously rises to the surface of consciousness to influence our actions.

Chit—The Desire for Unbounded Liberty
The *Chit* (consciousness and wisdom) characteristic of our

Divine identity is expressed through the human desire for unbounded Liberty. Every one of us deeply desires to possess knowledge and exhibit the liberty or freedom that comes from having knowledge. Every human being searches for wisdom in an effort to fulfill his or her potential. We believe that if we can just find the appropriate seminar or teacher, the truth we discover will set us free. It's because of this belief that you are reading this book.

We are all habituated to looking outside of ourselves for emancipation, but the sages of both East and West maintain that there is no seminar, book or teacher that can set us free. Instead, yoga science provides a road map for the inward journey to the ever-present Source of all wisdom and liberty.

Ananda—The Desire for Unbounded Happiness

Finally, the *Ananda* (bliss) characteristic of our Essential Nature is expressed through the deep, driving human desire for unbounded Happiness. "I want to be happy," we insist. "I just want to be happy." Did you ever meet anyone who wanted to be depressed? Of course not. We consider the question ludicrous because the desire to be happy is universal and so deeply ingrained. Even though all human beings intuitively recognize that we have the capacity for boundless Happiness, we mistakenly seek that Happiness from transitory objects and relationships that have no lasting capacity to make us happy.

Life, Liberty and Happiness are very familiar desires to every American, for "We hold these truths to be self-evident, that all men are created equal, that they are endowed by their creator with certain unalienable rights, that among these are Life, Liberty and the pursuit of Happiness." It is interesting that the Declaration of Independence names Life, Liberty and Happiness as humankind's most cherished, unalienable rights—the highest truths to be known and gained.

When you memorized the Preamble to the Declaration of Independence in grade school, did you ever stop to consider what an "unalienable right" meant? Was this mere poetry? No. An "unalienable right" can never be separated from you because on the highest level of consciousness Life, Liberty and Happiness *is* you. The desire for Life is an expression of your eternal nature, *Sat*. The desire for Liberty (the freedom to access knowledge and the freedom that comes from using that knowledge) is an expression of your intuitive consciousness and wisdom, *Chit*, and Happiness is the expression of your inherent fullness or bliss, known as *Ananda*.

By identifying Life, Liberty and Happiness as unalienable rights, the founding fathers served as a collective instrument for Divine intuition. This revolutionary political pronouncement clearly reflected the timeless yogic understanding that despite the apparent multiplicity of names and forms, bodies and minds, there is only one truth—One consciousness. The bliss-filled, eternal wisdom that *is* you, in the form of the reader of this book, is the very same that *is* us, in the form of the authors of this book.

Lesson of Las Vegas

This ever-present *Sat-Chit-Ananda* can be further understood when it is likened to the concept of space. Look around the room where you are presently seated. The space is definable because the room has four walls, a ceiling and a floor. Now, leave the room you're sitting in and become aware of the space in a second room. That room also has a definable space because of its four walls, ceiling and floor.

You've probably seen television news reports that showed the demolition of aging Las Vegas hotels. Each hotel that was imploded had hundreds of rooms, and each room represented an individual, definable space. However, when the dynamite charges were detonated and all the glass, bricks, steel, wood and plastic came tumbling down, what happened to the individual spaces of the individual rooms of that Las Vegas hotel? Of course, each individual space became what it always was: a part of the whole.

Any perceived identifiable space in a building exists for only a limited period of time. When circumstances cause the destruction of those four walls, ceiling and floor, the space of each room merely merges with the larger space. The essence of space itself never changes.

The Omnipresent One

All spiritual traditions have defined God as omnipotent, omniscient and omnipresent. The omnipresence of which all traditions speak is pure, bliss-filled consciousness—the eternal capacity to witness. Even though human, animal, plant and mineral forms are subject to change, death and decay, the sanctity of their essence is never compromised. God, the sages would say, is consciousness—with or without form, with or without name.

Through the ages, this underlying Eternal Divine Reality has been called different names in different traditions. Most of us would refer to the *Sat-Chit-Ananda* as the soul. In the Hindu tradition, it is spoken of as *Atman* or Self, and the collective *Atman* is known as *Brahman*. In Islam it is known as *Allah* or The Beloved. In the Jewish tradition it is called *Adonai*, or metaphorically referred to as *Eretz Yisrael*,[1] the land of *Israel*, the true *land of milk and honey*. In Buddhism, the word *Buddha* literally means the one who is awakened to his true nature. In Christianity, *Sat-Chit-Ananda* is called the Light of Christ. Jesus, for example, is known as the Christ (the anointed One) because he became One with the Father who is in heaven (the eternal "kingdom" beyond change, death or decomposition).

When you attempt to define any experience by giving it a name, the name is not what was being referred to. Words are

---

[1] *Eretz Yisrael* does not refer to a geographical location. As in the Biblical story of Jacob, it represents the result of the process of the individual ego wrestling with the angel of the Eternal until, following human effort, grace descends in the form of enlightenment. The true land of the Inner Dweller or Eternal Witness is within the cave of your own heart.

always less than what they describe. Words are merely a useful shorthand technique for communicating complex concepts or personal experiences.

Current scientific research indicates that it is the helpful habit of the left brain to represent complicated concepts with simple, easy-to-refer-to symbols. Such symbols save the time of re-examining in detail what is to be communicated. However, this inclination of the left-brain can be problematic. Its shorthand symbols never explain anything completely, yet, as a culture, we accept these symbols as reality.

There is a Zen injunction that advises, "If you meet the Buddha, kill him." The saying is meant to caution an earnest seeker against the common trap of deifying the teapot instead of drinking the tea. The Buddha, no matter how exalted and holy, is still a limitation on the Divine. Therefore, if you accept this limitation, you cut yourself off from experiencing the truth that lies beyond the word or form. In this Zen instruction, you are urged to "kill" (or surrender) the limitations that the mind tries to impose on that which exists beyond the mind.

Similarly, in Judaism, there is an injunction against writing the name of G-d, and against creating any "graven images." According to yoga philosophy, the reasoning is essentially sound. When the name of the Lord is written, the word is something less than the Lord. A word is a human being's narrow concept. The Absolute Reality includes the limitations, but also extends beyond the limitations of both the conscious and unconscious mind.

The purpose of all spiritual practice is to help you transcend the limited perspectives of the mind. *Sadhana* enables you to use the mind to go beyond the mind. It purifies your vision to help you see things more clearly as they are, rather than as they appear. By relying on the intuitive library within (the superconscious mind), you can gain access to the greater wisdom that is part of your Self. Once you begin to recognize and rely on that Divine Reality within, you increasingly find the capacity to discriminate between competing thoughts, desires and emotions. By identifying yourself with the Absolute Reality within, you begin to think, speak and act in ways that reflect the loving, creative and selfless choices of your Higher Self. As an instrument of Divine Providence, you are led for your highest and greatest good.

The real you is essentially spirit having a human experience. *Sat-Chit-Ananda* is the background of all reality—into which all gross and subtle objects appear. Therefore, consider: you have a body and you are aware of the body, but *you* are not the body. You have a mind and are aware of your thoughts, desires and emotions, but *you* are not the mind. *You* are not the thoughts, desires or emotions. The body and mind, with its thoughts, desires and emotions, are merely gross and subtle objects appearing in an all-pervasive, eternal consciousness.

In Chapter 15, I will describe how you can systematically begin this inner journey through seated meditation.

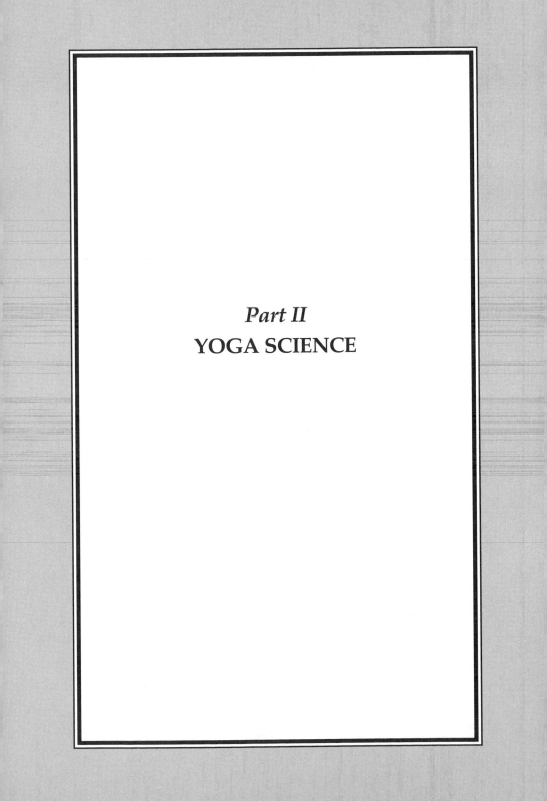

Part II
YOGA SCIENCE

CHAPTER 5

Preya or Shreya:
Passing Pleasure or Perennial Joy

To live for the physical, mental and sensual pleasures is like building a home on quicksand, or trying to cross a stream on the back of a crocodile, believing it to be the trunk of a tree.

SHANKARACHARYA

This above all:
To thine own Self be true.

WILLIAM SHAKESPEARE

If you were inspired to start a business, you'd probably write a business plan and survey the potential market to determine if people wanted or needed your product or service. You'd probably also interview several banks to line up adequate capital for your proposed venture.

Right now you want to be happy, healthy, creative, productive, nurtured and loving to the fullest extent possible. You want to be free from the pains, miseries and bondages you experience. Well, how do you propose getting from point A to point B? Buy a lottery ticket? You might get lucky, but there is a more reliable method.

The Compassionate Buddha reminds us that "You are what you think," and Swami Rama taught that "You are the architect of your life. You determine your destiny." What you are experiencing today is the consequence of your previous thoughts, and what you experience tomorrow will be the result of what you think today.

Your thoughts are the most powerful natural resource available to attain the purpose of life. As William Jennings Bryan observed, "Destiny is not a matter of chance, it is a matter of choice." The thoughts you choose to give your attention to, and your choice to withdraw your attention from others, will determine your destiny. But in order to determine which thoughts to pay attention to, you must first understand the nature and consequence of individual thoughts.

The ancient *Katha Upanishad* explains that every thought falls into one of two basic categories.

> *Passing pleasure or perennial joy? This is the choice one is to make always. The wise recognize these two, but not the ignorant. The first welcome what leads to abiding joy, though painful at the time. The latter run, goaded by their senses, after what seems to be immediate pleasure.*
>
> KATHA UPANISHAD[1]

Preya—Short-Term Ego or Sense Gratification

The first category of thought is called *preya*. *Preya* is defined as any short-term ego or sense gratification. Ah, *preya*! It's very pleasant, attractive, familiar, comfortable and extremely easy to give our attention to. In fact, our five senses of sight, smell, taste, hearing and touch constantly investigate the objects of the material world in search of the pleasant. When our senses identify something new and interesting, they immediately transmit the vital information back to our awareness (*Chit*).

Each of us is very familiar with *preya*. In the realm of food

---

[1]Translation of the *Katha Upanishad* from *Dialogue with Death*, by Eknath Easwaran, Part I, Canto 2. © 1981, 1992, The Blue Mountain Center of Meditation.

choices, it's the candy bar. Emotionally, the *preya* might be represented by fear, worry, anger or selfishness—directed toward yourself or others. *Preya* reflects a strong attachment; the ground upon which you currently stand. When you give your attention to the *preya*, you do experience a spike of passing pleasure or satisfaction, but ultimately the *preya* does not offer long-term benefit. In fact, the passing pleasure of serving the *preya* is always followed by some form of contraction, pain or dis-ease. Fortunately, yoga science provides another alternative.

Shreya—Highest and Greatest Good

The second kind of thought that appears in our awareness is the *shreya*, and its nature is expansive. Initially, the *shreya* may not be very pleasant, attractive, comfortable or familiar to us, but the choice of *shreya* inevitably becomes deeply satisfying because it always leads toward lasting joy. In the category of food, the *shreya* might be the choice of broccoli with dinner. Emotionally, it might appear as compassion or forgiveness.

Discriminating Between the *Preya* and *Shreya*

If the *shreya* always leads to the highest and greatest good, and the *preya* eventually leads to dis-ease, the choice for the yoga scientist is clear: every thought, word and action must be in service to the *shreya*. That is the black-and-white ideal, but in a world that appears in endless shades of gray, how, you might ask, can you identify which thoughts are *preya* and which are *shreya*?

The *Buddhi*

Twenty-four hours a day, seven days a week and three hundred sixty-five days of the year the reliable discrimination between *preya* and *shreya* is continuously broadcast, like a radio signal, into your awareness (*Chit*). In Sanskrit this invaluable function of the mind is called *buddhi*. In the West it is referred to as the conscience or discrimination, and in the early Christian tradition it was known as the Holy Spirit. The *buddhi* is analogous to a mirror because, when it is purified, it faithfully reflects the wisdom and will of the Divine Reality.

The *buddhi* allows the conscious mind to gain access to insight from the intuitive library of knowledge within—the superconscious mind. When such knowledge enters the conscious mind, no verification of its truthfulness is necessary. When your conscience speaks, you know what it says is true. The only question that remains is, do you have the will power to align every thought, word and action with the wise and good counsel of the *buddhi*?

The superconscious mind is not a figment of one's imagination. It is the same aspect of the mind from which Albert Einstein saw mathematical equations and Paul McCartney hears beautiful melodies. When you earnestly serve the *shreya* instead of the attractive and familiar *preya*, the doorway to the superconscious mind widens, allowing knowledge to flow into your conscious mind. It doesn't mean that you'll become a great mathematician like Einstein or a talented musician like Paul McCartney, but by purifying and exercising the *buddhi*, you will be able to access wisdom that will directly and positively impact every single relationship you have.

The word conscience comes from the Latin, and it means "with wisdom or knowledge." As a meditator, you are simply asked to make all your decisions consciously—based on the science of yoga and on the reliable advice of *buddhi*.

The *buddhi* allows the human being to transcend animal instinct in order to attain union with the Divine. When this occurs, humans are able to free themselves from the pains, miseries and bondages created by their learned habits of fear, anger and greed. The ancients tell us that the process of transcendence is the very reason each of us has been born with a human body-mind-sense complex. You have come to this plane of existence to take the next step toward Self-realization. By aligning every thought, word and action with the *shreya*, as defined intuitively by the discrimination of *buddhi*, you will transcend the animal, through the human, and unite with the Divine.

At first glance, *shreya* is generally not the more pleasant of the two choices. On the other hand, even though the *preya* may be more tantalizing to the senses and ego (*ahamkara*) initially, it will, over time, prove to be painful or destructive. Anyone who has ever experienced anger or fear knows they're not pleasant emotions, yet it's often difficult not to give the *preya* attention. Through repeated attention, even painful thoughts and emotions like worry, fear, anger, sadness and jealousy can become the familiar ground upon which each of us stands.

Very often the suggestions you receive from others blur the line between the passing pleasure and perennial joy. The gurus of our culture—Madison Avenue copywriters—are constantly repeating commercial mantras into your awareness. They suggest that if it looks pleasant, smells pleasant, tastes, sounds and feels pleasant, it's virtually guaranteed to be good for you. "Buy it," these commercials entreat. "You will become happy and your pain will be eliminated."

You should understand that these Madison Avenue gurus are not malicious, nor the cause of your troubles. In fact, the advertising industry is actually doing you a favor by acquainting you with available options. Admittedly, there are times when the pleasant and the good are one and the same. Yoga science has no admonition against the purchase of necessities and items that gratify the senses. You have a body equipped to experience pleasure and life is to be enjoyed. And, let's face it, everyone needs stuff. You need a car, a warm house, clothing, food and recreation. But ultimately you must be responsible for either accepting or rejecting the suggestions of the culture.

If you accept bold promises (from the culture or from your own senses, habits or ego) without exercising your discrimination, you will not always receive what was promised. No matter what your age, you already know that there are choices that yield strictly passing pleasure and others that serve your long-term interest. Your intuition and experience tell you that there is a difference between the *preya* and the *shreya*. The pleasant does *not* always equal the good.

The only way to know for certain if a particular thought will lead you for your highest and greatest good is to follow the wisdom of the *buddhi*. The more you align every thought, word and physical action with the expansive quality of *shreya*, your life will become healthy, happy, creative, productive and free of the dis-ease of stress, anxiety and pain. If, however, you continue to act exclusively on the contracting nature of ego and short-term sense gratifications by serving the *preya*, you will inevitably experience physical, mental, emotional or spiritual dis-ease.

It's always important to remember that at any moment the *shreya* can become the *preya* and vice versa. Suppose you've volunteered your services for a worthwhile organization or a friend. Definitely a *shreya*. But as you're leaving the house you receive a telephone call from a relative who has become ill and needs a ride to the hospital. In a split second, what was a *shreya* has become the *preya* to be surrendered, and a previously unforeseen circumstance suddenly has become the *shreya* you must serve.

CHAPTER 6
Creating the Software of the Mind

That the birds of worry and care fly above your head, this you cannot change; but that they build nests in your hair, this you can prevent.

CHINESE PROVERB

Samskaras and the Nature of the Unconscious

The mind is vast. Swami Rama of the Himalayas taught that "All the body is in the mind. All the mind is not in the body." Only a small portion of the mind is conscious. For most of our lives, the greater portion of the mind remains unconscious and is known in Sanskrit as *chitta*. The unconscious mind serves as the storehouse for attachments. It's a veritable catalogue of all pleasant and unpleasant memories, imaginations for the future and the experiences and information we have deemed vital to self-preservation. It also serves as the repository for fear, anger and unfulfilled desires.

Yoga science describes the character of the *chitta* as being analogous to wet sand. When you were a child playing at the beach and you pressed an object like a pail or shovel into wet sand, an impression was created. Similarly, when you repeatedly give your attention to any thought or desire, that subtle object is stored in the *chitta*—thereby forming an indentation in the topography of your unconscious mind. As you give continued attention to any thought, desire or emotion, the channel that is formed becomes deeper.

Each of these channels is known as a *samskara*, and consciousness (*Chit*) always flows through the sluice of least resistance. This means that the deepest, widest, most unobstructed channels in the unconscious mind become the software of the mind, the pathways through which consciousness travels. The deepest *samskaras* in the unconscious (*chitta*) link together to comprise our deepest tendencies (*vasanas*). These include both our creative, healthy habits and destructive, unhealthy habits, compulsions and addictions.

Because you have created these *samskaras* through your previous attention, you tend to think virtually the same thoughts, speak the same words and take similar actions every day. You are responsible for having created the software of your own mind through repeated attention to certain thoughts—both helpful and harmful ones. Your continued attachments to a variety of desires and emotions create the information highways in the unconscious mind. These, in turn, determine the development of the personality.

Nevertheless, *samskaras* are not permanent constructions. As Mahatma Gandhi wrote, "Humankind's greatness lies not so much in being able to remake the world . . . but in remaking ourselves." *Samskaras* are always works in progress. They can be altered. Many of them are very beneficial, but unless you consciously acknowledge and monitor their growth, debilitating *samskaras* can grow strong. Over a lifetime, these tendencies can increase bondage to pain and misery.

Remember, for every action, there is an equal reaction. When you consciously defer to the wisdom of *buddhi* in choosing which thoughts deserve your attention and which do not, you can prevent many painful consequences. The process is similar to tending a garden. If you want to grow highly prized varieties of flowers or vegetables, you must be diligent about pulling the common, vigorous weeds. If left to grow unattended, they will begin to crowd the more delicate plants and will eventually choke off the nutrient supply.

Changing Mental Software

The meditation process provides a reliable, systematic method for creatively rewriting the current limiting software of the mind. When you sit regularly for meditation and learn how to direct your attention consciously, you create new, healthy *samskaras* of love, fearlessness and strength.

Among all the practices of yoga science, only meditation requires you to define what is *preya* and what is *shreya* in advance of the moment. As you will learn in chapters 14 and 15, the process of seated meditation that we teach is called *mantra* meditation. This classical form of meditation trains the mind to direct its attention exclusively toward the sound of a *mantra*—a word or series of words containing the name of the Divine Reality. During your meditation the *mantra* is *always* considered the *shreya*—leading you for your highest and greatest good.

Any random and attractive thought, image or sound that competes for your attention during meditation is to be considered a *preya*. Therefore, when a thought comes forward from the unconscious mind into the conscious mind in meditation, you lovingly welcome and witness the thought and gently withdraw your attention from it, redirecting your attention back to the *mantra*.

When you consciously withdraw your attention from a competitive thought, two important things occur. First, because you have willingly given up your attachment to the *preya* in favor of the *mantra*, that same, subtle thought-object (*preya*) returns to the unconscious mind in a weakened state, and the depth of its *samskara* is subtly reduced. Second, as you replace your attention on the *mantra* (*shreya*), you're deepening this new, healthy *samskara* that will aid you in every relationship that comes your way.

Meditation is an engineering science. As the modern

Indian sage Eknath Easwaran often taught, "Meditation re-engineers the topography of the unconscious portion of the mind." It frees you from enslavement to unconscious fears, anger and self-willed desires by gradually bringing the elusive power of the unconscious under the direct control of the conscious mind. Learning to choose the *shreya* over the *preya* during seated meditation breaks the power of habit and prepares the meditator to make similar discriminating choices in daily life.

The Message of Pain

Whenever you give your attention to the *preya* instead of the *shreya*, you inevitably experience some form of physical, mental, emotional or spiritual dis-ease. Pain is a very important messenger in our lives. Unfortunately, the real meaning and value of pain is not well understood. Instead of learning from the lessons of pain, our culture has developed a wide variety of avoidance techniques including reliance on drugs, surgery and even consumerism. But pain presents invaluable guidance. As the Greek poet Aeschylus so profoundly observed, "Pain, which cannot forget, falls drop by drop upon the heart until, in our own despair, against our will, comes wisdom through the awful grace of God."

Pain is the shadow of the outstretched hand of Divine Providence. Pain is like the warning signs posted along the highway: Falling Rock Zone, Slow—Curve, Wrong Way—Do Not Enter. Pain provides essential telemetry to assure a safe journey. Pain advises when a mid-course correction is necessary. Pain lets you know when there is some form of friction in your life—friction between your self-willed attachment to the *preya* and the grace of the Divine Reality trying to lead you toward the *shreya*.

Yoga science advises that you heed the whispers of pain at a low decibel level. If you don't, the decibel level will only get louder and louder and louder—until your dis-ease turns into a full-fledged disease.

Pleasure can never have the same instructive effect as pain. A pleasurable experience just keeps you headed in the same external direction—away from the advice of your intuitive, discriminative guidance system, and toward the next object or relationship that you mistakenly believe will bring happiness or eliminate your dis-ease.

Pain, on the other hand, helps redirect your attention toward the *buddhi* so you can begin to consider a change in your life—a change that can eliminate the cause of the pain, not just ease its symptoms. True heart-centered yoga means swimming against the tide of our culture and the habits of a lifetime to rely on the power of love and eternal wisdom that already reside within you.

Because the overriding philosophy of our culture is based on commerce, messages selling the *preya* bombard us continually. Although no human being has ever been able to enjoy the short-term pleasure of the *preya* without eventually experiencing its unpleasantness, the messages from television, movies, radio, newspapers and magazines all suggest that the pleasant and the good are synonymous.

As Madison Avenue tries to convince you that objects and relationships will bring only the pleasant, its mantras often resemble the sign that flashes in big, red neon letters over the entrance to the local bar and grill: Free Beer! Free Beer! Free Beer! But just as you walk into that bar to claim your free beer, you spot a small, handwritten sign hanging beneath the neon. It simply says: "Tomorrow." There is no free beer today. That's the real message. No matter what day you arrive for free beer, it's always going to be served "tomorrow."

It's really quite amazing. The human spirit is so fundamentally optimistic that we continually pick ourselves up, dust ourselves off and reach for the next brass ring. But is that next brass ring you strive for the *preya* or the *shreya*? That's basically the only question you have to answer, and the *buddhi* will always guide you to the right choice.

Your discriminative faculty is always working, but its voice is often overwhelmed by the noise of the senses, the memories of the past, imaginations of the future and the self-serving advice of the ego. This can mean that the conscience ends up bound and gagged in the closet, attic or basement of your mind—while the ego and senses party on. Most of the time when you have an overwhelming desire to pursue the pleasure of *preya*, you'd prefer not to listen to your discrimination.

Have you ever visited a favorite restaurant to take advantage of an all-you-can-eat special? Madison Avenue gurus encourage you to over-indulge by consuming two or three meals for the price of one. As one national restaurant chain's advertising slogan directed, "Go overboard!" But the motivation behind this suggestion is hardly in service to your highest and greatest good.

After you consume the huge meal and experience the pain of indigestion, bloating, heartburn and acid reflux, you're probably eager to buy another product—that little white antacid pill that effectively shoots the messenger of pain. Sure, the damage to the body will continue, but Madison Avenue gurus cheerfully promise that within sixty seconds or so, you won't feel discomfort. And, should you experience a twinge of guilt for not having followed the advice of your conscience, Madison Avenue has yet another ingenious antidote. The manufacturers use calcium in their antacid recipe, and you are carefully reminded that "everyone needs calcium." This perverse logic would suggest that overeating can lead to strong bones. But with your innate powers of discrimination, you know differently.

CHAPTER 7

The Descending Force of Grace

*Everyone sees the Unseen in proportion to the clarity of his heart,
and that depends upon how much he has polished it. Whoever has
polished it more sees more—more Unseen forms become manifest to
him.*

JALALUDDIN RUMI

The message of the sages of all traditions is the same. If
you set your sails and navigate through every experience
attentively—moment by moment and thought by thought—
everything you need will come to you through *kripa*, the grace
of the Divine Reality. If you can rely on the *buddhi* when
deciding which thoughts to give your attention to, align every
thought, word and action with the *shreya*, and surrender your
attachments to the *preya*, you will never again be imprisoned
by debilitating fear, unnecessary worry or stress.

Grace is a natural force—always present and available to
each human being to assist in achieving life's purpose: Self-
realization and freedom from pain, misery and bondage.
In fact, grace is being offered constantly, but because it is
so subtly woven into the fabric of everyday occurrences and
relationships, its exquisite and beneficial powers often go
unnoticed.

When you earnestly do your daily *sadhana*, however, you

receive the material, moral and spiritual benefits of increased energy, will power and creativity that will always lead you for your highest and greatest good. Regardless of how seemingly insignificant the offering of *preya*, if you are willing to exercise the ascending force of human effort you will never be faced with circumstances beyond your capabilities. But if you fail to do your part and serve the *preya* through self-will, you effectively separate yourself from the Source of all and you will stagnate.

Path of Fire and Light

The human body contains psycho-energetic centers called *chakras*. These exist within the subtle body sheath known as *pranamaya kosha* (the body of *prana*) and are described as swirling patterns of the creative energy and consciousness known as *kundalini*. The seven major *chakras* lie along the *sushumna* channel—a central canal running from the base of the spine to the crown of the head. This primary energy pathway within the subtle body is roughly analogous to the spinal column in the physical body (*annamaya kosha*).

At each *chakra*, concentrations of nerves, muscles and glands become manifest, together with different levels of consciousness. For instance, two of the primary *chakras*, the navel and heart *chakras*, correspond to energy centers in the body commonly known as the solar plexus and cardiac plexus. The *chakras* below the heart center primarily represent expressions of energy and consciousness dealing with the basic animal instincts for survival of the individual. The consciousness of these lower *chakras* concerns notions of the individual *I*, *me* and *mine*. The higher *chakras* represent the increasing union of individual consciousness with the Absolute Reality.

Heart *Chakra* and the Star of David

The heart *chakra* (*anahata chakra*), found at the level of the physical heart, can be considered a demarcation between the animal consciousness of the lower *chakras* and the Divine consciousness of the higher *chakras*. Its symbol is two intersecting triangles—the same symbol that represents modern Judaism as the six-pointed Star of David.

The first triangle is turned upward—an ascending triangle symbolizing the fire, or resolve (*sankalpa*), of human effort. This ascending force is our conscious discrimination between the *preya* and the *shreya* in mind, action and speech.

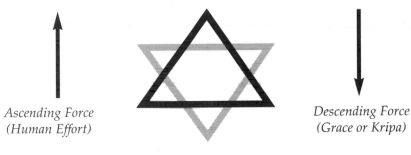

Ascending Force
(Human Effort)

Descending Force
(Grace or Kripa)

Symbol of the Heart Chakra

The second triangle depicted in the symbol of the heart *chakra* points downward. It represents grace (*kripa*). If you are consistently able to serve the *shreya* and surrender the *preya*, the *light* of the descending force of grace automatically appears in your life as love, fearlessness and strength.

But the sequence of events on the path of *fire and light* is critical. First and foremost, you must kindle your *fire* by taking the appropriate action based on the Divine wisdom of the *buddhi*. Then the *light* of grace descends. Jesus the Christ spoke of casting seeds on various kinds of soil, but only where the farmer had prepared the soil would those seeds sprout and prosper.

God is Great!

Many years ago there lived a king who relied extensively on the wise counsel of his best friend and most trusted minister for every major decision. One day, the king badly cut his hand. As court attendants scurried to help, the king's most trusted minister threw his arms toward the heavens and exclaimed with glee, "God is great!" This seeming insensitivity in the face of such physical and emotional trauma infuriated the king. To show his outrage, he immediately ordered the minister to be thrown into the dungeon. Upon hearing this decree, the minister once again threw his arms toward the heavens and shouted with great joy, "God is great!"

Several days later, when the king was feeling better, he went out from the castle on horseback for his weekly hunt. Upon spotting a deer, the king rode after it in chase. The deer eluded him for hours and, as dusk approached, the exhausted king dismounted to rest and fell into a deep sleep. In the middle of the night, he was awakened by a raucous band of tribal people who offered to bathe and feed him. As dawn approached, the tribesmen marched the king up to a high bluff overlooking their village and proceeded to tie him down on an altar. Now the king realized that his life was in danger, and he was filled with terror.

Suddenly, just as the king's head was about to be separated from his body, the wise man of the village unexpectedly stopped the human sacrifice. He explained that according to tradition only a "perfect man" could be offered as a sacrifice. Then, pointing to the unhealed wound on the king's hand, he ordered that the king be released.

With great joy and gratitude, the king rode back to the castle and immediately ordered his trusted minister to be released from the dungeon. The king told the minister of his harrowing experience and that he now finally understood why the minister had shouted, "God is great!" when the king had cut his hand. "However," the king said, "I still don't understand why you shouted 'God is great!' when I ordered you to the dungeon. Can you possibly explain this?"

"Well, your Excellency," the minister began, "if I had not been sent to the dungeon, I would most certainly have been riding with you on your weekly hunt, as I always do. Then, when the natives discovered that *you* were not the 'perfect man' . . . God is great!"

The moral of the story is this: If you are willing to surrender every thought, word and action to the will of the Divine Reality as communicated through the *buddhi*, you will always be led for your highest and greatest good. Despite the apparently unpleasant, despite the suggestions of the ego or the clamor of the senses, trustful surrender is the path of devotion that ensures your life will be filled with poetry and song.

Faith Born of Experience

If you should momentarily forsake your *sadhana* and take an action that serves the *preya* in thought, word or deed, no benefit accrues. Instead of receiving the bounty of grace, you experience some form of physical, mental, emotional or spiritual dis-ease. St. Francis de Sales put it this way: "God does not deprive us of the operation of His love, but rather, we deprive His love of our cooperation."

When the philosophy of yoga science guides your life you discover through your own personal experience that the light of Divine grace is often disguised as trivial, inconvenient, aggravating, worrisome or even painful thoughts or circumstances. If you fail to follow the advice of the *buddhi* in dealing with these thoughts or circumstances, grace cannot manifest. If you fail to recognize this, you may remain trapped in a whirlpool of delusion and conclude that real contentment in life comes about only by luck or by serving your own fear, anger or greed.

Initially, *sadhana* requires some discipline. As you experiment, however, the discipline soon yields to love because you experience the truth and pleasure of a practical, perennial wisdom that frees you from the bondage of habit and pain. Through personal experience, you cultivate *shraddha*—a faith that prepares you to rely on the teaching in ever more challenging circumstances and relationships. *Shraddha* is what the sages of every tradition refer to as trustful surrender to Divine Providence. Your highest and greatest good is always served when your actions serve Divine wisdom.

To verify this claim, begin working with the hypothesis that the thoughts, events and relationships in life are not mere accidents, but Divine manifestations perfectly suited to your own spiritual advancement. If you are earnest in your practice, you will begin to honor each and every thought as intrinsically valuable. As a yoga scientist, you are asked to consciously avoid any response that is injurious—not in harmony with *ahimsa*. By detaching yourself from the habits of fear, anger or self-willed desire, you are freed to consciously choose the thought, word or action that can fulfill your desires for unbounded Life, Liberty and Happiness.

Remember, grace is always flowing, but you cannot receive it by merely wishing for it. Rather, it manifests in the presence of the fire of human effort. Grace dawns when you do your actions with skill, love and full attention. The highest form of *kripa* is the grace of the Self. Only when your own conscience approves of your thoughts, actions and speech can you fully receive the blessings of grace.

Having a human body, mind and senses means that you have the instrumentation to venture beyond all the sorrow wrought by the limitation of animal consciousness and to live in the bliss-filled Reality of your own true Self. Do not delay. No one knows what the next moment of life will bring.

Grace, as the nineteenth century sage Ramakrishna taught, is a wind that is always blowing. If you really desire freedom in this lifetime and want to experience the full bliss of *Ananda*, set your sail today. As you skillfully navigate through life's many currents and crosscurrents with the *buddhi* as your sextant, the winds of grace will lovingly guide you through every challenging sea to a safe and bountiful harbor.

CHAPTER 8

Sacrifice:
A Mechanism for Transformation

It is more blessed to give than to receive.
JESUS THE CHRIST

The ritual of animal sacrifice was widely practiced in many early cultures. To be effective, the sacrifice had to represent a genuine loss—expressing the willingness to give up a real attachment. Only by consciously sacrificing the life of a healthy and productive animal was the offering considered meaningful.

In the ancient Indian scripture the *Bhagavad Gita*, Shri Krishna teaches Arjuna that duties performed as a sacrifice do not create bondage. "Whatever you do, make it an offering to Me—the food you eat or worship you perform, the help you give, even your suffering. Thus will you be free from *karma's* bondage, from the results of actions, good and bad." This kind of sacrifice is known as *yagna*. Real freedom, the *Gita* teaches, comes from mentally practicing the yoga of detachment— willingly giving up attachments by disciplining the senses and mind, and sacrificing the outcome, or fruit, of actions.

In daily life, the continued recurrence of certain *preyas* reflects strong attachments. Sometimes it seems almost impossible not to give these thoughts, desires and emotions your attention, but you can lessen the enslaving power of these deep *samskaras*. The surrendering of your attachment for the *preya* can begin by the fashioning of a small prayer in whatever form or tradition is most comfortable. No one knows better than you which attachments are the cause of your dis-ease. Simply make an offering of your fear, anger or selfish desire into the fire and light of eternal wisdom, ever-burning within the *cave of the heart*.

Silently repeat a meaningful prayer. For example: "Dear Lord, right now I am worried. This concern really has a hold on me. I'm attached to it, but I hear You through the *buddhi*, and don't want to continue serving this fear. I want to serve the *shreya*. Therefore, I offer this worrisome thought back to You, the Origin of all. Please accept this offering as the loving gift of a dedicated and humble heart. Consume it in the fire of your light and lead me for my highest and greatest good."

Your fear, anger and self-willed desires constitute an inherent power that belongs to you. Depending on your action, this power can manifest in either the contracting and debilitating form of *preya* or the expansive and liberating form of *shreya*. Whenever the *buddhi* advises you that what is appearing in your awareness is *preya*, welcome, witness and honor the *preya* and offer it back, as a genuine sacrifice, to the Origin from which it has come. This conscious act of renunciation and sacrifice effectively transforms the power of the *preya* into strategic reserves of energy, will power and creativity. At another time, when the *buddhi* suggests that you think, speak or act in service to a *shreya*, you'll find that you have the power at your disposal to do what is to be done.

Potential Versus Kinetic Energy

You learned in grade school science class that energy can appear in either the potential or kinetic form. The electricity in the wiring of your home is available for any use you choose. When you turn a light switch to the "on" position, energy appears in the form of light. This is the kinetic state because the energy is being used or expended. However, when you turn the light switch to the "off" position, the energy remains in the potential state—ready to be used at the flick of a switch.

The inherent power of fear, anger and self-willed desire can also be stored potentially or expended kinetically, and it is your personal attention that determines in which state the energy resides. If the *buddhi* defines a particular thought as *shreya*, it is suggesting that you transform the state of that thought energy from the potential into the kinetic by taking some appropriate action. In other words, you are encouraged to think about the *shreya*, speak in service to the *shreya*, and take some physical action in service to the *shreya*.

Such emotions as fear, anger and greed are not inherently bad or negative, for if they're handled skillfully, they can become helpful resources. If the *buddhi* recognizes them as *preya*, you are being asked to renounce your attachment to them so that their intrinsic power can be transformed and stored for your future use.

The Mind's Refinery

After years of practice in focusing the mind-field down to a point, and meticulous experimentation and observation, ancient sages understood the relationship between desire, action and consequence. In the *Brihadaranyaka Upanishad* they shared their insight:

> *You are what your deepest, driving desire is.*
> *As your deepest, driving desire is, so is your will.*
> *As your will is, so is your deed.*
> *As your deed is, so is your destiny.*
> BRIHADARANYAKA UPANISHAD

The laws of physical science state the same truth as the *Upanishads*: energy cannot be created nor destroyed, but it can be transformed. Viewing yoga as a sister science, the ancients experimented with controlling, conserving and transforming the energy of thought. Through trial and error they realized that when they renounced a single desire the energy of that desire manifested in a different form.

Recognizing this process, imagine what would happen if twenty gallons of crude oil directly from the fields of Saudi Arabia were pumped into your car's gas tank. It would wreck your engine. Crude oil is simply of no use in a combustion engine. To become an appropriate fuel for your automobile, the raw oil must first be refined.

Each of us has the capacity to employ a refining process that can transform the raw, inherent power of every thought, desire and emotion. When the *buddhi* intuitively advises that the unusable, destructive and constrictive power of a particular fear, anger or self-willed desire is appearing in your awareness in the form of *preya*, you, as a yoga scientist, have access to a mechanism for capturing and transforming that power. This refinement process is accomplished by consciously and willingly renouncing your attachment to the *preya*. In classical yoga texts, the employment of this discriminative faculty is referred to as *viveka*.

Remember, every gross and subtle object—including the *preya*—is a manifestation of the One Divine Reality. In every moment, the *buddhi* is always present to advise you that it's not in your best long-term interest to give the *preya* your continued attention. If you consciously or unconsciously choose to serve the *preya* in thought, word or deed, you will experience some form of physical, mental, emotional or spiritual dis-ease.

D = E + W + C
Desire = Energy + Will Power + Creativity

Through your personal *sadhana*, you will quickly learn that the transformative power of yoga science is a combination of conservation, ecology and banking. When you acknowledge that every relationship and action is actually a means for your spiritual unfoldment, great resources accrue to you in the subtle world.

Recognizing that desire is the fuel for human action, the ancient sages conceived a scientific formula that might well be called the spiritual equivalent of Albert Einstein's $E=MC^2$. The formula they discerned was $D = E + W + C$.

Every desire is composed of three basic components: energy, will power and creativity (consciousness). When you align every thought, word and action with the wise and good counsel of the *buddhi* by serving the *shreya*, you'll be led for your highest and greatest good. When you willingly and consciously surrender your attachment to the merely pleasant, comfortable, familiar and attractive *preya*, you really give up nothing of value. The intrinsic power of the *preya* is not lost to you. Instead, your voluntary act of renunciation and sacrifice (*yagna*) automatically transforms the *preya* into internal reserves of energy and will power and opens the doorway to the superconscious mind—your access to the Divine source of intuitive wisdom and creativity.

Conversely, when you go against the advice of the *buddhi* by serving the *preya* in thought, word and deed, your internal strategic reserves of energy, will power and creativity are diminished.

As Eknath Easwaran insightfully observed, the major crisis of our culture today is not one of IQ—intelligence quotient. Rather, the problem we face individually and collectively is one of WQ—will quotient. In twenty-first century America, countless people possess the intellectual capacity to make brilliant decisions, but because they are habituated to serving the *preya*, their reserves of will power have become bankrupt. Without sufficient will power to exercise discrimination, their reserves of energy and creativity are similarly diminished. The more these reserves are depleted, the more frequent and severe the tension, stress, anxiety and pain.

As in banking, our personal balance sheet always reflects whether deposits or withdrawals have been made. The choice of solvency or bankruptcy is up to each individual.

Fear, Anger and Greed:
Powerful Natural Resources

In modern life you need energy, will power and creativity to fulfill your many duties and responsibilities. You have obligations to yourself, your family, friends, business associates, society, the animal kingdom and the good earth Herself. You need a tremendous amount of energy, but where are you going to get all this energy? A certain amount comes from the food you eat and air you breathe, but the demands of modern life are tremendous, and you may sometimes find yourself without the reserves necessary to fulfill all your obligations.

Yoga science teaches that the creative energy you need is always available in the form of your thoughts, desires and emotions. A ready supply of power arises within you daily in the form of fear, anger and greed. If you do not expend this power kinetically in the present moment, you can consciously conserve and transform it for use at another time. Yoga science offers a systematic, practical method for conserving and transforming energy. It's very simple, and all it takes is knowing how to direct your attention appropriately, based on the intuitive wisdom already within you.

The Blues and Loss

Sadness, like fear, anger and greed, represents your inherent power. Everyone deals with an occasional case of the blues—what might be termed mild depression. When the blues start playing their sad, low-down melody, you have an opportunity to make great progress on the spiritual path. As a yoga scientist, honor and welcome the emotional dark cloud, surround it in the healing light of consciousness and ask the *buddhi* whether indulging this mood is a *preya* or *shreya*. Then, with all your strength, serve the wise counsel of the *buddhi*.

Remember, sometimes it's natural and helpful to feel sadness. It's part of being human. When we lose a loved one or face a major change in life, it's perfectly normal to mourn the loss. During those times, the blues can be a *shreya*—if you're also mindful to serve *ahimsa* and not harm yourself.

But there comes a time when the mourning period ends and continued grieving becomes an unhealthy *preya*. When the *buddhi* advises that singing the blues is doing you harm, it's time to sacrifice your attachment to the familiar and comfortable. This conscious act of renunciation can give you the courage to open your heart again.

Any mild depression begins with a desire that cannot be fulfilled. When the desire is repeatedly thwarted, the fiery emotion of anger arises. When that anger cannot fulfill the desire and can find no appropriate expression, it is repressed. Repressed anger becomes depression.

In the opening verses of the *Bhagavad Gita*, as the metaphoric battle at Kurukshetra is about to commence, Arjuna asks Shri Krishna to drive him onto the battlefield to survey the two opposing armies of the impending civil war. Arjuna was the greatest general of his time, but all his previous military engagements had been fought against foreign enemies. Now, however, Arjuna finds himself pitted against his relatives and revered teachers. His cause is undeniably just, yet because of his thwarted desire to protect those to whom he is attached, he is suddenly overwhelmed by a sense of deep despair that temporarily renders him incapable of fulfilling his duty.

The feeling of any loss or gain is the delusion of duality. It means that you have forgotten your true Self. True freedom comes only when you are willing to break out of the confines of a conditioned mind hobbled by limitation. Whenever you feel the blues draining your energy, focus and creativity, and your attention is locked on your own sorrow, remember to ask the question, "Who am I who is feeling this emotion?" Then, from the fullness of the Eternal Witness, seek the Divine wisdom of *buddhi* and place yourself in service to its judgment. At such times, it's especially helpful to undertake some selfless service by dedicating your efforts for the benefit of another. By sacrificing the *preya* of sad and hopeless emotions you can build reserves of energy, will power and creativity.

Attention Creates and Unlocks Vast Reserves

Your own attention—what you choose to give your attention to and what you choose to remove your attention from—determines your future. Attention is the engine of transformation. You already have all the necessary equipment. You don't have to buy anything. All you need is to be awake and to do what your discriminative faculty advises.

If you're a person who worries a great deal, and is often angered by situations and relationships, or besieged by desires for physical pleasure or material possessions, it means that you are a very wealthy individual. Your fears, anger and self-centered desires represent a powerful natural resource. Their latent power can bring you the health, happiness, creativity, productivity and loving, nurturing relationships you seek—if you are willing to make use of your attention as an internal mechanism for transformation.

Imagine for a moment that you've discovered a vast deposit of gold ore in your backyard. Without employing a mining operation and processing plant, you'd never benefit from your potential wealth. Similarly, without a philosophy of life that can turn your *preyas* into usable energy, will power and creativity, you will never realize your greatest potential.

Morning Tea Ritual

During the early days of our *sadhana*, Jenness had lingering doubts about the mechanism that transforms the power of desire into creativity, will power and energy. Could it really be so simple? As a yoga scientist, she decided to set up an experiment to determine if, by consciously giving up some small habitual indulgence, the energy of that habit could be transmuted into a creative resource in her life.

Jenness had developed the pleasant habit of enjoying a cup of hot tea with sugar and milk every morning. After consulting the *buddhi* regarding the effects of the sugar, caffeine and irritating tannins, she chose this as her test of the yogic formula **D = E + W + C**. She renounced her attachment to the gratifying tea ritual, began substituting the *shreya* of plain hot water and patiently watched for evidence of transformation.

Weeks later, Jenness had a conversation with a close relative who possessed precise knowledge of how to push her emotional buttons and always enjoyed doing so. During this particular exchange, however, Jenness suddenly found herself relaxed and loving, skillfully evading the usual pitfalls and frustrations. The meeting was actually quite pleasant and enjoyable—despite the fact that many sensitive issues were discussed.

Almost immediately, Jenness realized how the conversation had become so unexpectedly satisfying. Remembering her attachment to the tea ritual she had renounced, Jenness experienced an epiphany. "Aha," she humbly mused to herself, "now I know the transformative power of sacrifice through my own experience."

Consciously releasing the power tied up within small desires can increase your energy, will power and creativity—in ways and at times you most need help. The simple, yet courageous act of letting go, automatically activates a mechanism that transforms the mental energy of attachment.

Yoga science urges you to recognize that you always have choices, and that there are definite and specific consequences for each and every action. Moment by moment, the sages advise you to serve the *shreya* and surrender the *preya*. Only then will life become truly meaningful, creative and fulfilling.

Process for Transforming the Power of *Preya* Into Energy, Will Power and Expanded Creativity

1. While centering yourself in the Eternal Witness within, welcome, acknowledge and honor the thought, desire or emotion.

2. Consult the *buddhi* to determine whether the thought, desire, or emotion represents the *shreya* or *preya*.

3. If the thought, desire or emotion is *shreya*, serve it in thought, word or deed.

4. If the particular thought, desire or emotion is *preya*, after acknowledging, welcoming and honoring it, willingly and consciously surrender it back to the Origin from which it has come. Do this in whatever way is natural and comfortable for you.

By the willing and conscious removal of your attention from the *preya*, the inherent power of the *preya* is transformed in the subtle world into strategic reserves of energy, will power and consciousness.

Just Say "Yes!"

Sit quietly in a chair with your eyes closed. Bring your attention into the center of your chest and silently repeat the word "yes" ten times, making mental note of your emotional response. Then, with your attention still centered in the chest, repeat the word "no" ten times and evaluate the difference between the two experiences.

Most people find that giving attention to "yes" has an expansive, optimistic and liberating quality, while "no" feels heavy, contractive and burdensome.

Whenever you have a choice to make between the passing pleasure of *preya* and the perennial joy of *shreya*, just say "yes" to the Divine counsel of the *buddhi* and your thoughts, words and deeds will always lead you for your highest and greatest good.

The ego is likely to suggest that if you say "no" to an appealing *preya* you'll be denying yourself a genuine treat. So, don't say "no." Rather, view your sacrifice of *preya* as saying "yes" to the will of the Divine Reality. Saying "yes" to both serving the *shreya* and to surrendering the *preya* means never being deprived of anything worthwhile as you're led for your highest and greatest good.

CHAPTER 9

The Whitest Horse

From His Divine power comes forth all this magical show of name and form, of you and me, which casts the spell of pain and pleasure. Only when we pierce through this magic veil do we see the One who appears as many.

SHVETASHVATARA UPANISHAD

The sages of yoga science consistently remind us that if we are earnest in our *sadhana* and base our choices on the wise and good counsel of the *buddhi*, everything we need will come to us—like "a thief in the night." Because the vast majority of our choices relate to thoughts, desires and emotions, the fruits of these choices may require time and patience to be seen, understood and appreciated. A few precious experiences, however, are so immediate and dramatic that they're impossible to ignore. For us, the lesson of the whitest horse was both direct and profound and continues to inspire our spiritual practice to this day.

In ancient Indian scriptures, the term "white horse" appears in connection with the yogic practice of *pratyahara*—the withdrawal or purification of the senses. The name *Shvetashvatara* literally means "whitest horse" and refers to that sage who willingly and consciously surrenders the attractive, pleasant, familiar and comfortable allure of the *preya* in favor of the *shreya*—that choice that will always lead us toward our ultimate liberation—*moksha*.

A Lesson in Trust

In the autumn of 1993, Swami Rama left the United States and returned to Rishikesh in the foothills of his beloved Himalayan Mountains. At that time, rumors had circulated that this great teacher believed he had completed his life's mission and was ready to retire from the world in preparation for the final transition of death. Six months later, in March of 1994, we were invited to attend a one-month "spiritual journey" to study the *Shvetashvatara Upanishad* with Swami Rama in Rishikesh and to climb to the source of the Ganges River, high in the Himalayas.

Until that time, neither of us had felt a burning desire to visit India, yet we were suddenly drawn to this unique opportunity to study with Swami Rama for two reasons. First, we believed this would be Swami Rama's final public teaching, and since he had been our principal teacher for sixteen years, this trip presented an occasion for the respectful and sacred closure we longed for. The journey would be a way to say both "thank you" and "bon voyage." Secondly, since neither of us was even a novice mountain climber, the trek into the Himalayas represented a huge opportunity to confront our fears.

In discussing the possibility of making such a trip, however, cost quickly became a major issue. The $7,500 was an enormous amount of money for us at that time. As part of our spiritual practice we maintain a simple lifestyle, so withdrawing such a large sum of money from our long-term savings to travel halfway around the world seemed quite extravagant.

As the deadline approached, we were on an emotional seesaw. We knew the trip would be an important spiritual experience, but our concerns were real. We didn't have a lot of money and the cost represented a substantial sacrifice. Furthermore, there was the anticipated terror of entrusting our lives to allegedly sure-footed donkeys picking their way along narrow Himalayan rock ledges that, at any moment, might tumble us down into an unfathomable abyss.

Because our internal deliberations were so agonizing, we knew we were facing a major test of character. Witnessing our habit patterns, wrestling first with our fears and then with our desires, we earnestly tried to follow the suggestions of the *buddhi*—serving the *shreya* in thought, word and deed while surrendering our attachments back to the Origin from which they had come.

Finally, the day of reckoning was upon us. We had to make a decision—to go or not to go. And even though we had been struggling for weeks over the choice, that morning the answer was clear. There was no hesitation, no second-guessing. We both awakened that morning with a quiet certainty. We had passed beyond doubt. At 10:30 in the morning, with a calm deliberateness, we wrote a check for $7,500 and sent it off in the morning mail. The deed was done. Despite our fears and concerns, we were going to Rishikesh, India to study the *Shvetashvatara Upanishad* with Swami Rama.

As the confidence of our morning decision withstood guerrilla attack from deep-seated *samskaras*, we remained resolute. Worries did resurface, but we were steadfast in our efforts to witness and honor them while serving the wise and good counsel of the *buddhi*. At lunchtime, neither of us had very much to say. It seemed more appropriate to rest in our *mantra* as we prepared and ate our food rather than to rehash the long deliberations that had brought us to this peace.

Around 3:30 that same afternoon I received a momentous telephone call from a long-time art patron in Florida. He was calling to commission Jenness to create a traditional conformation portrait of his celebrated thoroughbred racehorse, Runaway Groom. Since the client had been a collector for many years and was familiar with Jenness's artwork, our conversation included none of the usual sales banter. Instead, we concentrated on where the horse was stabled in Lexington, the name and telephone number of the farm manager so we could schedule a visit and how long it would take to complete the commission.

When asked if he'd like to speak with Jenness personally to work out details of the painting, the client declined. "Jenness is a fine painter," he replied. "I have confidence that she'll create a magnificent painting." Then he added, "There is just one thing, however, that I'd definitely like you to tell her for me. As you know, I've been associated with the horse racing industry for many years. Please tell her that in all those years, this is the whitest horse I have ever seen."

With a chill at the back of my neck, the hairs standing straight up on my arm and my *mantra* resonating in my ears, I thanked the client and respectfully ended the conversation as quickly as possible—dashing out of my office and across the hall to Jenness's studio to recount the miraculous story. Choking a bit on the humbling events that had just transpired, I recounted the story. "Jenness," I said, "this morning, following the advice of the *buddhi*, we surrendered the *preya* of fear by sacrificing seven thousand five hundred dollars to travel to India to study the 'whitest horse' *Upanishad* with Swami Rama. Now, on this same afternoon, Don Dizney has just commissioned a painting of Runaway Groom, and he insists that I tell you personally that this is the whitest horse he has ever seen."

As if those coincidences were not enough to humble and inspire us, the price of the commission was, to the penny, the same as for the trip to India—$7,500! In other words, the portrait of the "whitest horse" was going to pay for our trip to India to study the "whitest horse" *Upanishad*.

We are still learning the great lesson of this amazing experience: that unimaginable and beneficial circumstances can, and do, come into our lives to guide us. But in order to receive this bounty of Divine grace, we must first consciously, willingly and lovingly serve the *shreya* and surrender the *preya*—preparing the soil for seeds of grace to sprout.

"Grace," the sages promise, "is always available," and the preparation for receiving is simple. The first step is abiding faith, *shraddha*. It is *shraddha* that provides us the will and resolution to surrender the *preya* in order to serve a higher good. *Shraddha* also prepares us to recognize Grace when it appears. If Grace falls directly into our laps, yet goes unrecognized, we do not truly receive it. We must be ready to see it for what it is and to gratefully accept and employ it.

For us, this story continues to be a straightforward and dramatic demonstration of a timeless law, one which is acknowledged in every tradition. Perhaps Jesus the Christ states it most succinctly in the Sermon on the Mount when He tells us, "seek ye first the kingdom of God, and all these things will be added unto you." This is the unforgettable message of our own experience with the grace of the *Shvetashvatara*—the whitest horse. Through continuous practice and the unshakable faith that is its reward, we prepare ourselves to know and receive the guidance and help that are already before us.

CHAPTER 10
Ahimsa is the Golden Rule

Thou shalt love thy neighbor as thy Self.
JESUS THE CHRIST

Ahimsa is the highest precept of yoga science. It is the first of the *yamas* and *niyamas*—constructive observances and disciplines codified in Patanjali's *Yoga Sutras*. *Ahimsa* means non-violence, non-injuring or non-harming, and it is the guiding yogic principle underlying every successful relationship—within and without, subtle and gross, with others and with yourself.

In practical terms, *ahimsa* is the same wisdom as the Golden Rule that instructs human beings to "Do unto others as you wish to have done unto you," or as Jesus the Christ teaches: "Love thy neighbor as thy self." Mahatma Gandhi always insisted that, "*Ahimsa* is an attribute of the soul—to be practiced by everybody in all affairs of life. If it cannot be practiced in all circumstances, it has no practical value." The logic behind all these instructions is one and the same: on the highest level of consciousness, thy neighbor *is* thy Self.

The sages of yoga science teach that every thought, word and action must be in harmony with *ahimsa*. If you serve *ahimsa* in mind, action and speech, you automatically will be in harmony with the universal law of *dharma*—that which maintains individual and social order by guiding humanity toward its highest destiny. If you practice *ahimsa*, you will experience a loving, healthy, creative and productive life. If you do not practice *ahimsa*, the consequence will be some form of physical, mental, emotional or spiritual dis-ease or pain.

Although yoga science acknowledges the multiplicity of changing names and forms, it recognizes only One Absolute Reality. Therefore, if you think, speak or act in a harmful or injurious manner, that injury will ultimately come back upon you. The Bible teaches that, "As you sow, so shall you reap," or, in modern parlance, "What goes around, comes around."

Your senses, ego and unconscious mind took control of the city of life many years ago. Yoga science helps you rectify that situation by placing them in service to a non-local intelligence greater than the mind and a truth that never changes. Even in the midst of a sea of change and turbulence, the wisdom of the eternal soul serves as a beacon leading you toward your highest and greatest good.

Our present world view has been formed by a culture that does not wholeheartedly embrace this philosophy, so it may take a little effort before you're able to practice *ahimsa* in every thought, word and deed. Because of the power of habit, you will need to exhibit a great deal of patience and kindness toward yourself. In fact, the successful practice of *ahimsa* always includes yourself. Charity must begin at home; it must include every relationship that involves you.

"Oh, no," you say, "if I indulge myself, others might think I'm selfish and that's not good." Well, yoga science explains that there's nothing wrong with being selfish—if the real Self being served is the Lord of Life. If you disregard the Divine wisdom of *buddhi* and you're not kind to yourSelf in mind, action and speech, you cannot truly benefit others—because there is no "other." When you serve the *buddhi* and make the effort to be gentle and kind to yourSelf, everything and everyone benefits—including you. Even the most simple and inwardly loving actions you take toward yourSelf (including your thoughts) have effects more far-reaching than you can imagine. When you drop a stone into a pond, the ripples stretch to the farthest edges.

The Tenth Man

Ten boys eagerly embarked on their first unsupervised overnight campout. As they crossed a wide and unexpectedly flooded stream, the ten were separated by the swift current. Upon reaching the opposite shore, the boys reassembled and one camper counted the others to make sure that all ten had made it across safely. Methodically pointing his finger to each boy, he began counting aloud. "One, two, three, four, five, six, seven, eight, nine." To his horror, he was able to count only *nine* campers.

In panic, each camper then took his turn in counting the others, but each could count only nine. Alas, someone was missing. As they wept for their drowned friend, a stranger passing along the same trail inquired as to the cause of their trouble. Upon hearing that one of the ten campers had drowned, the stranger arranged all the boys in a straight line—shoulder to shoulder—and began to count aloud. "One, two, three, four, five, six, seven, eight, nine, ten!" The stranger explained that the boys had erred in their count because each camper had failed to count himself as the tenth man. In fact, all the campers were—and always had been—present and accounted for.

It is essential that you always count yourself as an integral part of every circumstance. Remember this as you practice *ahimsa*. If, when trying to please others, you injure yourself, that act of "kindness" is to be forsaken. You are always the tenth man.

The *Sadhu* and the Snake

A wandering *sadhu* (holy man) entered a remote village in ancient India and found the streets strangely deserted. As he stood bewildered in the market place, a few villagers peeked out from shuttered windows, then hurried toward him asking for his help. They told him the story of their once happy community that had lost its joy when a huge and aggressive cobra made its den in their midst. The poisonous snake (*naga*) had attacked several people. Now all the children had to stay indoors for their safety and farmers feared to go into their fields.

"Please help us," they begged. The *sadhu* thought for a moment about what he could do, then answered, "Yes. I can help."

He went straight to the cobra's den and called until the powerful snake emerged. Then he spoke very sternly: "Now see here, Naga, it seems you have forgotten the first principle of yoga: *ahimsa*. This biting must stop! It's not kind." The *sadhu* proceeded to give the cobra a convincing lecture on the importance of *ahimsa*.

The snake saw the error of his ways and sincerely vowed to become gentle. Upon hearing this, the *sadhu* returned to the marketplace and confidently announced the cobra's reformation. Everyone cheered and thanked him, and he continued on his way.

Several months later, the holy man's travels brought him again to that same village. To his surprise, he found the cobra—now extremely thin and weak—lying in the middle of the road, badly wounded, bloody and barely alive.

"What has happened to you?" the *sadhu* asked with great concern. "I did as you told me," the snake gasped. "But the boys, knowing they had nothing to fear, threw stones at me and beat me with sticks. I remembered to practice *ahimsa* and did not harm them. Now, see what has become of me because of your advice."

As the *sadhu* began to attend compassionately to the cobra's wounds he quietly explained, "I told you not to bite, but I never told you not to hiss!"

Practicing *ahimsa* never makes you a doormat for someone else's insensitivity. In fact, you must apply *ahimsa* to yourself first before it can become an effective force in relationships with "others." By respecting yourself and others, you learn to reach deep into your inner creative resources to fashion the skillful response that is appropriate to the circumstance.

Lesson of the Dinner Plates

As children, Jenness and I often watched Ed Sullivan's "Toast of the Town" television show on Sunday nights. Among the performers we saw over the years, one old-time vaudevillian's act always held our attention, and we've thought about it often in relation to yoga science.

This performer had a rather simple act. Before him stood three long banquet tables. Secured to the tables were upright wooden dowels, each measuring about three feet in height. The performer proceeded to balance a spinning dinner plate atop one of the dowels on the table and kept it balanced by twirling the dowel. Then he balanced a second and a third plate. By the time he started to balance the fourth one, he had to run back to the first and re-twirl the dowel. And then he'd run to balance the fourth plate and a fifth plate and a sixth plate—until there were twenty or so! By the end of the act, to keep all his plates in the air simultaneously, he was dashing back and forth like a madman. Needless to say, it was a riveting sight.

That vaudevillian was a great teacher—a true *guru*. His act has taught us a lot about our own habits. When we were twenty, we said to ourselves, "We can do that," and we balanced a few plates in the air. When we were thirty, we said to ourselves, "We can do that, too," and up went a few more. When we were forty, "We can do that." When we were fifty, "We can do that."

But as we entered middle age, we began to realize that a lot of our time was being spent just rushing to keep all those plates in the air. We had taken on so many obligations, it sometimes felt as though we were enslaved to tiring and stressful expectations, disappointments and hassles. We had become so busy keeping all our plates in the air that we hardly had time or energy for nurturing ourselves and our loved ones.

To help us end our bondage, yoga science poses this question: "Who is it who is choosing to balance all these plates?" In other words, "Who am I?" That is always the key! "Who am I, who has all these plates in the air? Who am I, who desires to have these plates in the air? Am I practicing *ahimsa* by keeping so many plates in the air?" Remember, each and every thought is merely a suggestion of what to give your attention to; it is not an imperial command. You can always have control over your actions.

Swami Rama of the Himalayas always marveled at the intelligence of his Western students, but he also recognized our lack of patience. He likened our condition to that of a first-time gardener. The novice tills and fertilizes the soil, carefully plants the seeds, covers them gently, waters them, says a prayer and retires for the night. Waking the next morning filled with exuberance, he races to the garden to survey his new crop, only to be emotionally devastated because nothing has sprouted. Concerned that the seeds might have been defective or eaten by some pest, the gardener digs up the seeds, trying to discover the problem. Of course nothing is really wrong with the seeds. The problem is a lack of patience and under-standing of the process. Anything worthwhile takes love and self-discipline.

Remember: be kind to yourself; put some conscious effort into learning to love yourself. Be patient, and try not to take on too much too soon. Throughout your entire *sadhana*, start with what's easy and the choice will be exactly right for you. In order to be the right choice, it must be easy. If you wanted to become a body builder, you wouldn't rush into the gym and, with no prior experience, begin to bench-press two hundred pounds. You'd start by lifting just the bar with no additional weight. Then, you'd gradually add five pounds, then ten pounds, then twenty—until you reached your ultimate goal.

Ahimsa must begin with you, and in order to apply the precept of *ahimsa* to every thought, word and action, you must exhibit patience and love. In the words of William Shakespeare, "How poor are they that have not patience! What wound did ever heal but by degree?"

Give your *sadhana* a little time, but continue to test, experiment, evaluate and trust the teaching. Slowly, slowly, you will begin to recognize that there is a perfectly compassionate and benevolent wisdom beyond the mind—always eager to lead you for your highest and greatest good.

Gandhi's Experiment with Anger

Early in the 1920s, when Mahatma Gandhi was working to promote civil rights in South Africa, he was traveling on a train. He was a highly educated young attorney, well-dressed and seated in first-class accommodations. As he sat on the train, a British conductor approached him and announced that because of his dark skin he would have to move to the rear coach. Gandhi insisted that he had appropriate first-class passage, displayed his ticket and refused to submit to the racist indignity. Despite his protestations, however, young Gandhi was summarily thrown off the train.

That night in a cold, dark, abandoned railroad station, Gandhi was battered by a relentless storm of rage. He endured wave after wave of fury as he strode up and down the platform, fuming. Mighty, righteous anger roared in his awareness throughout the night, raising the level of his fury to volcanic proportions.

Gandhi could have reacted in a destructive manner. He could have chosen to serve the *preya*. He could have picked up a club or found a gun. He could have injured or even killed someone. Instead, recalling the truth of yoga science, Gandhi had a profound realization that night. Anger is power! He suddenly recognized the tremendous power that existed in the anger of the Indian people—enough power, if it were focused, to cast off the shackles of the world's greatest military force. In one great flash of insight, Gandhi knew that his vision for Indian independence could be realized by transforming huge reserves of mental energy through the disciplined practice of *ahimsa*.

Slowing Down

The speed at which our culture is operating makes moment-by-moment decisions extremely challenging. Rushed judgments are generally based on our reactionary habits of fear, anger and self-willed desire, rather than a conscious evaluation of alternatives and consequences.

Yoga science, however, encourages us to consider possible choices that we otherwise might overlook. The prevailing tide of our culture suggests that to be happy or successful we should be driving at one hundred miles per hour in the passing lane of life. But yoga science teaches us that true happiness can be found by driving comfortably in the far right-hand lane at a slower and safer rate of speed. Each of us can do it, of course, if we are aware that we have a choice, and if we can rely on the wisdom of our discriminatory faculty rather than the suggestions of others. Certainly, there are circumstances that occasionally require us to drive in the fast lane, but we don't have to make it a dangerous habit. The decision is ours, and must be made consciously moment by moment.

Training the Senses

Learning to train the senses is an important step in attaining real freedom and happiness. In yoga science, this form of discipline is known as *pratyahara*.

Like school children, our senses are without the capacity to discriminate. Anyone who has ever worked in a business environment knows that if all the employees were seventh graders, running a successful operation would be impossible. And yet that's very much the situation we find ourselves in when the untrained senses reign. "Let's look at something pleasurable," sight clamors. "Let's smell something pleasant," the nose butts in. "Let's hear something delightful," the ears insist. "Let's taste something delicious," the mouth suggests. "Let's touch something lovely," the hands propose. Very little of lasting value and no real fulfillment results from satisfying this crew's constant demands. For instance, you may love chocolate ice cream, but if you followed the taste buds' suggestion and ate only chocolate ice cream at every meal, you'd quickly grow quite sick of it and your health would suffer.

Based on our personal experience, we can assure you that the life of a yoga scientist is never dull or drab. Remember that we're not asked to give up sense pleasures, only our attachment to them. This life is to be enjoyed. However, to fully appreciate the world without regrets, you must establish balance—choosing your actions with mindful attention and discrimination.

Karma Yoga:
Placing the Welfare of Others First

Putting the welfare of others first (*karma yoga*) is a practical application of *ahimsa*. The sages tell us that only One reality exists—consciousness itself: *Sat-Chit-Ananda* (eternal existence, consciousness/wisdom and bliss). Yes, countless names and forms do exist. Duality exists, but only relatively. Absolute Reality is One.

Yoga science helps us to annihilate the perceived separation between "me" and any "other" by teaching us how to focus our attention on the One Absolute Reality—in all creatures, objects and situations. In many Asian cultures, people traditionally greet one another with their palms together in the prayer gesture and with a slight bow. In India, the spoken greeting is *Namaste*: "I pray to the Divinity in you." You and I are One.

Yes, each of us has a different name, form and capabilities, but the Absolute Reality *(Sat-Chit-Ananda)* is the very same within each of us. So, to offer the fruit of your action to an "other" means that somewhere in space and time, something will be added to you. To hold on to the fruit of one's action—to be attached to the result of the action in a self-willed and judgmental manner—means that somewhere in space and time something will be detracted from you. Each of us reaps the fruits of his or her actions according to the universal *law of karma*, "As you sow, so shall you reap."

The Company You Keep Is Stronger than Your Will

Do you remember when your mother or father warned you against associating with certain acquaintances? "Don't hang around with those kids," they warned. "They're not a good influence." The sages give the same loving parental advice: the company you keep is stronger than your will. It's a version of the law of physics that states a liquid assumes the shape of the container in which it is held.

On the subtle level, if you keep company with thoughts that your discriminative faculty recognizes as *preya*, this association gradually influences you to pay increasing attention to such thoughts. The more attention you give these subtle objects, the more likely you are to take actions based on the influence of *preya*, and the more you diminish your will power. Remember, all power flows from the subtle to the gross.

Children, as we know, are sometimes inclined to go against the advice of their parents. In childhood, a certain amount of experimentation is necessary. Sometimes a child may have to touch a stove to find out if the burners are hot, but as an adult you do not have to touch every burner on every stove. In determining what company to keep in our lives and in our minds, the mature human being utilizes the *buddhi's* capacity to discriminate rather than personal experience alone. With practice, the yoga scientist becomes increasingly decisive and fearless.

Inspirational Reading and *Satsang*

Ancient scriptures, as well as the writings and biographies

of the great mystics of all traditions, also become positive companions in our lives. A suggested reading list can be found in the *Resources* section at the end of this book. This company is a great support and inspiration because these human beings have already dealt with the very same issues you are facing today. At the turn of the twenty-first century, our culture would have us believe that our modernity makes us different from our predecessors. After all, we've taken trips to the moon and have computers, cell phones, television, fancy automobiles and air conditioners. On a very basic level, however, no difference exists between us and the cave dwellers who lived twenty thousand years ago. When the caveman was sharpening his one-and-only stone knife and the point broke, the anger and fear he had to deal with were no different from the anger and fear you feel today. Names and forms have changed, but when your computer software program crashes, you face the same emotions as the caveman.

Throughout history, the highest goal of life for humankind has remained the same: in the face of fear, anger and selfish desire, to remember the wisdom of the Divinity within; to recognize that a choice exists; to learn to discriminate between the *preya* and the *shreya*; and to align each thought, word and action with the *buddhi*.

This scientific process can transform the consequences of powerful emotions and desires and empower you to live each moment in harmony with the first precept of yoga: *ahimsa*. For this reason, the practice of *satsang*—enjoying frequent contact with like-minded spiritual seekers and teachers—will strengthen your will power and enhance every aspect of your *sadhana*.

CHAPTER 11

Are You a Reactionary?

*As irrigators lead water where they want, as archers make their
arrows straight, as carpenters carve wood, the wise shape their
minds.*

THE COMPASSIONATE BUDDHA

Each of us receives varying measures of praise and blame
every day. Yoga science reminds us that both are really only
suggestions. We can choose to accept any suggestion or
to reject it. There is no reason to remain enslaved to the
suggestions of another.

Good Boy or Bad Boy?

From the age of two, Swami Rama was raised in the cave
monasteries of the Himalayan mountains. When he was seven
or eight years old, a monk he greatly respected sternly told
him, "You're a very bad boy!" Following this mystifying and
unpleasant encounter the boy was crestfallen and grew
depressed.

A few days later a second monk, whom the young boy also
respected, greeted him with a big smile on his face. Hugging
the child, he exclaimed, "You're a wonderful boy!" Following
this praise, the child's spirits soared.

After some time, he began to ponder this perplexing

situation. One monk he respected greatly had told him he was a bad boy, and he grew depressed. Then a second monk he also respected told him he was a good boy, and he felt happy. The conflicting pronouncements were confusing. To solve the dilemma, he went to his master. "Sir," he asked, "am I a good boy, or am I a bad boy?"

After considering the boy's confusion, the master replied, "My son, you are neither a good boy nor a bad boy. You're a stupid boy—for accepting the suggestions of others so freely!"

Buddha's Begging Bowl

A similar story is told of the Buddha, who was traveling with his disciple Anand. In those days, as in modern India, renunciates wandered with begging bowl in hand, asking for food. However, in the Buddha's village renunciates began to outnumber the householders who were bound by custom to support them.

One morning the Buddha and Anand approached a farm where a woman was busy in the barn milking her cows. She was already exasperated after tending to a long procession of begging renunciates. Upon seeing the Buddha and his disciple, she burst into an angry tirade against the useless band of beggars who constantly interrupted her work. She shouted, "You're a strong, healthy man. Why do you beg? You're a blight on society and a disgrace to your family! Why don't you get a job?" With that, she picked up some cow dung and, extending her hand as if to fill the Buddha's waiting bowl, shouted, "You want something? Take this!"

Reacting to her wrath, Anand became just as enraged, and in an attempt to protect his master's dignity, began to loudly berate the woman's vulgarity.

But the Buddha, serene as ever, simply bowed respectfully, pulled back his empty bowl and kindly whispered to the woman, "No thank you, Mother. I have no need of your offering."

For the enlightened Buddha, the woman's anger was

merely a suggestion. Because he was centered in a state of equanimity (*nirvana*) and awake to his own true nature, he could not be forced into an angry reaction. The Buddha was a free man. He was able to choose the *shreya* over the *preya*.

Even if the Buddha had momentarily experienced a desire to react with anger, it would not have meant that he had to be enslaved to that suggestion. Remember, thoughts that evoke anger, fear or greed come to everyone. There's no crime in having a thought. But continually serving the *preya* in mind, action and speech only assures dis-ease. By willingly and consciously surrendering the *preya*, even habitual angry thoughts can be transformed into reserves of energy, will power and creativity—available for use when needed most.

The important lesson to remember is that when people or circumstances offer you their anger, negativity or anything else that is not in harmony with the Divine counsel of a purified *buddhi*, you are under no obligation to accept it. The choice is yours.

These stories are reminders that our every thought, word and action has certain distinct consequences that can lead us either closer to fulfillment or farther away. If we embrace this philosophy of life that helps us steer a determined course, we can skillfully navigate the unpredictable currents and crosscurrents of life. Otherwise, we unconsciously remain reactionaries to whatever suggestions come our way.

When we earnestly pursue our *sadhana* and contemplate the question "Who am I?" we begin to hear the *buddhi* quite clearly. Then, by consistently following this intuitive wisdom we find ourselves capable of keeping our balance—even in tremendous flux and travail.

The key to successful living is learning to base our worldly actions on the intuitive wisdom within. By cultivating one-pointed attention, we are free to see things as they are, rather than as they appear. We stay open to our Inner Source of well-being—to the exclusion of the mind's random suggestions—and creative ideas flow from the superconscious mind.

You already possess your own unique key to the library of knowledge within. It can unlock your own unique wisdom. The wonder and challenge of this lifetime is that if you can remain awake in the present moment and use your key to intuitive wisdom, you will realize your fullest potential. In other words, you will live in unbounded Liberty and Happiness—no matter what.

Lesson of Motion Pictures

Watching a good movie can be very entertaining. In a darkened theater, a well-produced film can capture your attention and transport you to another reality. A classic movie like "Gone with the Wind" can leave you with the feeling that you know Rhett Butler and Scarlet O'Hara and that you remember what it was like to live in the South during the Civil War.

Technically, a motion picture is nothing more than a series of individual frames of celluloid spliced together. Because the frames of the movie are projected onto a screen in a darkened theater in such rapid succession, the viewer experiences the illusion of reality.

The same can be said about individual thoughts that come into your awareness. Eknath Easwaran taught that a thought is analogous to an individual movie frame. When a thought comes into your awareness, it is your continued attention that splices one thought to a second thought, to a third thought and a fourth. Just as with a rapidly projected movie, it is your attention that creates the illusion of reality. As you give continued attention to any subtle or gross object, your attachment to it grows until you have created one powerful, overwhelming, seamless desire.

Between and surrounding two thoughts, however, there exists a silence. In that silence there is consciousness, the sea of eternal consciousness into which all objects appear. In yoga science, this omnipresent sea of consciousness is known as the Eternal Witness.

If you are awake to the presence of the Eternal Witness within, Its perfect wisdom will come forward into your awareness to help you see the infinite possibilities existing in that silence between two thoughts. If you consciously serve that Eternal Witness in thought, word and deed you will create new, healthy *samskaras* that lead you for your highest and greatest good. However, if you ignore the possibilities, your mind, action and speech will remain enslaved to the self-created mental software of habit and familiar emotion. The consequence is inevitable pain and limitation.

If a thought comes into your awareness, view it as a suggestion of what to give your attention to. As your *sadhana* becomes more consistent, you will be increasingly free to consciously choose the *shreya* over the *preya*. Real freedom is knowing how to direct your attention with discrimination. You can act consciously, creatively and lovingly, even when confronted with the temptation of the comfortable, attractive and familiar.

Remember, thoughts, desires and emotions are forms of raw power coming to you through the grace of the Divine Reality. What are you to do with that power? The answer to that question can determine whether you have a rewarding life, lived free from worry, or the life of an enslaved reactionary.

CHAPTER 12
Who is Your Guru?

Who is wise? He who learns from all men.

THE TALMUD

I have learned silence from the talkative, toleration from the intolerant, and kindness from the unkind; yet strange, I am ungrateful to these teachers.

KAHLIL GIBRAN

Since the 1960s, many North Americans have traveled to the East in search of a *guru* who might liberate them from the painful trials and tribulations of everyday life. During the same time, a succession of spiritual teachers have visited the West to teach the ancient science of yoga and to guide seekers along the path of Self-realization.

Tradition dictates that when a relationship is established between student and teacher, the teacher becomes responsible for the development of the student, and that the greater the student's adherence to the teaching, the quicker his or her progress will be. This interaction and commitment is known as the *guru-disciple relationship*, and for many earnest students this is a time-honored path to the personal liberation known as *moksha*.

Contrary to popular cultural myth, *guru* is not a person. *Guru* is a principle—a universal force of light that dispels the darkness of ignorance. As fundamental as the elements of space, air, fire, water and earth, the *light of guru* is also a naturally occurring element, or *tattva*. But unlike the elements that make up the material world, the *guru* principle exists as a teacher within each of us—always available to help correct our ignorance and cure our dis-ease.

Since our Essential Nature already exists in a state of perpetual light, the darkness spoken of here—that which is in need of enlightenment—is a condition of the mind. The mind and its habit patterns of fear, anger and greed keep us groping in a state of darkness, ignoring the light of our own Divine nature. The confused mind does not realize its own self-imposed limitations. The function of the *guru* principle is to purify the mind so it can recognize that it must find the light and, ultimately, surrender and merge with the light. Enlightenment refers to an enlightened mind—an instrument of *guru* continuously reflecting the discrimination of *buddhi*.

> *Guru is timelessly present in our heart. Sometimes the guru principle is externalized as an uplifting and reforming factor in our life—a spiritual teacher, mother, father, wife, friend, or adversary, or as an inner urge towards righteousness and perfection. All we have to do is to heed the suggestion of guru and we will be led for our highest and greatest good. What guru asks each of us, in return, is quite simple: learn self-awareness, self-control and self-surrender. This may seem arduous at times, but it is easy if we are earnest—and quite impossible if we are not. Earnestness is both necessary and sufficient. Everything yields to earnestness.*
>
> NISARGADATTA MAHARAJ

Yoga philosophy explains that the *light of guru* appears in every relationship, if we are willing to look beyond our *raga/dveshas* (likes and dislikes). As we become detached from our own fear, anger and self-willed desire, the mind is purified and we are open to important lessons for growth and expansion. Regardless of whether our relationship is personal and intimate, or one as distant as those facilitated by the media, every relationship is an expression of Divine Providence—a means to our spiritual unfoldment.

To receive this grace we must first learn to include *all* and exclude *none*. We must be willing to accept and welcome the fact that every relationship has something beneficial to bring us, as well as something unique to receive from us. Whether the situation appears pleasant or unpleasant to the *ahamkara* (I-maker or ego), we can learn to be present with whatever appears—welcoming, honoring and observing it without being controlled by it. Centered in the fullness and equanimity of the Eternal Witness (*Sat-Chit-Ananda*), we can invite the *light of guru* to dwell within us and shine forth through us in the form of selfless love. Eventually, this love is returned to us because when we give love we give to our Self.

In daily life we all encounter relationships that we perceive as being either pleasant or painful. The sages remind us, however, that pairs of opposites are not what they seem. That which appears as pleasant eventually will become unpleasant. For instance, we may love to hear a certain song on the radio, but if that song were played twenty-four hours a day, the pleasure would inevitably yield to dis-ease. And that which appears as unpleasant will just as inevitably yield a special blessing.

The key, of course, is to be present in each moment—paying attention and knowing that the *light of guru* reveals itself at the point of equanimity. If we are open and attentive, every relationship provides a unique and beneficial teaching of *guru*.

Elvis is *Guru*

An acquaintance once asked, "Wasn't Elvis Presley's life a tragedy?" The question opened a floodgate of memories. My relationship with Elvis Presley had begun in 1956. As a teenager, listening to Elvis's music was one of my first experiences with meditation. Every time I listened intently to his music I felt happy—so happy in fact, that I began to associate Elvis and his music with my happiness. As Paul McCartney similarly observed, "I always knew that no matter how I felt, if I played an Elvis record it would make me happy." Because of this experience, over the years I continued to freely give my attention to Elvis Presley.

For me, Elvis had charisma. To some extent, each of us has experienced the power of charisma. When someone has charisma, we feel an overwhelming, magnetic attraction that demands our attention. But from a yogic perspective, it's interesting to question the *karmic* purpose of such a phenomenon. What is to be learned from an individual who commands our attention, our love, or even our anger?

Before responding about the tragedy or non-tragedy of Elvis's life, I began to process some memories of him from the *chitta*. Because I had given Elvis my attention over the years, I actually knew quite a bit about his desires, choices, achievements and some of the painful consequences he experienced—many of which appeared to result from serving the *preya* of ego or sense gratification. Elvis Presley was obviously a generous and loving man, yet many of his actions were not in harmony with the *guru* in the cave of my own heart. Observing all this, I knew that as a yoga scientist, Elvis Presley's life was not a tragedy for me. Because I had been attentive to Elvis's life, I was able to receive many important lessons that instructed me what to do—and what *not* to do. Yes, even Elvis can be a vehicle for *guru*.

The Child is *Guru*

Swami Hariharananda, a contemporary sage who lived twelve years as a hermit in the Himalayan mountains, tells a charming story of the time he participated in a teaching conference in India. On the first morning of the meeting, torrential rains postponed the opening session. Not wanting to waste an opportunity to teach, Swami Hari approached a young boy who stood holding a candle inside the darkened building.

Inspired by the candlelight and the knowledge that all light is One, Swami Hari intended to explain a very basic lesson of yoga science: that the light of a candle is the same as the light in a boy's eye and the light of the sun. Pointing to the flame, Swami Hari asked, "Son, do you know where that light has come from?" As he pondered his answer, the boy alternately looked at the flame, then toward Swami Hari, then back to the flame, and again to Swami Hari. Gazing intently at the flame, he took a deep breath and vigorously blew out the candle. "Sir," he asked, "do you know where the light has gone?!"

As Art Linkletter often mused, "Kids say the darndest things"—and profound things as well. In this story, the child unexpectedly becomes the teacher and a vehicle for *guru*. His penetrating response reminds us that Swami Hari's original question cannot be answered by the intellect. Instead of trying to hedge or ineptly answer the question, the child simply redirects the Swami's own attention back to *guru* and even beyond—back to the Source of truth.

In order to be open to the ever-present *light of guru*, in whatever form it may appear, each of us must be willing to be as innocent, open and non-judgmental as a child. When the outer *guru* reflects the truth of the inner *guru*, the advice is to be heeded and served. When a suggestion from the outer *guru* is not in harmony with the inner *guru*, as reflected by the purified *buddhi*, the advice is to be honored, respected and lovingly rejected, with gratitude—for your teacher has just taught you what not to do.

The Teacher and Teaching are within You

Your every thought presents an opportunity to choose what to give your attention to and what to withdraw your attention from. As a yoga scientist, you cultivate skills that enable you to be consciously present to serve the *shreya*—moment by moment—as suggested by the *buddhi*.

Each human being possesses the capacity to consult the discriminative faculty of *buddhi*. We all have intuitive access to the knowledge that can answer life's most perplexing questions—if we can only learn to quiet the mind and look within.

The *Chandogya Upanishad* teaches, "*Tat tvam asi.*" It means: Thou art That. In other words, you are what you have been seeking. And when you actually experience this truth through your *sadhana*, Thou and That literally become One.

In practical terms, each imagined distinction and every space between you and the objects of your perception is annihilated, and you become "One with the Father." You really are not a woman nor a man. You are neither black nor white, rich nor poor, fearful nor fearless, angry nor forgiving, stressed nor calm, happy nor sad. You may be aware of a male or female body. You may be aware of poverty or wealth, stress or calm, anger or forgiveness, but You, on the highest level of consciousness, are none of these. You are the Eternal Witness—pure Consciousness having a human experience.

Being aware of that Eternal Witness and abiding in the Self, you always have access to the wisdom of *guru*. The more you rely on that *light* within, the more you become free to transform the contractive nature of *preya* skillfully into an ever-expanding, creative resource.

It's all so very simple. Logically, it must be simple. In order to be available to every human being on an equal basis, the pathway to Happiness must be the common denominator, and that common denominator is pure consciousness—awareness within. You don't have to be of a certain race. You don't need a high school diploma or college degree, or to be the follower of any particular religion. You are merely asked to be awake, like every great sage, to hear and to serve the wisdom of *guru* in mind, action and speech.

CHAPTER 13

Renunciation

No one is free who is not master of himself.
WILLIAM SHAKESPEARE

The concept of *renunciation* is often misunderstood in our modern culture. The idea of giving up anything attractive is often defined as the misdirected and unhealthy suppression of normal desires. Just look at the media. Our culture continually encourages us to embrace any thought, object or relationship that gratifies the ego or senses. If an object looks, smells, tastes, sounds or feels pleasant to us, Madison Avenue says it is good and encourages us to indulge our senses and to buy it.

In reality, the *renunciation* of short-term ego or sense gratification can become a tremendous opportunity for growth. If you learn to give your attention to only those thoughts, words and acts that are compatible with the advice of the *buddhi*, the possibilities for a healthy, happy, loving and nurtured life are boundless. The concept of *renunciation* is simple, yet profound: you must let go of something of value in order to receive something of value. It is in giving that you receive.

Just for a moment, think about how precious your breath is to you. Without breath, human life is impossible. The ancient Hebrew sages taught that life is breath and breath is life. With that in mind, what is it that makes it possible for you to inhale your next blessed breath of life? It is your exhalation!

You have to give away your precious breath through exhalation before you can inhale the vital force that maintains the city of life.

To understand, practice and benefit from the teachings of yoga science, you must be willing to give up some lesser desires. In order to contemplate the question, "Who am I?", to sit for meditation, or to determine which word to speak or action to take, you are going to have to give up something that habit would prefer you hold on to.

To practice *renunciation*, center yourself in the fullness of the Eternal Witness and remember that *renunciation* must always be in harmony with *ahimsa* for the transformative process to be effective. That which is to be renounced could be something of seemingly little consequence. For example, you might give up a second cup of coffee or the last chapter in the novel you're reading when it's time for your evening meditation. If the *buddhi* defines the desire as *preya*, willingly offer it back to the Origin from which it has come. Giving up small things like these is the perfect beginning practice.

Do not try to renounce attachments that are beyond your current comfortable capacity to give up. Deep-seated attachments, like addictions to tobacco or alcohol, are best left alone until smaller triumphs have strengthened your energy, will, creativity and confidence. When the time is right, however, and the choice is clear, even a long-standing dependency can be renounced joyfully for your highest and greatest good.

Lesson of the Oil Lamp

Once, long ago there was a dedicated student who desired Self-realization more than anything else in life. Toward that end, he implored his master to give him an advanced practice that would help him attain the final truth. The master agreed and sent the young seeker to visit King Janaka to receive the counsel of a great sage.

King Janaka was not only the ruler of his country—busy with all the duties such a post requires—but was also highly regarded as a Self-realized master of great wisdom. When the young man arrived at court, he was escorted to the king's chambers where Janaka greeted him warmly and asked how he could help.

The seeker spoke eagerly to King Janaka: "My teacher has said that you can show me the secret of living happily and successfully in this world, while at the same time experiencing the presence of the Divine in each moment. I humbly request that you share this teaching with me."

Impressed with the student's sincerity, the king instructed him to fill a lamp to the top with oil and to walk through every one of the scores of rooms in the palace without spilling even one drop of the precious oil. After finishing his practice, he was to report back to the king.

With great care and purpose, the student did exactly as he was directed. He did successfully visit every room in the palace without losing even one drop of oil, yet he was not satisfied that the effort had yielded its intended purpose. He felt no more enlightened than before.

When the student returned to the king's chambers to report his success, Janaka asked the seeker what he remembered about the extraordinary palace and the many wise people he met on his way. "I'm afraid I can't remember much about the palace, Sir, nor do I recall anything notable about the people I encountered. I couldn't take notice of anything beyond the lamp and the level of the oil."

"Fine," the king responded, and continued the teaching. "Now, once again fill the lamp to the top with oil and walk through every room without spilling a drop, and at the same time, appreciate and enjoy all the beauty and insight you encounter."

Discipline and *renunciation* by themselves do not necessarily lead to happiness or enlightenment. Real liberation (*moksha*) means that, while remaining centered on the Divine Light within, you are also present to appreciate, enjoy, serve and learn in every relationship and circumstance that comes your way while living in the world.

Abraham and Isaac

The Bible tells us that the Divine Reality instructed Abraham, who had waited one hundred years for a child, to offer his son as a sacrifice. This story concerns a question more profound than whether or not young Isaac would lose his life at his father's hand. Rather, Abraham, the man who would become the patriarch of the Hebrew people, was being asked if he could, and would, give up his greatest attachment. He was being asked if he would give up that which he might hold more dear than his love for the Lord.

The story prompts us to consider our personal attachments to both objects and relationships. Are habitual attachments more dear to us than our desire to be free from pain, misery and bondage? The story of Abraham and Isaac also dramatically illustrates that for profound results, a real sacrifice must be made internally on the subtle level. For his part, Abraham was willing. He took the young boy up to the mountaintop, bound his hands, placed him on an altar and then, knife in hand, raised his arm aloft.

Only after Abraham's arm began to descend—ready to plunge the blade through the boy's throat—did the angel of the Lord intercede. Why? Because at that moment the Lord had already received what He asked for. The devout Abraham had fully surrendered his attachment and was purified by his sacrifice. Then, now, and for generations to come, the story of Abraham and Isaac teaches the real meaning of sacrifice.

In twenty-first century America, we've been taught that the path to happiness lies in the acquisition of honors, objects and wealth. It is by taking, we are told, that we receive.

Despite that prejudice, *renunciation* remains a necessary practice in establishing a balanced, healthy and contented life. If we want something new and beneficial to come into our lives, we have to make a space for it. To move from point A to point B, we must renounce the place upon which we stand. Otherwise we can't move forward and we experience stagnation. When Jesus the Christ taught that, "It is easier for a camel to pass through the eye of a needle than for a rich man to enter the kingdom of God," He was not asking us to deny ourselves the necessities of life. He was suggesting that if we can give up our attachment to *preya*, we will be free to experience true Happiness.

If we want to swim from one end of a swimming pool to the other, we have to renounce the water and push it away. That act allows us to move forward. It makes sense. However, we are taught just the opposite. The tide of our culture makes the irrational suggestion that our happiness (continuing the swimming pool analogy) will be the result of drawing the water toward us. But experience teaches us differently. If we do nothing but pull objects and relationships toward us, we can actually drown ourselves.

Lesson of Sarcasm

After my mother and father, I consider my maternal grandfather to be my first spiritual teacher. When I was less than a year old, Papa recognized that his grandson was "a very comical fellow."

It's hard to say why some people are funny and others are less so, but as early as I can remember, I was aware that I could make people laugh. As I grew, it became a talent I increasingly relied on. Whenever I needed to break the ice in a relationship, my good sense of humor came to my assistance. As this skill developed, I came to rely on humor and later, sarcasm, as a defensive tool in stressful situations. All those years Bob Dylan was hearing beautiful poetry, I was hearing funny one-liners. In school, however, my timing often got me into trouble. While most of my classmates considered me extremely amusing, the teachers rarely shared such unbridled enthusiasm.

There's no doubt that humor, and especially sarcasm, is most effective when the punch line is unexpected, surprising or even shocking. Really successful sarcasm often bears a poisoned tip. The laugh that follows a sarcastic punch line is frequently at the expense of someone's well-being or self-esteem.

Practicing yoga science has changed my humor, and, in effect, my personality. Now, I try not to utter sarcastic comments that might be upsetting or hurtful to another person. Rather, I make use of my desire to verbalize sarcastic thoughts as part of my *sadhana*. I still hear funny, often sarcastic one-liners, but instead of habitually verbalizing them, I now chuckle to myself as I ask the *buddhi*, "Should I give enough attention to this joke to let these words pass my lips? Do I want these potentially injurious words to become manifest? Does the Divine Reality want them to be manifest? Is this thought in harmony with *ahimsa*?" Many times, the reply from the *buddhi* is, "No. This thought is not in harmony with *ahimsa*. It is the *preya*."

Centered in the fullness of the Eternal Witness and guided by the power of the *mantra*, I must admit that I silently appreciate the humor. Then, exercising self-discipline, I follow the judgment of the *buddhi*. I take my attachment to the joke (and to all those potential smiles on the faces of those within earshot) and I sacrifice it back to the Origin from which it came. As part of my *sadhana*, I willingly and consciously renounce the little zing, the passing ego pleasure I would have experienced by making people laugh at the expense of another.

This *renunciation* of sarcasm as a *preya* should not be confused with the therapeutic value of humor. "Cheerfulness," Swami Rama's master taught him, "is the most powerful *mantra*." Very often humor is the *shreya*. It has the capacity to nudge us away from our involvement in self-will, bad moods and debilitating relationships.

But when the *buddhi* clearly defines sarcasm as the *preya*, I fashion a personal prayer as a mechanism to facilitate my sacrifice. As I mentally place the sarcastic joke into the fire in the *cave of the heart*, I pray:

"Dear Lord, O my Inner Dweller, while I am attached to the humor of this sarcastic one-liner, I hear the *buddhi* leading me toward the *shreya* and away from the *preya*. While the old personality desires to verbalize this humor, I willingly and consciously offer it back to You. Please accept this offering, consume it in the fire of your *Light* and transform its energy. Help me to purify this instrument that I may be of service and lead me for my highest and greatest good."

This simple, conscious act of renouncing the *preya* in favor of the *shreya* facilitates the transformation of the power of desire for the sarcastic humor into strategic reserves of energy, will power (resolve) and creativity (consciousness).

Part III

MANTRA SCIENCE

CHAPTER 14

The Mantra is Your Leader

Blessed be the name of the Lord from this time forth and for evermore. From the rising of the sun to the going down of the same, the Lord's name is to be praised.

PSALMS

Oh, the charm of the Name! It brings light where there is darkness, happiness where there is misery, contentment where there is dissatisfaction, bliss where there is pain, order where there is chaos, life where there is death, heaven where there is hell. He who takes refuge in that glorious Name knows no pain, no sorrow, no care, no misery. He lives in perfect peace.

SWAMI RAMDAS

In any new endeavor you need a guide to help direct your energies toward the attainment of your chosen goal or desire. In the transformative science of yoga, the *mantra* is your leader.

For every action there is an equal reaction. When you continually give your attention to the *mantra*, there *will* be an effect. You may not be aware of the *mantra's* effect immediately, but its subtle power is continuously stored in the potential state—available to you when it is most needed.

According to the sages of the world's great spiritual traditions, the *mantra* reduces physical, mental and emotional dis-ease (stress, anxiety and pain); strengthens will power; facilitates the freedom to become an instrument of love, forgiveness and compassion (even in the face of your own fear, anger and self-willed desire); and slowly transforms your consciousness.

While the words of some *mantras* have no literal meaning, all *mantras* can be considered compact prayers. A *mantra* may be a single word or a series of words, usually including the name of the Divine Reality. *Mantras* are most effective when heard mentally from within rather than spoken or perceived through the external auditory sense. Some *mantras* are "unstruck" sounds. They are not the result of two objects coming into contact with each other, like two hands clapping or the vibrating of the vocal chords. Rather, they were discovered in deep meditation.

Every sound has a form. An oscilloscope is a scientific instrument that visually depicts the shape and design of sound waves. The *mantra* is considered a subtle seed that will grow into a concrete form through our continued, one-pointed attention. Remember, the *mantra* contains the name of the Divine Reality. Therefore, in subtle terms, the *mantra* is the Divine Reality in an as-yet unmanifest form. As you meditate on the sacred sound of the *mantra*, its Divine form gradually becomes a manifest force in the world through your thoughts, words and actions.

In ancient times, many women and men devoted their entire lives to meditation—evaluating the physical, mental, emotional and spiritual effects of certain sounds. Through these studies, *mantra* science revealed that specific words had a powerful and beneficial effect on the health of the entire body-mind-sense complex.

An understanding of the word *mantra* can be found in its etymology. The word *mantra* joins the Sanskrit words *man*, "the mind," and *tri*, "to cross." When used regularly and earnestly, the *mantra* can help a meditator cross over the turbulence of the mind to the sea of peace and bliss. The *mantra* is also an instrument that purifies and calms the mind by altering its software.

Even though as Americans we are free women and men living in the greatest democracy in the history of the world, each of us is enslaved to our habit patterns. We have created the software of our own individual minds by what we have chosen to give our attention to and what we have chosen to withdraw our attention from. Because of these habit patterns, we think the same things, say the same things and do the same things—with few exceptions—every day.

According to yoga science, it is the mind that separates individuals from the unbounded Life, Liberty and Happiness of their Divinity. Ignorance of the true Self is the real cause of physical, mental and emotional dis-ease. Without awareness of the Absolute Reality within, human beings cannot see the possibilities available to them when an action is required. They remain enslaved to their deepest *samskaras*. Human beings tend to behave like racehorses that run around the track with blinkers on. They get around the track all right, and they might look successful, but, in truth, they're leaving a universe of possibilities unobserved and unexplored.

As the mind becomes habituated to serving the *preya*, attention dwells on familiar, contractive thoughts, desires and emotions. The consequences inevitably affect both the physical body and subtle energy body. In other words, enslavement to *samskaras* of fear, anger and self-willed desire perpetuates a consciousness that can give rise to physical, mental and emotional dis-ease in every cell, in individual organs and in entire bodily systems like the cardiovascular, digestive, respiratory, neurological and reproductive systems.

Mental repetition of a *mantra* introduces a powerful vibration of purifying spiritual energy. Over time, the expansive vibration and consciousness of the *mantra* supercedes competitive and contractive vibrations in the unconscious mind. With consistent attention to *sadhana*, the healing wave of the *mantra* stills all other contending vibrations.

It's not unlike the singer's practice of striking a tuning fork and placing it next to her ear in order to synchronize her voice with middle C. When you listen to the *mantra* repeat itself silently in your awareness, the vibratory quality of the name of the Divine Reality influences your unconscious mind (*chitta*). This re-engineering, or purification, of your mind-field predisposes you to choose the *shreya* over the *preya* with ease.

During deep meditation, the *mantra* can bring consciousness to the state of stillness known as *samadhi*, in which the individual Self unites with the Absolute Reality and the entire body-mind-sense complex abandons its usual habits and vibrates in tune with the peace and bliss represented by the *mantra*. As twentieth century mystic Meher Baba taught, "A fast mind is a sick mind. A slow mind is a healthy mind and a still mind is Divine."

By giving your conscious attention to the *mantra* throughout the day and during seated meditation, you will begin to discover—experientially, rather than intellectually—that the Supreme Reality rests at the innermost center of your being. This discovery is the greatest of treasures, and the *mantra* stands as a perpetual reminder that perfection is both within you and *is* you—waiting to flow through your thoughts, words and deeds.

You may not recognize the results immediately, but as you repeatedly direct your attention to the sound of the *mantra*, there is a very real effect. The cause and effect are as certain as the law of gravity that causes an apple to fall from its tree to the ground. In physics, the *Law of Action* states that "for every action there is an equal reaction." The law is at work on the subtle level as well. Continuous repetition of the *mantra* deposits reserves of love, fearlessness and strength in your personal, subtle bank accounts, available for your use when you need them most.

The Subtle to the Gross

A second law of yoga science states that all power resides in the subtle world. A change must take place on the subtle plane of existence before it can occur on the gross level. It is the nature of the Divine Reality to endlessly manifest from the subtle to the gross. Just as all of the tree exists in the seed, the very chair you are sitting on right now was originally an idea in the mind of a human being. The first and most basic manifestation of your chair appeared as a subtle thought. The mind moves first and the body follows. You cannot even raise your hand without first entertaining a thought. Simply acknowledging this relationship between the subtle and the gross yields great power.

Modern American culture, however, has little understanding of the subtle. You can't see the subtle. You can't smell, taste, hear or touch it, and you certainly can't buy or sell it. Yet every word and action has its origin in a thought. This book you're holding in your hands was first a thought in the minds of its authors. As we gave more attention to the idea of a book, we began to speak to each other about it, and the desire to write it began to grow. Then, with concentrated attention, that desire grew into the act of writing. Only then did the book take material form.

Remember, in Genesis it is written: "God said, 'Let there be light,' and there was light." The Buddha taught how the law works for human beings: "You are what you think." Your destiny is the consequence of those thoughts, desires and emotions you choose to give your attention to and those you choose to withdraw your attention from.

Japa—Prayer without Ceasing

Many Christians are familiar with the injunction to "pray without ceasing." In yoga science, *japa* is the name given to the practice of silently and lovingly listening to the *mantra* throughout the day. *Japa* is the same practice the ancient Hebrew, Christian and Muslim sages observed in following the Old Testament commandment to "Love the Lord thy God with all thine heart, all thy soul and all thy might."

Each spiritual tradition prescribes a way of remembering—a mechanism for centering your awareness on the Divine Reality. In Judaism, a *mezuzah*—scriptures encapsulated in a small decorative container—is placed on the doorposts of a building, so that when people go out or come in they are reminded of the One God. Catholics use the rosary beads as an aid to practicing "prayer without ceasing." The *mala* for the Hindus and Buddhists, and prayer beads for Muslims serve the same goal—constant remembrance.

The practice of *japa* is simple, easy and pleasurable. Just rest your attention silently, lovingly and continuously on the sacred sound of the *mantra* as if you were listening to beautiful music. Attend to the *mantra* with the same emotion that parents feel as they communicate to their newborn baby. Learn to speak the language of love with your *mantra* as if it were your beloved. Remember: all power lies in the realm of the subtle. As you think, so you become, and for every action there will be an equal reaction. Therefore, whenever you have a few moments, take the opportunity to practice the silent, loving repetition of your *mantra*.

Your moods can have all the force of an intense weather pattern, yet you always have a choice of how you direct your attention. In every circumstance, simply do what is to be done when it is to be done, and the stored power of the *mantra* will come forward when you need it most in the form of love, fearlessness and strength.

Paradoxically, despite this promise, it's essential not to anticipate specific results as the consequence of your *japa* practice. Being omnipotent, omniscient and omnipresent, the Absolute Reality is eager to provide precisely what you need—if you can simply accept that you are an integral part of the One beneficent intelligence and are ready and willingly to do your part.

Jesus the Christ spoke of this understanding in His Sermon on the Mount found in St. Matthew.

> *And why take ye thought for raiment? Consider the lilies of the field, how they grow; they toil not, neither do they spin: And yet I say unto you, That even Solomon in all his glory was not arrayed like one of these. Wherefore, if God so clothe the grass of the field,*

which today is, and tomorrow is cast into the oven,
shall he not much more clothe you, O ye of
little faith? Therefore, take no thought saying, What
shall we eat? or, What shall we drink? or, Wherewithal
shall we be clothed? For after all these things do the
Gentiles seek: for your heavenly Father knoweth that
ye have need of all these things. But seek ye first the
kingdom of God, and his righteousness; and all these
things shall be added unto you. Take therefore no
thought for the morrow: for the morrow shall take
thought for the things of itself.

When and Where to Practice *Japa*

With all your heart, try to establish an intimate relationship with your *mantra*. Once you choose a *mantra*—following the guidelines provided at the end of this chapter—the *mantra* should become your default thought, constant companion, and Divine background music of your life. Whenever you're not being asked to fulfill some specific duty or responsibility, listen to the *mantra*. Lovingly direct your attention to the reverberating sacred sound of the *mantra*—just as if you were tuning in a radio station playing your favorite melody.

When you wake up in the morning, begin the day by listening to your *mantra*. While falling asleep, listen to the sacred sound of your *mantra*. In fact, if you fall asleep listening to the *mantra*, it will repeat itself throughout the night—sowing seeds of wellness and strength in the unconscious mind. When you're taking a shower, listen to the *mantra*. When you're preparing your meals or eating, silently listen to your *mantra*. When you are sick, listen to the healing vibration of the *mantra*. When you have an appointment with the doctor or dentist, listen to the *mantra*. When you're unexpectedly stopped by a red light during your morning drive to work and a thought that evokes anger appears in your awareness, witness the anger and willingly substitute your *mantra*. The more you listen to the *mantra*, the more you benefit.

Suppose you're running late and need to pick up a quart of milk on your way home from work. You dash down the dairy aisle of your local supermarket and locate the express checkout only to find a man in front of you with thirty items in his grocery cart. Posted overhead is a sign clearly stating that this register is only for customers with ten items or less. In the midst of your frustration, just lovingly surrender your anger and relax with your *mantra*.

As long as you are not being required to concentrate your attention in furtherance of an action, any time is an appropriate time to listen to your *mantra*. It is neither necessary nor advisable to wait for a crisis situation. Whenever you think of it during the day, give your attention and listen to the sacred sound. Then, in the face of fear, or anger, or self-willed desire, the *mantra* will come forward into your awareness with the courage, love and strength you need.

Jesus the Christ taught his disciples, "Where your treasure is, there will your heart be also." Your greatest treasure does not lie in objects and relationships that are subject to change. These have no power to make you happy or to eliminate your pain. To experience true Happiness, learn to center your attention on the Absolute Reality within and grease all your actions with love. To accomplish this, just give your continuous, loving attention to your *mantra*. Remember, the *mantra* is the Absolute Reality. With the *mantra* in your awareness, you will be able to choose the thoughts, words and deeds that will always lead you for your highest and greatest good.

You need not fear that *japa* will diminish your capacity to respond instantaneously and creatively. You will definitely not be turned into an automaton by repeating your *mantra*. In fact, you'll find that under certain circumstances, the *buddhi* heartily endorses the *mantra*'s receding into the unconscious mind while you plan some future action, enjoy a good joke or attend to some responsibility that needs all your attention. When the action is completed, the *mantra* will come forward again to gently reclaim your attention.

Your entire *sadhana* is essentially an internal and uniquely personal process. No other person hears the thoughts you think. No other individual knows the choices you face moment to moment as you deliberate whether to serve the *preya* or *shreya*. Essentially, your freedom and happiness depend only on what you choose—what you think, what you say, and how you act. Making every thought a means for your liberation is the only way to prove the efficacy of this wisdom for yourself. You cannot control what comes to you, but you can become free to always respond lovingly and wisely.

In life, each person seeks guideposts and direction. If you were visiting a friend in a distant city for the first time and you had only her address, you'd seek direction from someone who was familiar with that city. You might download a map from the Internet, call the American Automobile Association for a trip plan or perhaps ask a policeman for directions once you arrive.

In the process of becoming free from pain, misery and bondage, the most accurate and beneficial direction comes from within. The advice that will always lead you for your highest and greatest good comes from the superconscious mind, and the power of the *mantra*—realized through both seated meditation and *japa*—makes that library of Divine wisdom more accessible.

Mantra Walk

A brisk, silent, twenty-minute walk with your *mantra* echoing in your awareness is one of the healthiest and kindest practices you can undertake. Whether you're feeling on top of the world or totally overwhelmed by the stress of the day, just leave your CD player at home and go for a *mantra* walk. As competitive thoughts, desires or emotions vie for your attention, lovingly welcome, witness and honor them. Then willingly surrender them back to the Origin from which they have come. This practice has an extraordinary revitalizing, calming and centering effect. Try to make morning and evening *mantra walks* a regular part of your *sadhana*.

David and Goliath

You're probably familiar with the Bible story of David and Goliath in which the young boy defeated the powerful giant with an ordinary slingshot. But first, in preparation for their historic encounter, David must have entered into a deep contemplation. During that spiritual practice, the young shepherd boy probably became aware of two powerful thoughts.

David's first thought was that he must journey from the Israelite position to the Philistine encampment. Listening to the inner voice of the *buddhi*, young David, the spiritual seeker, recognized that this particular thought was a *shreya*—one that would lead him and the Hebrew nation for their highest and greatest good. He therefore gave it his attention and began walking toward his appointment with Goliath.

The second thought David surely had in preparing for Goliath was fear. As a human being, David was susceptible to thoughts and emotions very similar to our own. In fact, based on his situation, David was probably bombarded by many fearful thoughts—one after another after another. Yet, by consulting his *buddhi*, he knew the fear was a *preya*.

The Old Testament reports that on his way through the "valley of the shadow of death," David stopped to pick up five smooth stones. Biblical commentators agree that these stones were used in David's slingshot to slay Goliath. While this is no doubt true, there is another, more yogic interpretation of the story. Yoga science suggests that, although tempted by fearful thoughts, David made a conscious decision to withdraw his attention from the *preya* of fear and to redirect his loving attention to the "five smooth stones"—the five words of his *mantra*. Instead of serving fear, David chose to serve the name of the Divine Reality—over and over again.

Rocks that are tumbled together become highly polished and precious stones. The five smooth stones that David picked up in the face of his fear were the powerful words of his beloved *mantra*. Certainly, as he walked through the "valley of the shadow of death," he could have succumbed to the temptation of fear. If he had, however, he would have likely lost the battle against Goliath—paralyzed and defeated by the power of his own fear. As President Franklin Roosevelt noted during the depths of the Great Depression, "The only thing we have to fear is fear itself."

Being present in the moment, David did not yield to the allure of fear. As a yoga scientist, he recognized that he had a choice. He was awake every step of the way and was free to choose the *shreya* of his *mantra* over the *preya* of fear.

In doing so, David's fear was transformed into energy, will power and creativity. By listening to the *mantra*, his healthy *samskaras* of love, fearlessness and strength were deepened in his unconscious mind. When David finally came face to face with Goliath, he was fully prepared to accomplish his mission. He had at his disposal everything he needed to act skillfully and to attain success.

Flying to Indiana

Once, when we were flying from New York to Indiana to visit family, our plane encountered a series of violent thunderstorms. The trip became quite an ordeal. We were jostled around severely as the plane flew through one stretch of turbulence after another. While we endured the bumpy ride, persistent and fearful thoughts kept calling our attention. "What if we get struck by lightning? What if this plane goes down? What if we're injured, or worse?"

But in the midst of that fear, the stored influence of the *mantra* also came forward to remind us that we had a powerful option. Like David, we recognized that we did not have to be enslaved to the debilitating suggestion of fear and worry. The appearance of the *mantra* in our consciousness freed us to remember the perfection of the One Reality from which everything emanates. And so, re-centering ourselves in that eternal fullness, we began to welcome, honor and then lovingly offer the fear back to its Divine Origin as we repeatedly directed our attention back to the sound of the *mantra*.

When the plane landed safely, we felt a tremendous elation. But attachment to that excitement would also have meant continued enslavement to the fear. In fact, the alluring highs of life, known as *sukha*, very often are more seductive and enslaving than the painful and unattractive lows, known as *dukha*. Successful living depends on acting skillfully from a state of equanimity, no matter what the circumstance. "Quiet minds," Robert Louis Stevenson wrote, "cannot be perplexed or frightened, but go on in fortune or misfortune at their own private pace, like a clock during a thunderstorm." *Japa* is a valuable tool for developing this capacity.

Choosing Your *Mantra*

We offer you the choice of the following *mantras* because sages from the world's great spiritual traditions testify that they work. Certainly there are many beautiful words in the English language, like peace, harmony, love and joy. These words and their equivalents in other languages have positive, uplifting sentiments, but there is no indication that they work as *mantras*. With that in mind, we suggest you choose a proven *mantra* from the list provided—one that speaks to your heart.

Every *mantra* has a powerfully unique vibratory quality. Each human body also resonates with a certain specific vibration. In fact, every object in the universe, no matter how solid it appears to be, is actually a shimmering dance of particles. It is on this level of vibratory energy that the *mantra* operates.

To begin the process of choosing your own personal *mantra*, please read through the following list of great *mantras*. As you read the individual *mantras*, quietly bring each one into the *cave of the heart* (midpoint between the two breasts) to find which *mantra* resonates there most lovingly.

While reviewing the *mantras*, you may discover that you have an allergy to *mantras* from your own tradition or religion. This is not uncommon. When choosing your *mantra*, be certain you feel a strong affinity for the sound. With that in mind, we present the following *mantras* for your consideration.

World's Great *Mantras*

From the Christian tradition:
Jesus
Isha (Sanskrit for Jesus)
Yeshua (Hebrew for Jesus)
Lord Jesus Christ, Son of God, have mercy on us
Lord Jesus Christ
Hail Mary
Ave Maria

From the Hebrew Tradition:
Barukh attah Adonai (Blessed art thou, O Lord)
Ribono shel olam (Lord of the Universe)
Shema Yisrael Adonai Elohanu Adonai Echad
    (O, Inner Dweller, the Lord our God, the Lord is One)
Shiviti Adonai l'negdi tamid (I hold God before me always)

From the Islamic Tradition:
Allah
Allahu akbar (God is great)

From the Hindu Tradition:
So-Hum (I am That)
Hare Rama, Hare Krishna
    (Hare means loving praise. Rama is the the highest
    ideal of mankind. *Krishna* is the power that draws you
    to the Divine Reality in the cave of the heart.)
Rama
Om namaha Shivaya
    (Nothing is mine, everything is Thine. Everything I
    need is here for me to use and enjoy, but not to possess
    nor to be possessed by.)

From the Buddhist Tradition:
Om mani padme hum (Jewel in the lotus of the heart)

Read through the list of *mantras* slowly and choose the *mantra* that speaks to your heart. You might base your decision on the fact that (1) the *mantra* comes from your own religious or spiritual tradition; (2) the word (or words) simply feel right and good as you listen to it; (3) you may be strongly attracted to the meaning of the *mantra*. Any of these reasons is a good one, provided you are sincere in your deliberation and choice.

Once you have carefully chosen a *mantra*, listen to its sound for a day (as often as possible for twenty-four hours) to feel how it resonates in your heart. If it has not begun to feel comfortable after the first day, change your *mantra*. However, if the *mantra* you've selected feels right to you at that point, continue to use it lovingly.

Establishing an intimate relationship with the *mantra* is an essential ingredient in practicing meditation. If you were digging for water, you wouldn't drill two feet in one place, quit your effort and drill three feet in a second location, then move off to a third site to begin the process all over again. If you wanted water, you'd choose a likely spot and keep drilling—displacing everything that is not water until you reach the water-bearing strata. That's the key to success in finding water and in using your *mantra*. Once you have identified your *mantra*, stick with it and it will serve you well.

Fake It Before You Make It

Initially, listening to the sound of your *mantra* is likely to feel like discipline, but soon it will become comfortably familiar and, with earnestness, the familiarity will soon yield to love. In modern parlance, fake it before you make it. It might seem like a strange instruction, but this sentiment works well in the early days of *sadhana*. Even though the practice of *japa* (or any other practice) might seem uncomfortable initially, continue to give it your attention. The more you base your thoughts, words and deeds on the teaching, the more the truth of the teaching will be revealed to you. Once you experience the truth of the teaching, that truth will set you free from your pain, misery and bondage. Then you won't need to fake it. Your discipline will have become love.

To appreciate the degree of difficulty in starting a new habit, try this experiment right now. Fold your arms comfortably in front of you. After five or ten seconds in this position, fold your arms the other way.

You probably noticed that the first time you folded your arms it was natural and easy—because you did it on the basis of habit. However, when you tried to fold your arms another way, it was probably more difficult. It may have taxed your brain to imagine how you were going to position your arms. Habits are difficult to break, but change can be a creative force that leads you beyond your present limitations.

I knew a man who suffered many years with lower back pain. Because our *Easy-Gentle Yoga* exercises had helped eliminate my own back pain, I offered to teach these stretches to my acquaintance. "If *Easy-Gentle Yoga* has helped me so much," I said, "the program might just help you, too." Despite the sincere offer, he declined. "If I didn't have the pain in my back," he quipped, "how would I know who I am?" The man's humorous, but very telling response, reflects a sentiment that many individuals rarely verbalize but privately harbor, either consciously or unconsciously.

Even though it's easier and more comfortable to do things by habit, many of our unexamined habits are not serving our best interests. Habits, however, are not necessarily bad. Our ability to form them and to act on them consistently is very valuable. The same mechanism that formed your "bad" habit can be employed to form new, healthy habits. If you have a thorn in your foot, the traditional yoga story teaches, you may need to use another thorn to remove it. Then, both thorns can be thrown away. The habit of the *mantra*, and the habits of other yogic practices, are not ends in themselves, but are extremely effective tools for realizing unbounded Life, Liberty and Happiness.

If you have difficulty in establishing a strong and intimate relationship with your *mantra*, have patience and be persistent. If you listen lovingly and continuously to your *mantra*, it will become your best friend—a better friend than your mother, father, spouse, child, sister or brother, priest, minister or rabbi. Why? Because the well-established *mantra* will always serve you with love, fearlessness and strength when you need it most. Even when the body and senses begin to fail in preparation for the great transition of death, the stored power of the *mantra* will come forward to guide your attention and to lead you from this shore to the next.

Choosing to give your attention to the *mantra* represents the *shreya*. Habits of fear, anger or self-willed desire represent the *preya*. Simply recognizing that you always have a choice is an important breakthrough. When you can remain centered in the Eternal Witness, it becomes easier to observe your thoughts and to choose between them according to the *buddhi's* advice.

The choice is yours. Consciously or unconsciously, you constantly make decisions and take actions—all of which have consequences that can lead you to either fulfillment or further dis-ease. Work with your *mantra*. As a yoga scientist, experiment with the power of your *mantra*. The more you listen to the *mantra*, its protective vibration—like the grooved pavement along the side of the highway—will come forward as a gentle reminder that you need to pay greater attention to the course you are steering. The sages promise that with sincere effort, your choices and actions will yield profound results.

As you begin the practice of *japa*, it's important not to expect specific results. That's not the way the *mantra* works. Repeating the *mantra* to gain a particular, mundane outcome is futile and a misuse of its power. You probably won't win the lottery as a result of listening to your *mantra*, but if you're conscientious in your effort, the power of the *mantra* will provide just the right mix of love, fearlessness and strength to bring you exactly what you need, when you need it—not just once, but in every moment for the rest of your life.

Since every action produces an equal reaction, listening to the *mantra* will definitely produce an effect. Even though the consequence may not be initially apparent, the sages promise that your consistent practice of *japa* will lead you for your highest and greatest good—perhaps in ways far beyond your imagination.

As with all practices of *sadhana*, in order to give your attention to the *mantra*, you're going to have to withdraw your attention from something else that's calling you. Only you will know what that something is. It might be the thought of a second piece of apple pie, your concern about a bill or a thought that evokes anger toward your spouse. In the Bible, Abraham was asked to give up his attachment to Isaac. Certainly, you won't have to make such an enormous sacrifice, but you will definitely be asked by your own conscience (*buddhi*) to renounce something familiar—something that represents the ground upon which you stand.

About English *Mantras*

It is important that you learn to listen attentively to the sound of the *mantra* rather than simply repeating it in a mechanical manner. Remember, the power of the *mantra* resides in its vibration or sound, rather than its literal meaning. This is particularly pertinent when an English language *mantra* is chosen, since, for most of us, English is our native tongue. *Mantras* composed of English words carry an associated meaning that competes for our attention. If you've chosen an English *mantra*, concentrate on listening to the sacred sound of each syllable, rather than thinking about its literal meaning. If language presents any disturbance, it will soon disappear as the repeated vibration transcends the literal meaning.

Personal *Mantra* Initiation

Your experiments with the practices set forth in this book may lead you to a desire to further deepen your *sadhana*. When you're ready to make an intensified commitment to learning more about yourself and the science of yoga, plan to attend one of our many courses or retreats at the American Meditation Institute in Averill Park, New York. At that time, if you so desire, please contact me to discuss the value of a personal *mantra* initiation. In any event, it's quite likely that the *mantra* you choose from the list provided will become the friend and support you rely on for a lifetime.

Directing the Genie

In an ancient time there lived a queen who enjoyed collecting objects of art. One day she visited an antique shop in her kingdom and was immediately drawn to an exquisitely jeweled box. When she asked the shopkeeper about the beautiful item he was oddly hesitant to discuss it. Instead, he tried to draw the queen's attention to other items on display. This tactic only fueled her interest in owning the box.

"Your Majesty," the shopkeeper forewarned, "a dangerous legend surrounds this box. The box, some say, contains a genie. If the box is ever opened, a genie will materialize as a loyal servant to fulfill every desire the owner of the box expresses. The legend warns, however, that if there is no desire to be fulfilled, the genie will then kill its master!"

Intrigued by the story, the queen demanded that the shopkeeper sell her the box. When she took it home to her castle, she could not resist opening it. To her amazement, a genie instantly appeared and humbly declared, "Your wish is my command. Whatever you direct me to do, I will accomplish."

The appearance of the genie and the promise of his powers delighted the queen, and she began ordering him to perform all sorts of tasks around her huge estate. With incredible speed, the genie completed each assignment and instantly reappeared, demanding yet another chore. Initially, this collaboration between the queen and the genie was congenial, but after only a few days it became increasingly difficult for the queen to think of new assignments. The tyranny of the genie's constant demand for work became exhausting. With each passing hour, Her Royal Highness grew more concerned about the potential threat to her life if she could not continue to find desires for the genie to fulfill.

Desperate for a solution, the queen asked the advice of her most trusted minister. This wise man had, indeed, heard the legend of the box and also knew the antidote that would save the queen's life. He advised her that the very next time the genie asked for an assignment, she must instruct him to chop down the tallest tree in the forest, remove all its limbs and bury one end of the pole in the lawn behind the castle. Then, whenever there was no particular desire to be fulfilled, the queen should instruct the genie to climb up and down the tree-pole continually . . . until she called again for his help.

In our lives, the mind is our genie. The more indiscriminate attention we give to our thoughts, the more they grow into desires. The more we act on our self-willed desires (by serving the *preya*), the more we experience dis-ease and pain in our lives. The *mantra*, however, is like the tree-pole in the fable. Whenever we are not being called to serve the *shreya* in thought, word or action, we can always generate reserves of love, fearlessness and strength by giving our attention to the *mantra* through the practice of *japa*.

Part IV

MEDITATION

CHAPTER 15

Starting Your Meditation Practice

Close your eyes and you will see clearly.
Cease to listen and you will hear truth.
Be silent and your heart will sing.
Seek no contacts and you will find union.
Be still and you will move forward on the tide of the spirit.
Be gentle and you will need no strength.
Be patient and you will achieve all things.
Be humble and you will remain entire.

TAOIST CONTEMPLATION

Human beings have been able to put a man on the moon, build powerful supercomputers, construct magnificent bridges spanning enormous bodies of water, cool hot air in the summer and heat cold air in the winter, and yet, if someone asked us who we are, we'd probably admit we don't really know. This is an interesting paradox: how can we reliably know anything else if we don't first know who we are? We are born, go to school, marry, have children, earn a living, take a few vacations and then pass away—without truly knowing who we are, from where we have come, why we are here and where we will go. It's a thought-provoking commentary on our culture and the kinds of knowledge we prize.

Unlike the education you received in high school or college, the practices of yoga science provide first-hand, experiential knowledge of your true Self. In knowing who you are and understanding your inner dimensions, you are free from the constricting nature of the unconscious mind and are able to fulfill the supreme purpose of your life.

During the normal waking state, your mind continuously employs the five senses in search of pleasant experiences. In meditation, however, your relationship with the senses changes. You sit quietly with your head, neck and trunk straight. You gently close your eyes and mouth, and willingly close off the senses: the normal avenues through which information comes into your awareness. In meditation, you are not looking, smelling, tasting, hearing, or touching. Instead you are focusing all your conscious attention on the *mantra*.

As you begin to sit in meditation, something very interesting happens. Imagine for a moment that someone firmly grips your hand and pulls you toward him with great strength. What happens? Because the hand and body are connected, the body comes forward as your hand is pulled—even though you intended to stay in your chair.

Similarly, the conscious and unconscious mind are also connected. As you sit in meditation, you intend to give all your conscious, one-pointed attention to your *mantra*. That works well for twenty or thirty seconds, but since the mind is habituated to varied and changing stimulation, it very quickly gets bored with only one solitary thought to observe.

As you deliberately reduce sensory input from the external world, many engaging and competitive thoughts begin to bubble up from the unconscious mind into your conscious awareness. "Hey," the mind might ask—interrupting your meditation—"how long have I been meditating? Do I have enough money for my child's college education? Why is my spouse so insensitive to my needs? Why haven't I seen any flashing lights or had some mystical experience?"

Before you begin to meditate, however, you pledge to yourself that for whatever length of time you sit (one minute, five minutes, ten minutes or fifteen minutes), you are going to give your complete attention to your personal *mantra*. No matter what other thought, image or sound comes into your awareness, no matter what charm, attraction or temptation begins to call your attention, you resolve to give your undivided attention to your *mantra*.

Through this process you learn to assume the perspective of a witness. Meditation teaches you how to observe your thoughts, desires and emotions in a detached manner—without becoming involved with them. In meditation, as your worrisome, fearful, angry, entertaining, frivolous and desirous thoughts are bathed in the light of consciousness, you learn how to willingly and consciously withdraw your attention from the *preya* and how to skillfully redirect your awareness back to the *mantra*.

Within a few days, your meditation practice will accomplish several things. First, it will minimize your susceptibility to the temptation of the competitive thoughts arising from the unconscious. This skill helps you avoid being a reactionary. Second, as you willingly return your attention to the *mantra*, the love, fearlessness and strength it generates will be increased. You will also be building three beneficial skills: detachment (*vairagya*), discrimination (*viveka*) and will power (*sankalpa*), all of which will be discussed later in more detail.

Meditation is a Barometer

As your meditation practice becomes consistent, you're likely to encounter certain physical and mental obstacles. Don't allow them to inhibit or prevent your meditation, but rather, consider them a form of barometric reading—providing helpful information about the present state of your mind.

The kinds of impediments to meditation that you might encounter are: (1) an illness, such as a cold; (2) physical, mental or emotional discomfort that makes it difficult to sit comfortably; (3) the effect of too much or too little sleep; (4) anxiety or tension resulting from the day's internal or external relationships; and (5) the effect of eating too much or too little food.

Despite your intention to give complete and undivided attention to the *mantra* during meditation, your awareness may become commandeered by a crowd of uninvited and quite unruly thoughts. If your mind is not as focused as you had intended, ask yourself (during a quiet contemplation *after* meditation), "What kinds of relationships (thoughts, words and actions) have I had during the past twenty-four to forty-eight hours? What opportunities were presented to me? What were the circumstances? How did I respond?" Remember, for every action there is always an equal reaction.

Be specific and don't ignore the little things. For example, consider what you ate yesterday. What time did you eat? What kinds of emotions and thoughts were you experiencing during mealtime?

Through contemplation you may conclude that your difficulties in meditation could have resulted from previous choices you've made. For instance, even though you may normally eat your largest meal at 6 P.M., yesterday proved to be an exception. The events of your day were off-schedule because relatives were visiting from out of town and you celebrated the reunion at a favorite restaurant. You ate much too late, skipped your evening meditation, went to bed with a full stomach and had a difficult time sleeping. You woke up late, feeling tired and distracted, and during morning meditation your mind was quite unruly.

Experiences like these will affect your meditation practice. As a yoga scientist, evaluate relationships, experiences and the choices you make to discover their impact on your daily meditation. If your meditation seems difficult, it could mean that some of your recent decisions were not in harmony with the *buddhi*. Therefore, like a scientist, begin to isolate and experiment with different variables you wish to test. Perhaps tomorrow you'll have your largest meal around 1 P.M. or eat a light dinner. After making changes, evaluate your evening and morning meditations, and if your meditation seems more settled and focused you'll know you're headed in the right direction.

You Can't Avoid Actions

Every aspect of life requires action. Even inaction is an action. As long as you are alive, you cannot avoid taking actions, and every action has a consequence. Even a serious spiritual seeker who renounces worldly possessions and relationships to live in a remote monastery must still maintain relationships with his or her mind and habit patterns. Renunciates consciously or unconsciously continue to make decisions concerning their own body, breath, senses, thoughts, desires and emotions.

Since there is no escape from performing action, why not choose those actions that cause the least amount of friction in your life—the least amount of pain, misery and bondage? A regular meditation practice prepares you to know the peace, happiness and bliss of the Absolute Reality within. Then, as you center yourself in the contentment of your Essential Nature, you will become free to choose consciously the thought, word and action that will lead you for your highest and greatest good.

Place for Meditation

Meditation can be practiced almost anywhere that is quiet and uncluttered, but it is essential that you make every effort to meditate in that space at the same time every day. Within a few days you will begin to identify your meditation practice with your meditation space.

Whether you're able to dedicate a spare room exclusively to your meditation practice or simply designate a corner in your living room, bedroom or den matters little, but it is important that the space be comfortable and have good air circulation. It is best if your meditation space is separate from those areas that are identified with your household duties and responsibilities. Choose a location that is away from heavy traffic areas (like the kitchen) and away from the television, telephone, children and pets. Find a setting where you are not likely to be interrupted. While it's not necessary to decorate your meditation space lavishly, a beautiful painting or picture of an influential spiritual teacher can provide inspiration.

Time to Meditate

Your meditation will progress best if you meditate at the same time every day. Establishing this habit is an important step in deepening your practice. Remember that each of us has an ongoing relationship with the animal body. Anyone who has ever trained a puppy, for instance, knows that animals are most comfortable and cheerful when activities take place according to schedule.

The best times for meditation are early morning (just prior to and during sunrise) and late evening, when your commitments are fewer and you're least likely to be interrupted. At first, try to select one or two brief periods (two to three minutes) when you can meditate without inconveniencing others, being disturbed, ignoring your duties, or feeling rushed or preoccupied by other tasks.

If you rise a little earlier in the morning or meditate just prior to sleep at night, you can easily incorporate meditation into your daily routine. As your practice deepens, try to extend your meditation time by increments of one or two minutes. Sitting for twenty or thirty minutes may be a worthwhile goal, but only if it's in harmony with *ahimsa*. Remember, be patient and kind with yourself. It's more beneficial to sit for five minutes every day, with some preparation, than to sit for thirty minutes one day, then skip the next two.

Evening Meditations

After your work, homemaking or child-rearing responsibilities, you may find yourself too tired to sit as long as you could in the morning. That's fine. Remember two things in this regard. The first, as always, is *ahimsa:* non-injury, non-harming. Do not overburden yourself. The second point to remember is that everyone's practice is going to be a little bit different.

Your practice will be shaped by your own unique circumstances and relationships. You're not competing with anybody else. Whether you have one minute, two minutes, five or fifteen minutes to meditate, that's perfect. Start off with a short period of time—something manageable. Be aware of your present limits, honor them and respect the differences between you and others. No matter what amount of time you commit to your meditation, be regular and consistent. As in all of yoga, your intention and honest effort are always the most important aspects of your practice, not how much you accomplish. "Blessed are the pure of heart," Jesus the Christ taught, "for they shall see God." The key is your intention.

Budgeting Your Time

Once you've established a regular schedule, you'll begin to experience the phenomenon of unconscious preparation. As your meditation time approaches, your body and mind will begin to prepare for that regular, anticipated event. Even when you are caught up in some unusual, demanding or simply entertaining activity, your body and certain levels of your mind will begin to prepare for your meditation so that when the time actually comes, the meditation proceeds with relative ease. If, on the other hand, you have to make a decision each day about when and where you're going to meditate, you introduce a great deal of conflict and confusion and you deny yourself the helpful factor of unconscious preparation for your practice.

In order for meditation to become a regular part of your daily life, it must be made a priority. When you create a financial budget for yourself you define certain priorities and fixed costs like food, mortgage, automobile and vacation. In the same way, meditation must be made one of the fixed commitments within the time-budget of your daily schedule.

Without commitment and self-discipline, the benefits of meditation will forever remain elusive. However, overcoming inertia and procrastination is not as difficult as you might think. The transformation process of yoga science recognizes that within every desire lies the requisite amount of will power to fulfill that desire. Every time you renounce the *preya*, you are building reserves of energy, will power and creativity that can be used at another time when you're called to do an action in service to a *shreya*—like sitting regularly for meditation.

Music, Incense and Alarms

During the preliminary procedures leading up to your meditation, feel free to burn incense, light a candle or listen to inspiring music: hymns, gospel, *bhajans* or any calming or centering music. You may find these additions helpful as you bathe, pray and complete your *Easy-Gentle Yoga*. But before you sit down for your breath exercises, survey of the body and meditation, please turn off the music and extinguish the incense. Since your eyes will remain closed during your meditation, you may keep the candle burning if you like.

Please turn off the music and extinguish the incense because the practice of meditation is training your attention to a single point of focus, to the exclusion of any other thought, image or sound. If only on a subtle level, music and incense call the senses and divide your attention—leading you away from union with the Absolute Reality in the silent sea of bliss that is your true abode.

Remembering *ahimsa* (non-injury), please do not use an alarm to end your meditation. Such an abrupt transition from meditation into the normal waking state can be a shock to your nervous system. You have the capacity to end your meditation at a time of your choice. You've probably already had the experience of going to bed knowing that in order to catch an early morning plane you have to be awake at 5 A.M. Maybe you worried that you'd oversleep, but you were wide awake even before the alarm sounded. Similarly, when you sit for meditation and pledge to yourself that you're going to listen to the *mantra* for a predetermined amount of time, that same Inner Dweller that operates the autonomic nervous system will remind you when it's time to conclude your meditation. Simply look at the clock before you meditate and tell yourself that you're going to sit for five, ten or twenty minutes and you will soon be able to end the meditation at the chosen time—almost to the minute. As your practice deepens, you won't even need to refer to the external clock before you sit.

Loose-Fitting Clothing

Wear soft, non-restrictive clothing. Any comfortable exercise pant or pajama with a loose-fitting waist will do. Wear nothing tight around the torso—nothing that could restrict the breath. If you are wearing everyday pants, unbuckle your belt and open the top button and zipper. Do not wear tight shoes during meditation. Bare feet are best, but socks, light sandals, or house slippers are also fine.

Eyeglasses

Remove eyeglasses during meditation. Even though you might not be consciously aware of them, the weight and constriction of the glasses on the temples and nose should be avoided. They are also cues to the mind to direct attention outward.

Creating Love for Your Practice

The more you listen to the sacred sound of the *mantra*, the more you will be free from your limiting and debilitating habits. The *mantra* generates love, fearlessness and strength to help you do what is to be done, when it is to be done. After meditating for just a few days, you'll begin to experience the pleasure of being centered in the silence of your eternal Source, and your sense of discipline will yield to love.

Therefore, be patient and persistent! As you begin your meditation practice, it's quite acceptable to sit out of a sense of duty. At first, that may sometimes be necessary. Just remember that your *mantra* has the power to lead you to the attainment of your deepest driving desire—freedom from physical, mental and emotional dis-ease. In a very real sense, the meaningful, creative and joyful Life, Liberty and Happiness you seek are the consequences of having a focused and discriminating mind.

CHAPTER 16
Systematic Procedure For Meditation

Still your mind in Me, still your intellect in Me, and without doubt you will be united with Me forever. If you cannot still your mind in Me, learn to do so through the regular practice of meditation.

SHRI KRISHNA (BHAGAVAD GITA)

Since the early 1970s, Jenness and I have been experimenting with the practices of yoga science. During these many years we have added or subtracted preparatory practices based on what was comfortable and effective for us at each stage of our developing *sadhana*. It's not that we weren't disciplined. We were. Even so, in the very beginning, we found it nearly impossible to meditate every day. Instead, we began with *japa*. Then we learned *pranayama* and *Easy-Gentle Yoga* and eventually committed to daily morning meditations. It was not until a few years later that we added evening meditation.

Before you read the entire systematic procedure for meditation, remember that *ahimsa* is the highest precept of yoga science. This means you should not take on too much too soon. Without question, your meditation will be enhanced by some preliminaries to help calm and focus both the body and mind. Yet, above all else, you must be kind to yourself. Because of its length and specificity, it would be unreasonable and unkind of us to expect you to memorize and practice this complete procedure immediately. Instead, we suggest that you familiarize yourself with the instruction we present. Then begin with whatever portions of the procedure you enjoy and that come easily to you. Over time, your personal practice will develop on its own.

Each preliminary practice prior to your meditation is intended to progressively narrow the range of distractions that come into your awareness. Collectively, these practices engage your body, mind and senses while focusing your attention down to one point.

Systematic Procedure for Meditation

1. PREPARE THE BODY PHYSICALLY

It's always a good idea to prepare the body physically prior to meditation. When the body is refreshed, comfortable, relaxed and clean, you have taken positive steps to assure an effective meditation. Washing your face, hands, wrists and feet, or taking a shower will give you a fresh feeling and clear the mind. Your body will be more comfortable in meditation if you empty your bladder. Also, if it is your custom, empty your bowels after you rise, in preparation for morning meditation.

2. PRAYERS

If prayers are part of your tradition, include them at this time. Remember that you are following your own path. This systematic procedure is merely a group of suggestions. If the suggestion feels comfortable and fits into your lifestyle, then by all means make it a part of your practice. Every aspect of your systematic procedure for meditation must resonate in your heart. So, consider these suggestions and then fashion your own path. (See *Contemplation, Repentance and Prayer*, Chapter 39).

3. RELAX AND STRETCH THE MUSCLES

It's important to stretch the body prior to your meditation. The longer you sit still for meditation, the more movement your body will require at other times of the day. Chapter 37 will present *Easy-Gentle Yoga*—a complete program to stimulate and massage the joints, glands, lymphatic system, muscles and internal organs. Once learned, these exercises can take as little as fifteen minutes to complete and will create a vast improvement in your overall health and meditation practice. If you already are committed to your favorite *hatha* or stretching exercises, feel free to substitute your current program for ours.

Always consult with your health care professional before starting any new exercise program.

4. *PRANAYAMA*
Alternate Nostril Breathing (*Nadi Shodhana*)

Seated in your chosen meditation posture with your head, neck and trunk straight, eyes and mouth gently closed (see step 6), complete three cycles or rounds of *Alternate Nostril Breathing* (see Chapter 29). This practice clears and purifies the subtle energy channels from the base of the spine to the crown of the head. It enhances one-pointed attention, calms the mind, oxygenates the blood and energizes your entire body.

5. SURVEY THE BODY

This relaxation practice is unlike common stress-reduction exercises that ask you to consciously relax certain parts of your anatomy. While that kind of practice can ease bodily tension, it also reinforces the duality of a subject-object relationship. When you ask the shoulders to relax, you are the subject, the shoulders are the object, and an expectation is created that the shoulders will, or should, relax as directed.

The form of relaxation practice that we recommend reminds us of the 1960s science fiction movie *Fantastic Voyage*. In that film, scientists were treated with a secret serum that reduced their bodies to microscopic size. Then, through hypo-dermic injection they were sent off on a "fantastic voyage" through a living human body. Similarly, we ask you to travel through your own body—just to witness it in its entirety, with-out expectation or preconceptions. You are asked to become an explorer (the Inner Witness), visiting and observing new worlds within your own body.

On this mental journey, allow yourself to be open to what-ever appears and all that it may concern. For instance, when you visit your shoulder, imagine that you are actually deep inside your shoulder joint observing whatever presents itself.

As you are fully present to each part of the body, you may perceive a color, texture, heat or cold. You may become aware of a thought, memory or emotion. Or nothing at all. There is no correct or incorrect observation. Simply maintain your obser-vation until the location no longer calls your attention and then move systematically to the next area of your anatomy that beckons.

Consciousness exists within every cell of the body. By attending to your body's messages you will find that energy has been blocked in certain areas. Remember, attention means love. As you give your attention freely without intention or expectation, you are expressing unconditional love. This process of bathing the body in unconditional love (attention) often unblocks energy that has been entrapped in muscles, joints or organs by the habits of an undisciplined mind.

Consider the crying baby. When Mom or Dad picks up the crying baby and bathes the child in loving attention, the baby stops crying. Similarly, the body subtly seeks relief from dis-ease by inviting your attention, and pain is its means of communication. By merely giving the body your attention, without judgment or criticism, you become a participant in the healing process.

Your unconditional love, or attention, (together with other yoga therapies we will discuss later) can effectively remove obstructions in the subtle energy body, allowing the physical body to manifest its natural tendency to good health.

But remember, your attention must be free of expectation or judgment.

Depending on the amount of time you have available, feel free to abridge the suggested itinerary below. Perhaps one day you'll have just enough time to travel from the head to the toes without the return trip. That's fine. Remember, it's better to be regular and do less than to eliminate the practice altogether.

The following sequence is meant only as a suggested itinerary for your survey of the body. Do not begin with a preconceived itinerary in mind. As you mentally travel through the body, allow the Inner Dweller to guide you systematically—moving progressively down the body from the crown of the head to the toes, and if you have time, back up again.

Sample Survey of the Body

Following *alternate nostril breathing*, keep your eyes gently closed while remaining in your chosen meditation posture with your head, neck and trunk straight (see step 6). Begin inhaling and exhaling through the nostrils slowly, smoothly and deeply in one continuous, unbroken movement. Allow the belly to swell gently as you inhale and contract gently as you exhale. Try to eliminate any jerks, pauses or sounds in the breath and keep the body motionless. Exhale from the crown of the head down to the bottom of the feet, then inhale from the bottom of the feet to the crown of the head. Exhale all the day's anxiety, tension, worries and stress. Inhale the healing energy of the infinite and universal life force.

Now bring your attention to the crown of your head. Visit the right hemisphere of the brain, beginning at the forehead and traveling to the back of the head (to the cerebellum). Then visit the left hemisphere in a similar manner. Visit your right temple, then the left. Be an explorer, observing whatever comes into your awareness. Have no intentions. Remain free of judgments, conclusions or opinions of what is being witnessed. Now, visit all the small muscles around your eyes, eye sockets and eyebrows. First one eye and then the other. Go deep into the eye socket and visit the optic nerve of each eye. Come down into your nose and then the sinus cavities. Just observe—without expectations. Visit one ear and then the other. Next, come into the mouth. Visit the inside of the cheeks, gums, tongue and teeth. Visit the throat, thyroid and neck.

Then come into your right shoulder joint and rest deep inside the center of that joint.

Is there a color that appears? Is there a pattern? Do you sense warmth or coolness? Are you aware of some thought or emotion? Is there nothing appearing? Remember, there is no right or wrong answer. If something does call your attention, welcome and observe whatever appears and all that it may concern. Then allow the Inner Dweller to guide you on to the next logical part of the body.

Come down the right arm to the elbow, forearm and wrist joint. Visit your right hand: each finger, joint and finger pad—one by one. Now, come up the arm and visit the left shoulder joint. Come down the left arm and explore the left elbow, forearm, wrist joint and your entire left hand. Now move into the heart center and visit your heart. Visit the right lung and the left. Visit the right breast and the left.

Visit your stomach, gall bladder, liver, spleen, pancreas and appendix.

Come into your kidneys, first one and then the other. Visit your bladder. Visit your large and small intestines. Visit your reproductive organs. Now, settle into the small of the back and visit the complex connections of nerves and muscles there.

Notice whatever appears to you without any intention.

Go deep into your right hip joint. Come down the thigh into your knee.

Remember: no judgments, no conclusions, no opinions.

Come down your leg into your calf, Achilles tendon, ankle and foot. Visit the bottom of your right foot, the instep, each toe, each joint, and the pad of each toe. Next, come up the leg and over to your left hip. Be inside the joint. Explore the left knee, ankle, foot and toes in the same manner.

Remember, throughout your entire journey simply give your attention and let the Inner Dweller guide you.

After you complete this practice, imagine your body is a hollow reed. Gently exhale as though your entire body is exhaling and inhale as though your entire body is inhaling. With each exhalation, release all your tensions, worries, fears, expectations, anticipations, opinions and anxieties. With each inhalation, breathe in the vital energy of consciousness. Exhale like a wave from the crown of the head to the toes and out through the floor—releasing your stress and anxiety back to Mother Earth. Next, inhale from the toes, through the body, back to the crown of the head. Exhale and inhale completely four times. Allow the inhalation to gently yield to the exhalation and allow the exhalation to gently yield to the inhalation—no jerks, no pauses, no sounds.

6. CHOOSING YOUR MEDITATION SEAT

Now, you're ready to meditate. You may select a traditional floor posture for meditation or you may sit on a firm, slightly cushioned straight-back chair (see pages 146-147). In either case, sit erect with your head, neck and trunk straight. Whatever posture you choose must be *stable* and *comfortable* and encourage proper spinal alignment. Choose a comfortable posture that allows you to sit erectly, free of bodily distractions and pain.

Unless you have some physical handicap or are recovering from a serious illness, you should never meditate on your bed. Although the bed may be comfortable, your established mental associations between the bed and sleep will make it very difficult to remain alert. Remember, meditation is accomplished in the wakeful, conscious state—not in sleep.

Meditating in a Chair

When you sit for meditation in a chair, choose a firm, comfortable, slightly cushioned seat and position yourself away from the back support of the chair. You may want to consider a chair with arms, if falling asleep becomes a factor (which it should not).

To establish a comfortable and stable meditation posture, sit forward and tuck a thin pillow or the edge of a folded blanket just under your buttocks, making sure the support does not extend underneath your thighs. Proper placement of the pillow or blanket will tilt the pelvis slightly forward and help to establish a balanced posture with the head, neck and trunk straight. It also provides the increased comfort of sitting with your hips slightly higher than your knees. Depending on your particular anatomy, adjust the height of your seat with a cushion or pillow so that from the knee down your leg is perpendicular to the floor. If needed, a firm cushion or folded blanket on the seat of your chair will accomplish this. Your feet should be parallel and approximately shoulder-width apart. Comfort will determine the exact placement. Rest the hands comfortably on your thighs.

Sitting in this firm, stable posture permits all of your internal organs to rest unencumbered rather than being compressed by a rounded spine. A meditation posture is correct when your relationship with every internal organ and all limbs is non-injurious—in harmony with *ahimsa*.

Meditating on the Floor

Although Westerners are most familiar with the image of meditators sitting cross-legged on the floor, there's no magic in that posture. In fact, for many of us it would never be truly comfortable—especially for longer meditations. Most Americans have less flexibility in the hips and knees than do our Eastern counterparts who grew up in cultures that required sitting on the floor to eat, entertain, study and play.

If you feel you can be comfortable meditating on the floor, begin by sitting cross-legged on a carpeted floor or meditation rug. Position each foot on the floor underneath the opposite knee—resting the knees gently on the opposite foot. Place a thin cushion or the edge of a folded blanket just under your buttocks. Experiment with position and thickness of blankets or pillows to relieve pressure on the knees and feet, and to keep a slight inward curve in the lower back. If your thighs, calves or hips are tight and disturb your meditation, give extra attention to those muscle groups in your daily stretching exercises.

Proper Posture

To align your head, neck and trunk, begin by rolling your shoulders forward and backward three times. Then, raise your shoulders up toward your ears, squeeze them gently for a few seconds and let them drop quickly by their own weight into a comfortable position. There should be a slight inward curve at the small of the back and the head should be held upright rather than forward. Avoid sitting in a stiff, military posture. Keep the head, neck and trunk straight by establishing a relaxed balance.

Lower Back Support

If you have a weak lower back, don't be shy about using pillows to fill in the space between your back and the back of the chair. Make yourself as comfortable as possible while keeping your head, neck and trunk straight. You may consider extra pillows as training wheels, but don't be overly concerned if you continue to feel the need for additional support as your meditations deepen. (On the other hand, don't become so dependent that every time you travel you need an extra suitcase for your favorite pillows!)

Positioning Elbows and Hands

As you sit firmly in your meditation posture, place your hands on your thighs. The exact placement will depend on the length of your arms. If you have long arms, your hands will rest closer to your knees. If your arms and torso are of average length, your hands will rest at mid-thigh. Hand placement can

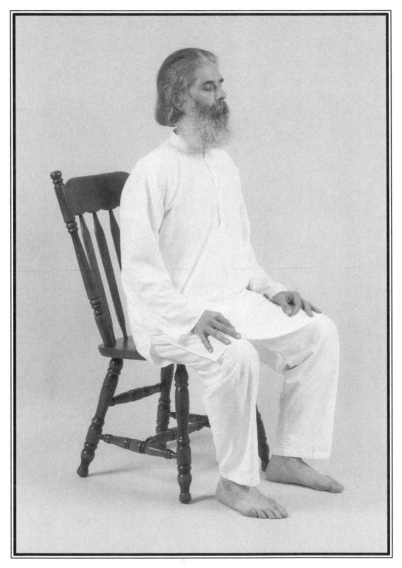

Meditating in a Chair

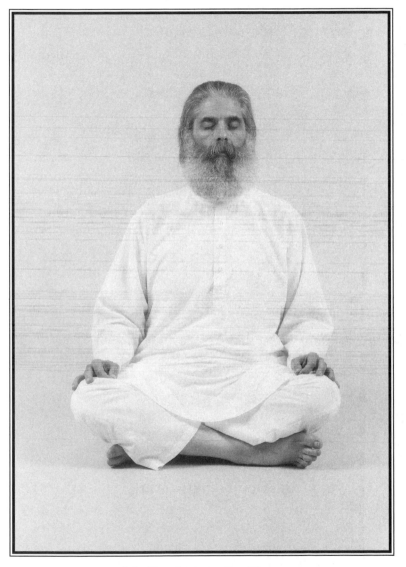

Meditating on the Floor

affect overall posture. Although the exact placement of your hands will depend primarily on comfort, the line of your head, neck and trunk must remain vertical.

Finger Lock

We continuously lose subtle energy through the fingers. In order to conserve and direct this energy during meditation, gently join the thumb and index finger of each hand, forming the traditional okay sign. Then, rest your hands on your thighs. Positioning your fingers in this manner effectively completes a circuit of magnetic energy traveling through the body. This position is called the *finger lock*. Your hands should rest on your thighs with palms facing down or up—depending on which position is more comfortable. Your fingers should remain stationary in the *finger lock* (the thumb and index finger together) throughout your meditation.

Root Lock

Just as energy is dissipated through the fingertips, subtle energy is also lost through the base of the spine. When preparing for meditation, engage the *root lock* by gently tightening the anal sphincter muscle. Squeeze gently, and once the lock is established, withdraw your attention and disregard it. This practice helps creative energy rise to the higher *chakras* (energy centers) in preparation for meditation. (See step 10).

7. ACKNOWLEDGING THE ETERNAL WITNESS

With your eyes and mouth gently closed and your head, neck and trunk straight, gently direct your attention into the *cave of the heart*—the mid-point between the breasts, at the level of your physical heart—where the Eternal Witness resides.

When we refer to "me" in conversation, we often intuitively gesture with our index finger toward the *cave of the heart*. We never point to our head, elbow or ear to communicate who we really are. Therefore, prior to meditation, visit the *cave of the heart,* acknowledge the Eternal Witness—your true Self—and fashion a brief prayer asking for guidance in your meditation. For example, you may use the traditional prayer of yoga science:

"O, Inner Dweller,
Lead me from the unreal to the real.
Lead me from the darkness to the light.
Lead me from mortality to immortality."

If you prefer using a prayer from your own tradition, or one that spontaneously arises in your heart, feel free to substitute. Infuse your prayer with love as you call upon the Divine Reality to guide your meditation. If you like, ask the mind to quiet down its habitual chatter and call on the body to cease its constant activity. Both reminders will help you become less identified with the body and the mind and more centered in the Eternal Witness.

8. *SANKALPA* (RESOLVE)—PLEDGE OF ATTENTION

After you've decided how long you will sit, enter meditation with joy and devotion in your heart and determination in your mind. With your awareness centered in the *cave of the heart,* pledge to yourself that no matter what thought, image or sound appears in your awareness, you will continue to give your complete and undivided attention to your *mantra.* Repeat this essential *pledge of attention* to yourself just prior to your meditation:

"I want to do it. I can do it. I have to do it. I am going to do it—no matter what! No matter what charm, attraction or temptation appears in my awareness; no matter what thought, image or sound comes into my awareness—I am going to listen to the sacred sound of my mantra and offer my love."

Even if you plan to meditate for only one or two minutes, it's helpful to express your determination mentally. Why? Because it is the nature of the mind to think. As long as you live, the mind will generate thoughts into your awareness. While you cannot stop the mind from thinking, you can quiet it by choosing what thoughts you give your attention to. In fact, one of the main purposes of meditation is to train the mind to give complete attention to a solitary object of consciousness—in this case, the *mantra*. By making the pledge of *sankalpa* to yourself before meditation, you are defining the *mantra* as the *shreya* (highest and greatest good) and relegating any other thought, image or sound to the status of the *preya* (ego or sense gratification) for the duration of your meditation.

9. VISUALIZING THE BREATH

After the *pledge of attention*, mentally acknowledge your body and the space the body occupies. Then begin the following breath awareness practice that systematically focuses your attention.

Along the Spine with the *So-Hum Mantra*

Visualize your breath moving within the spinal column for approximately five breaths. Imagine the breath as it rises from the base of the spine to the crown of the head and as it descends from the crown of the head to the base of the spine. All breathing is done through the nostrils, with the lips gently touching.

As you complete your inhalation, smoothly begin your exhalation. As you conclude your exhalation, lovingly start your inhalation. Visualize your breath moving in a continuous ellipse, so that your inhalation gently yields to your exhalation, which gently yields to your inhalation, which again yields to your exhalation. Your breath should flow without a pause between exhalation and inhalation or between inhalation and exhalation (see *Diaphragmatic Breathing*, Chapter 28).

As you inhale, visualize your breath rising from the base of the spine to the crown of the head while you mentally (silently) hear the syllable SO. Elongate the sound of the letter "o" as you visualize the inhalation.

As you exhale, follow your breath from the crown of the head to the base of your spine with the syllable HUM. As you visualize the exhalation, the sound of the letter "m" is elongated. In Sanskrit, the *So-Hum mantra* means "I am That," referring to the *Sat-Chit-Ananda.*

So-Hum is the natural *mantra* of the breath. *So* is the *mantra* of the breath's inhalation and *Hum* is the *mantra* of the breath's exhalation. If you gently place your index fingers in your ears and listen to the interior sound of your breath for a few seconds, you can hear a resonance approximating *So-Hum* with each complete breath.

At the Bridge Between the Two Nostrils

Place your attention on the bridge between the two nostrils, at the point where the upper lip meets the nose. As you exhale from the nostrils, mentally hear the *Hum*; as you inhale through the nostrils, mentally listen to the *So*. Be aware of each inhalation and exhalation until your breath relaxes, lengthens and becomes a smooth, slow and steady stream. Eliminate all jerks, pauses and sounds in the breath. Your limbs should remain motionless. Inhale and exhale five times with your attention at the bridge between the two nostrils using the *So-Hum mantra.*

From the Nostrils to the Eyebrow Center

Next, inhale and exhale five times with your attention moving up and down from the bridge between the two nostrils to the space between the eyebrows. As you inhale, visualize the breath moving upward to the space between the eyebrows, and mentally hear the *mantra So*. As you exhale, visualize the breath from the space between the eyebrows moving downward to the bridge between the nostrils, and mentally listen to the *mantra Hum*.

10. MEDITATING AT THE EYEBROW CENTER

Now, rest your attention in the space between the two eyebrows, slightly inward toward the brain. For most students, this is the place at which you will meditate. It is called *ajna chakra* and is traditionally referred to as the *third eye*. Sit quietly and focus all your attention in this space. The eyes are gently closed and relaxed—as if looking straight ahead. You are not *looking* at the space between the two eyebrows with your eyes; rather, you are totally inside that space.

When you are comfortable in the space between the two eyebrows, abandon all attention to the breath. Do not entertain any thoughts. Do not entertain any images. Do not attend to any sounds from your external or internal environment. Disregard all visual suggestions. Let go of your expectations, intentions, judgments, conclusions and opinions. Resting in the presence of the Eternal Witness within, lovingly invite your *mantra* into your awareness at the space between the two eyebrows.

Avoid mechanical repetition of your *mantra*. Instead, lovingly and patiently wait for your *mantra* to appear. Within a few seconds, when you begin to hear the *mantra*, let the focus of your mind silently and continuously flow toward the sound and vibration. Give your complete, undivided attention to the *mantra*. Give the *mantra* more and more attention, remembering that attention is love. As this process deepens, the sound you hear at the space between the two eyebrows will envelop your total awareness.

Lovingly surrender yourself to the *mantra*—the name, subtle form and power of the Divine Reality. When the mind and the *mantra* become one, the *mantra* will lead you beyond the sound to its Origin—the Center of Consciousness—the sea of peace, happiness and bliss that is your true nature.

Initially, if you find it difficult to hear the *mantra* as you would listen to a song on the radio, repeat it silently to yourself. As you observe yourself repeating the *mantra*, ask yourself several times what the *mantra* sounds like—until you can hear each syllable distinctly. Then, concentrate your attention exclusively on the sound of the *mantra*. This process withdraws your attention from body and mind consciousness and enhances your witnessing capacity.

10A. MEDITATING IN THE CAVE OF THE HEART

Alternatively, if you are primarily ruled by your emotions, your meditation should take place in the *cave of the heart*, rather than at the space between the two eyebrows. If you are inclined to meditate in the *cave of the heart*, follow the same systematic procedure through step number 9 (VISUALIZING THE BREATH: At the Bridge Between the Two Nostrils Using the *So-Hum Mantra*). Then, follow the breath between the nostril bridge and the *cave of the heart*. As you inhale, visualize the breath as it moves upward from the *cave of the heart* to the bridge between the two nostrils and mentally listen to the *mantra So*. As you exhale, visualize the breath from the bridge between the two nostrils downward to the *cave of the heart* and mentally hear the *mantra Hum*.

Now, rest your attention inside the *cave of the heart*. This space is called *anahata chakra*. This is the place at which you will meditate. Sit quietly and focus all your attention in this space as you remember your *mantra*. (For a detailed description, please review step 10).

11. *GURU CHAKRA*

In the center of the forehead, above *ajna chakra*, lies the *guru chakra*, depicted as an ascending triangle. It is the center of intuition, where the human being gains access to the superconscious mind.

Within the *guru chakra* rests an eternal flame. While you are in seated meditation, you may offer any distracting thoughts, images or sounds (*preya*) into the *guru chakra* to be consumed. After you have offered the distraction into the *guru chakra*, return to the eyebrow center at *ajna chakra* (or the *cave of the heart* at *anahata chakra*) and continue directing your attention to your *mantra*.

At other times during the day when you are not sitting for meditation, you may offer thoughts of *preya* into the flame at *guru chakra*, inside the *cave of the heart* (*anahata chakra*) or to another representation of the Divine that you hold most dear.

12. CONCLUDING YOUR MEDITATION

When you are ready to conclude your meditation, gently bring your awareness into the *cave of the heart* and acknowledge the Eternal Witness, the Divine Reality within. For a brief time, observe the *I-amness* as you allow consciousness to observe consciousness. Then, contemplate the question, "Who am I?"

Remaining motionless with the eyes closed, acknowledge the body and the space the body occupies. "I have a body, but I am not the body." Acknowledge the mind with its thoughts, desires and emotions. "I have a mind. I am aware of the mind with its thoughts, desires and emotions, but I am not the mind."

Make the transition to external awareness by abandoning the *finger lock* and placing your closed, cupped hands over your eyes. Gently open your eyes into the darkness and rest there for a few seconds. In the darkness, silently address the Divinity within the *cave of the heart* as follows:

"O, Inner Dweller, lead me from the unreal to the real."
As you slowly separate the fingers to permit light and form to enter your awareness, silently repeat:
"Lead me from the darkness to the light."
Position your hands in the prayer position, palms together in front of the *cave of the heart*, as you silently repeat:
"Lead me from mortality to immortality."
Finally, with your hands in the prayer position, repeat the

following short prayer silently (or aloud if you are participating in a group meditation):

"Om, Shanti. Shanti. Shanti." (Peace. Peace. Peace.)

Each repetition of *shanti* represents a prayer for peace: peace within your own mind, peace within your personal relationships and peace throughout the universe. It also calls for peace to permeate your three states of consciousness: waking, dreaming and deep sleep.

Pillar of Light[1]

You seem a little jumpy today, breath. Eyes, you are like straw tossed on a flood. Fingers, you are blades of grass in a storm. My beloved body, why are you blown like a leaf in the wind? Ah, mind, my familiar mind, you amaze me: how you squander all that energy, how you shun all that love, how you close the inward floodgates, how you sporadically spill into the reservoir outside you. You are like a mirage in the desert.

But I think it is time we had a conference. Come brethren, let us form a circle around a pinpoint of celestial light. Settle down on this sacred seat of meditation, draw yourself to yourself. Each of you, my body, breath and mind, let us be in harmony and worship together the pillar of light that reaches up through the spine and further to the heights of heaven.

The sun shines from one side of this pillar, the moon from the other. They circle around it day and night, borrowing their light from its heavenly splendor. When all others sleep, He, in whose light the sun and the moon share, remains awake sending out the rays of wakefulness.

Brother breath, settle down. My body, go still. What is this, twitching fingers? Tongue, cease this twitter. Echoes of my mind, now subside. Here enters stillness, the beginning of silence. Purity now shares this dwelling with us.

I wish you this day a glimpse of the cosmic pillar of light.

Swami Veda Bharati

---

[1]Reprinted from *"The Light of Ten Thousand Suns,"* © 1998, Published by Yes International Publishers, St. Paul, MN, www.yespublishers.com.

CHAPTER 17

Diminishing Distractions

An uncontrolled mind is like a bird with broken wings that falls into the river of passion and is carried with the current to the deep ocean of sorrow.

SWAMI RAMA OF THE HIMALAYAS

The philosopher is Nature's pilot.
And there you have our difference:
To be in hell is to drift; to be in heaven is to steer.

GEORGE BERNARD SHAW

It's hard to avoid hearing about the benefits of meditation. Even mainstream publications like *Time* magazine and *Reader's Digest* have reported that meditation can reduce stress, boost immunity, lower blood pressure, increase energy and enhance creativity. But when you sit for meditation and you're assaulted by unrelenting whims of the mind, it may feel as if you're adding stress to your life instead of subtracting it.

If your meditation practice is not the enjoyable and energizing experience you anticipated, remember that meditation is first a method of training and calming the mind. In truth, meditation alone does not create a healthy body and mind, yet a healthy body and mind are the consequences of skills you learn in meditation. When you disempower potential distractions by exercising detachment, discrimination and will power, the mind is free to serve the wise and nurturing advice of the *buddhi* whenever a decision is required. These decisions, in turn, have healthy, energizing and creative consequences.

In seated meditation, the *mantra* is always considered to be the *shreya*—that which will lead you for your highest and greatest good. During this time any competing thought, image or sound—no matter how important or alluring—is always considered the *preya* (short-term ego or sense gratification).

The totality of mind is vast, but at any given moment only a small portion is conscious. Most of the mind rests in the unconscious—an immense storehouse of merits and demerits, attachments, memories, emotions and unfulfilled desires created by your previous attention.

During meditation, you close off the normal avenues by which information comes into your awareness. However, the mind is an instrument of thought, habituated to the stimulation of new and varied information. When the mind is required to give attention to only one object, in this case the *mantra*, it quickly becomes bored and yearns for greater stimulation. After all, that's its habit, and you've rarely deprived it before.

As you try to focus your attention on the *mantra*, the unconscious mind (*chitta*) will issue forth from deep storage all sorts of attractive thoughts and images to satisfy the habit of thinking. "How will I pay my bills at the end of the month?" or "My children's lack of respect makes me furious!" or "I have a wonderful idea!"

Although your attention may repeatedly wander away from the *mantra* to some visual or conceptual imagination or an external sound, this behavior poses no problem for the detached Eternal Witness. Meditation is the practice of continually redirecting attention from the *preya* to the *shreya*. Do not confuse this process with the state of *samadhi* (union with the Divine), which occurs when the mind has learned to focus attention continuously like an unbroken stream of oil poured from one container to another.

It is the nature of the mind to think. Anyone who tells you that meditation will stop you from thinking does not completely understand the process. Meditation teaches you how to manage your thinking by developing the skill to determine which thoughts deserve your attention.

Chain Reaction

As you slowly, lovingly and attentively listen to the sacred sound of the *mantra*, a competitive thought may come forward from the unconscious. If attractive enough, this single thought can set off a dialogue within your mind. This one thought can give rise to many successive thoughts—creating a veritable chain reaction. The sequence might sound like this: "Hey, what's for dinner?" the first thought asks, moving the *mantra* off the radar screen. "That's a good question," a second thought chimes in. "What did I eat last night?" a third thought asks. "Chinese food," a fourth thought fondly remembers. "Well, maybe I'll have Italian food tonight," a fifth thought suggests. "But before I decide, I really should check to see what's in the refrigerator," a sensible sixth thought recommends.

As you're mentally rummaging through the refrigerator in search of the perfect food, a very important seventh thought alerts you that . . . "I'm not listening to my *mantra!*"

Even though you intend to give your attention only to your *mantra*, other thoughts may come into your awareness. If that occurs, do not try to reconstruct the chain of thoughts that brought you to the refrigerator. Simply acknowledge that the thought in your awareness right now is not the *mantra*.

Remember, as the highest precept of yoga science, *ahimsa* requires your response to be non-injurious. Therefore, do not follow the distraction; it is the *preya*. Instead, after you have respectfully witnessed the thought, gently and willingly withdraw your attention and offer the distraction back to the Origin from which it has come. Then return your attention to the *mantra*. Do not resist the thought, image or sound by pushing it away. Do not dismiss it in frustration. Do not become angry and do not criticize yourself for being a poor meditator. Such reactions are not kind and they are not in harmony with *ahimsa*.

Instead, remain patiently centered in the Eternal Witness during meditation and you will increasingly exhibit *vairagya* (detachment). When you discover that you're not listening to your *mantra*, calmly acknowledge that it's simply not appropriate to give attention to the contending thought. If the thought is important, trust it to reappear later, when you can address it.

This is the process of meditation. It will occur again and again, but as you become more skilled, the mind will become more concentrated and one-pointed as it repeatedly chooses the *mantra*. In effect, you are creating a global skill: learning how to redirect your attention masterfully from the *preya* to the *shreya*.

Two-Track Effect

As you meditate, you may be listening to your *mantra* when you suddenly realize that you're also attending to a second thought, image or sound. The distraction may have been present for some time before you noticed. A fantasy, a sound, a bodily sensation, or any number of habitual or attractive thoughts may distract you from the *mantra*. Simply welcome and acknowledge it, then gently withdraw your attention and redirect it back to your *mantra*.

Through such respectful *renunciation*, you automatically increase your internal reserves of energy, will power and creativity. As the rival thought returns to the unconscious mind, its *samskara* becomes shallower. Furthermore, as you redirect your attention to your *mantra*, the *samskara* of the *mantra* deepens—generating love, fearlessness and strength.

In effect, meditation reduces the constrictive power of fear, anger and self-willed desire while it increases your access to the expansive qualities of the *mantra*. Meditation is the process for transforming debilitating power into serviceable energy, will and creativity. The key is learning how to direct your attention so that the power of the unconscious mind comes under your conscious control.

Consider the *preya* of your fears, anger and selfish desires. Each represents a valuable portion of your own personal reserves. Nevertheless, for the human being, these attachments are rarely beneficial forms of energy. They must first be refined into a useful form, and meditation is the refinery. Through meditation, a potentially hazardous form of energy can be transformed into a beneficial reserve for performing any action the *buddhi* suggests that you undertake.

Thoughts of Physical Harm

An anxious thought may suddenly burst into your awareness during your meditation. For example, you may think you feel a spider crawling up your leg, or you may imagine that you've stopped breathing. In the first days of meditation, check to make sure there's no spider or that you are indeed breathing. Then, simply welcome and witness the intruding thought, surrender it, gently withdraw your attention and consciously replace your attention on the *mantra*.

Unbearable Itch or Sleeping Foot

During the early days of your meditation practice, the body is the most likely source of distraction. The unbearable itch or the suspicion that you have lost all sensation in your foot or hand may call your attention away from the *mantra* by their perceived urgency.

Before you scratch or wiggle, acknowledge the itch or thought calling your attention. Gently withdraw your attention from it and replace your attention on your *mantra*. Such distractions will fade as the mind recognizes and accepts the benefits and pleasures of meditation. Within a few weeks, you'll be able to sit comfortably.

Dangers Lie Only Outside YourSelf

Thoughts that reflect a *samskara* of fear may also distract you. For instance, you may imagine that your heart is beating too slowly or too fast, or that you're breathing improperly. The sages assure us, however, that there is no danger along the path of inner exploration. We have a body, yet we are much more than the body. We are aware of thoughts and yet we need not be enslaved to our thoughts. We are pure awareness, the Eternal Witness (*Sat-Chit-Ananda*), and when our attention is directed to our union with that Divine Reality, the consciousness within every cell of our body enjoys a state of peace, contentment and healthfulness.

The only real dangers lie in the external world of duality. When human beings believe themselves to be separate and incomplete entities they inevitably become fearful that they will be unable to secure the object of their desire, or that they may lose what they have. These are the fears that invite danger into our lives.

Ego—The Great Impostor

Remember the sage advice of Swami Rama of the Himalayas: "All the body is in the mind." The mind always moves first and the body follows. The body will not become animated unless and until there is a movement in the mind. We cannot even scratch our head without first entertaining a thought. When thoughts concerning the body come forward during meditation—and they will—your body will not move from your still posture unless you give attention to the thought that suggests an action.

The mind is capable of many disguises: an imagined mosquito on your cheek, a foot that's asleep, a smoldering resentment, nagging fear about money, some overwhelming desire or a flight of fancy.

The thoughts that come forward from the unconscious mind during meditation reflect our many attachments. They represent things we like or dislike (*raga/dveshas*). That's why it's essential to develop *sankalpa* (resolve) prior to meditation: "I want to do it, I can do it, I have to do it, I am going to do it, no matter what charm, attraction or temptation might call my attention."

Before you meditate, pledge to yourself that even if an overwhelmingly attractive or important thought, image or sound demands your attention you will be firm in your focus on your *mantra*. No matter what the competing thought may be, it is always only a suggestion. It may be significant, delightful, frightening or anger-provoking, but your meditation is simply not the appropriate time to think about it.

The thoughts, desires and emotions arising during daily meditation often represent issues of importance to be addressed during your contemplation practice. Contemplation (practiced at another time—not during your meditation) helps you review the habitual ways your sacred energy is being used. It allows you the insight to make conscious choices that will lead you to freedom from pain, misery and bondage. (See *Contemplation*, Chapter 39).

Distractions in your meditation practice are not something "bad" to be summarily dismissed or filed away for future retrieval. By patiently practicing *ahimsa* when sacrificing the *preya* in seated meditation, you diminish distractions and establish a quiet, contented and relaxed mind. When you experience that profound peace, your consciousness will begin to flow in new, creative ways that motivate you to make different choices. The consequences of those actions will bring you the unbounded Life, Liberty and Happiness you deeply desire and richly deserve.

CHAPTER 18

Training One-Pointed Attention

The mind is a mischief-maker. It jumps from doubt to doubt; it puts obstacles in the way. It weaves a net and gets entangled in it. It is ever discontented; it runs after a hundred things and away from another hundred.

SATYA SAI BABA

The prevailing tide of our culture encourages multi-pointed attention. Today each of us is encouraged to multitask, to become the proverbial short-order cook by frying the eggs, toasting the bread, brewing the coffee and serving everything simultaneously and on time—without breaking yolks, burning toast or serving coffee that's less than piping hot. Then it's immediately on to the next order and the next. It's no longer enough merely to be good at what you do. People are urged to develop expertise in many different areas—and often asked to report to more than one boss during the workday.

Such demands are quite opposed to the single-pointed attention of *dharana*, cultivated through the practice of yoga science. When your mind is one-pointed, you have access to the superconscious mind from which all wisdom flows.

Each of us has our own distinct spectrum of potentialities, so the knowledge received from the superconscious mind impacts our every relationship in unique and positive ways. To use the limited analogy of the radio, each individual mind is a receiver that can be tuned to receive a continuous program of personalized wisdom.

The greatest artistic, creative and productive achievements in history have been facilitated through minds exercising one-pointed attention. Similarly, at the pinnacle of any Olympic competition, the gold medal is won by the athlete whose mind has been made one-pointed. The gold medalist possesses the skill to remain focused regardless of competitive thoughts, desires or emotions that could steal energy and attention.

Never undervalue the power of your own attention! Attention means interest, and interest means love. To thoroughly know anything, to discover or create anything, you must give your heart to it—which means your ATTENTION. The greater the focus of attention, the more profound the blessing.

It's commonplace to complain that in our modern civilization people don't believe in anything anymore. However, upon deeper examination, it appears that the opposite is true: people will believe in almost anything. In our culture, multi-pointed attention and the pursuit of short-term sense gratification are constantly encouraged. Instead of leading to Happiness, however, the fulfillment of every desire inevitably leads only to yet another desire.

One goal of meditation is to make us response-able. If we train the senses, manage our desires, strengthen our will power and coordinate the functions of the mind to reflect the Divine wisdom of *buddhi*, every response will be appropriate to the circumstance. These practical skills help us unite the power of all our assorted and unrelated desires to fulfill our one, all-consuming passion—our desire for unbounded Life, Liberty and Happiness.

The creation story found in the Bible is poetic and thought-provoking, but you may understand it differently after you consider its yogic interpretation. According to yoga science, the Divine Reality continuously manifests from the undifferentiated, subtle state to the gross, material level of existence through the mechanism of one-pointed attention and will. God merely willed light into existence, thus beginning the process of creation. This mechanism for creation is constantly operating through the consciousness of human beings. When we give sufficient one-pointed attention to a particular thought, it becomes more concrete—taking the form of the words we begin to speak. When we direct even more attention to the thought, desire or emotion, we're likely to take some physical action in the material world in furtherance of that original thought. In other words, every human being actively participates in the ongoing process of creation by choosing the focus of his or her attention.

The key to contentment lies in understanding that although we have little or no control over the thoughts that come to us, we always have a say over whether or not we continue to give them the attention that will empower them to shape the events of our lives. As the Compassionate Buddha taught, "You are what you think." What you think today determines what you experience tomorrow.

Subtle thought objects that come into our awareness are similar to the gross objects we perceive every day through the senses. In the terminology of yoga science, these subtle and gross objects with which we interact are called *prakriti*. They are generated by our habitual likes and dislikes (*raga/dveshas*) and are the consequences of our previous actions. This very logical relationship of action to consequence is known as *karma*. By cultivating one-pointed attention and employing the discrimination of *buddhi*, we can reliably choose which thoughts to give our attention to and thereby realize our highest and greatest good.

Power of the Laser

Laser technology provides an apt analogy to illustrate the benefits of concentrating available energy. The elementary unit of light energy is a photon. Incandescent and fluorescent light bulbs are designed to produce ambient light by scattering photons in many directions, bouncing them off the ceiling, walls and floor. This disorganized light energy serves to illuminate low-light environments. By directing all the photons in one direction simultaneously, however, scientists create a laser beam powerful enough to cut through steel and precise enough to perform micro-surgery.

When you learn to cultivate one-pointed attention, you apply the principle of laser technology to the energy field of the mind and produce similarly profound results. By learning to focus your entire attention (mental energy) toward a single object of consciousness (like a *mantra,*) you are able to expand your consciousness by tapping into a library of intuitive wisdom.

Understanding the Subtlest Form of Relationships

Suppose a new thought, a suggestion, appears in your awareness. If your mind is entertaining memories from the past or is off somewhere in the future, you will most likely respond unconsciously. Without conscious, one-pointed attention, you are likely to react from the conditioning of a *samskara* in your unconscious mind. This translates into the unconsidered choice of the *preya* over the *shreya* (which would have led you for your highest and greatest good).

When a student of the Buddha asked him if he were a god, prophet or angel, the Compassionate Buddha replied that he was none of these. And when asked what he considered himself to be, the Buddha simply replied, "I am awake!" That is the meaning of the word Buddha—"the awakened one." By his answer, the Buddha referred to being present every moment to the choices that continuously present themselves to us. Consumed neither by memories of the past nor imaginations for the future, the yoga scientist mindfully welcomes each thought individually as a mere suggestion of what to give his or her attention to. With regular practice, you too can develop the skills necessary to "wake up" from the restless night of ignorance into a higher state of conscious living.

Power of a Glass of Water

A brilliant young student, feeling proud of his great knowledge, once asked his teacher, Narada, to explain to him why it is that everyone can't see the Eternal truth, cultivate one-pointed attention, make discriminating choices and thereby end their sorrow. Having both a great love for the disciple and an understanding of his limitations, the master agreed to share this knowledge, but only after the young man fetched a glass of water from a nearby house to quench Narada's thirst.

Eager to please his master, the disciple approached the house and knocked. To his amazement, when the door opened the most beautiful woman he had ever seen stood before him. As he gazed into her eyes, he fell deeply in love and the two soon married. In the years that followed, he and his wife found joy in one another, were blessed with healthy children and amassed considerable wealth and property.

But eventually his fortunes changed. Death snatched away the lives of his wife and children, and floods destroyed his property. He was left alone, poor and old. One night, as he sat brooding in his hut, there came a knock at the door. When he opened it, his master, standing before him, asked, "So? Where's my glass of water?"

The mind, ignorant of its true nature, habitually moves amidst desire, fear and anger. When the mind operates in this manner, the decision-making process is corrupted, and the human being sacrifices the discriminative faculty of *buddhi* in favor of the rapid-fire reaction of deep-seated, unconscious habit or compulsion (*samskaras*).

In principle, however, the training of attention is simple: when the mind wanders after a *preya*, gently redirect it toward that which will lead you for your highest and greatest good. Problems arise when a distraction is not just a stray thought, but the product of a deep *samskara*—a compulsive resentment, worry or desire. The power of such thoughts is often overwhelming because there's nothing the ego likes more than to think about itself and to rejustify your dualistic orientation.

Here again, your leader is the *mantra*. Whenever a selfish, contractive thought appears in your awareness, welcome, witness and honor the *preya*, withdraw your attention and consciously redirect your attention toward the *mantra*. When the *mantra* takes hold, the connection between the *preya* and your attention is broken. An overwhelming, compulsive thought or a powerful sense craving has no real power of its own. All its power comes from the attention you give—and when you withdraw your attention, the thought or desire will be powerless to compel you to act.

In Sanskrit the point of fully focused attention is called *bindu*—a seemingly insignificant dot vibrating with awesome possibility. This concept can be easily grasped by considering its parallel in physics: the process of nuclear fission. When concentrated energy penetrates an atom it causes the atom to split, releasing enormous amounts of energy, enough power to destroy—or to illuminate—a major city.

As the training of your attention grows, you'll observe a similar, more subtle process occurring again and again in your own consciousness. When you cultivate a concentrated, one-pointed love for the *mantra*, its power will effortlessly manifest, granting you the freedom to choose thoughts, words and actions for your highest and greatest good.

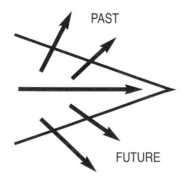

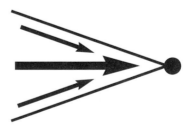

Dissipated Attention
An undisciplined mind, rarely in the present moment, randomly misdirects potentially creative energy by serving fear, anger and self-willed desire.

One-Pointed Attention
A focused mind directs its energy to a single point, *bindu*, and experiences pleasure, clarity and creativity.

Take Small Steps to Train Your Mind

Certain relationships that require an action may seem insignificant and unrelated to your *sadhana*, yet they can be powerful opportunities to bring you closer to fulfillment—if you can practice one-pointed attention. For example, while you're eating, don't watch television. By doing both at the same time, you're training the mind to divide its attention. As a consequence, your body will neither digest as thoroughly nor assimilate the nutrition of the food as completely as it could if you were mindfully eating with one-pointed attention. Furthermore, you simply cannot fully enjoy the pleasures of the flavor, texture, scent and colors of your food while half of your attention is devoted to the evening news.

Remember that the body, *annamaya kosha*, is composed of food and water. Your physical body is a shrine that houses Divinity. The body is a church, a temple, a mosque. When this is understood, the act of consuming food to maintain the shrine becomes a sacrament. Choosing what, where, when and how to eat is an important aspect of *sadhana*, and yet we seldom think of it in quite that way. Most of our decisions concerning food choices are based solely on input from the senses, ego and *samskaras*.

The training of attention can continue in all your activities. For instance, when you're at work trying to complete a task and the phone rings, you may have a great desire to continue what you're doing while you talk on the phone. "I can do both," you tell yourself. "This conversation is not particularly demanding." It's probably true that you could accomplish both tasks—at less than full efficiency—but we urge you to experiment.

As a yoga scientist, ask the *buddhi* which desire represents the *preya* and which is the *shreya*. If the telephone call is the *shreya*, try to witness and surrender the desire to continue working, then give one hundred percent of your attention to your conversation. Place your pen on your desk and direct your complete and undivided attention to the person who wants to speak with you. No one else will ever know the mental deliberation you've made, but by exercising this kind of detachment and discrimination, you'll develop a sharp focus of your mind-field for the benefit of every upcoming relationship.

As you look for opportunities to unify your everyday desires, the power of the *mantra* will help you remember your true nature as the Eternal Witness. Once centered in that fullness you will come to realize that by dividing your attention you are actually working counter to your highest and greatest good. Learning to make even this kind of seemingly insignificant act an integral part of your *sadhana* can become a means for your liberation.

In truth, Divine Providence is bringing you a telephone relationship with a specific individual for a specific reason. You just might be uniquely qualified to give that person something she needs: insight, encouragement, comfort or love. Or it's equally possible that the other person can give you something you need. Relationships do not exist without purpose. Even if another person is offering only anger, yoga science says the anger is meant to help you develop qualities like patience, forgiveness and compassion, or to lead you to self-examination.

Performing more than one task at the same time may seem like an efficient use of energy, but the habit takes its toll on your health. Recent scientific studies conclude that multitasking asks the brain to function beyond its capacity. The brain simply cannot process more than one piece of information at a time. It might appear to your casual observation that you can drive and talk on the cell phone simultaneously, but to accomplish both, the brain has to run back and forth between activities. When faced with the demands of multitasking, the brain actually becomes overloaded, slows down and sends an S. O. S. to the adrenals to release stress hormones into the body. Prolonged release of adrenaline eventually leads to sleep deprivation, anxiety and depression.

Metaphoric Soaker Hose

You have probably seen or used a soaker hose. A soaker

hose is like an ordinary garden hose with one small but important difference. A multitude of tiny holes allows water to escape all along the fifty or so feet of its length. This provides gentle irrigation for plants and shrubs, but because the force of the water is dissipated along its span, there's very little water pressure at the far end.

Just like a soaker hose, the untrained mind dissipates a tremendous amount of creative energy by indulging a host of little desires and entertaining a legion of habitual thoughts. If you're in the habit of multitasking, you're likely to find yourself with inadequate supplies of energy, will power and creative ideas when life makes an important demand.

Now, imagine taking a roll of duct tape and carefully sealing all the holes along the length of the soaker hose of your mind. Closing those countless outlets will give you a tremendous force with which to work. If you learn to conserve and transform the energy of small, petty desires of *preya*, you'll have access to endless resources.

So, begin today to look for new and creative ways to develop your one-pointed attention. Don't eat and watch television at the same time. If food is important, turn off the television. If a specific television program is important, postpone your meal until an appropriate time. If you're washing the dishes, don't entertain distracting or annoying thoughts. Instead, give your attention to the sensual pleasure of immersing your hands in warm, sudsy water. Watch mindfully as the soft, wet sponge caresses the smooth porcelain and the newly sparkling glassware catches the light. You'll find that you actually enjoy the experience. Every activity, completed with full attention, will be more pleasurable and rewarding—added benefits as you skillfully hone your one-pointed concentration.

CHAPTER 19

One-Minute Meditations

Before embarking on important undertakings, sit quietly, calm your senses and thoughts and meditate deeply. You will then be guided by the great creative power of Spirit.

PARAMAHANSA YOGANANDA

The *one-minute meditation* practice may be used as a preliminary centering exercise before seated meditation, as an occasional substitute for your seated meditation when time is short or whenever you feel the need to focus and calm yourself during the day.

Even if you're in a business meeting at work and cannot sit in privacy, the benefits of this practice will be profound. A *one-minute meditation* will calm your mind, center your attention, give you access to your reserves of energy and send wonderfully beneficial and reassuring messages to the entire autonomic nervous system.

In a social situation you don't even have to draw attention to yourself by closing your eyes. Merely sit or stand with your head, neck and trunk straight, bring your attention to the breath at the bridge between the two nostrils and listen for sixty seconds to the *So-Hum mantra*. Nobody else should even be aware of your practice.

One-Minute Meditation at the Nostrils

Remember that it is important to invoke your *sankalpa*, (resolve or determination) prior to every meditation practice. Before you begin a *one-minute meditation*, restate your *pledge of attention*. "I want to do it. I can do it. I have to do it. I am going to do it—no matter what charm, attraction or temptation comes into my awareness." Pledge to yourself: "For sixty seconds, I will give my complete attention only to the inflow and outflow of the breath at the bridge between the two nostrils while silently listening to the *So-Hum mantra*." Breathe diaphragmatically—allowing the belly to expand gently as you inhale and contract gently as you exhale. The breath should be full, but not beyond your normal comfortable capacity. Ideally, you should wear clothing that fits loosely around the waist. (See *Diaphragmatic Breathing*, Chapter 28.)

Bring your attention to the bridge between the two nostrils and attend to each inhalation and exhalation. As you inhale, silently listen to the sound SOOOO. As you exhale, silently listen to the sound HUMMMM. If distractions come into your awareness, patiently welcome and witness them respectfully, gently withdraw your attention and focus on the breath at the bridge between the two nostrils while continuing to listen to the *So-Hum mantra*. At the end of one minute, you may extend the meditation for a second minute or conclude the practice.

One-Minute Meditation
Listening to Your *Mantra* at the Eyebrow Center

As an alternative, practice a *one-minute meditation* using your personal *mantra* at the space between the two eyebrows (*ajna chakra*). Follow the same preliminary instructions as above, but place your complete attention on the sacred sound of your *mantra* at the space between the two eyebrows. At the end of one minute, you may extend the meditation for a second minute or conclude the practice.

Following the *one-minute meditation*, take a few moments to make the transition into the activities of your day. Let your *mantra* accompany you, in the form of *japa*, as you meet the needs of each moment with calm attention and the skills you've developed in meditation.

In our culture, we rarely experience the joys of stillness. Even when we sleep the body remains restless. Regardless of hectic personal and business schedules, you can always make time for a *one-minute meditation*. The important point to remember is to be consistent with your meditation practice. Regular meditation, even a *one-minute meditation*, will calm, center and energize your mind and body. And all it takes is an investment of sixty seconds!

Student Testimonial

Several years ago I had a student who benefited greatly by consistently practicing *one-minute meditations*. Julia had a high-pressure job and lifestyle. She was a wife, mother and a professional troubleshooter working on the computers of a high-level government office. Her job was to quickly diagnose the problems and to rectify them in the shortest possible time.

Her anxiety from both home and work situations had contributed to a serious problem with hypertension. Before learning to meditate, Julia's blood pressure consistently registered 130/90. Because of her medical condition, her doctor monitored Julia's pressure twice a week. Although she had tried medication, the side effects seemed worse to her than the disease. She also had restricted the amount of sodium in her diet, but this had little or no effect.

As a computer programmer, Julia brought a scientific approach to her meditation practice. When she started meditating, she changed no other variable in her life except to add the daily practices she learned in our classes. These included meditation, breathing practices, *Ayurveda* and *Easy-Gentle Yoga*.

Although Julia's family and career responsibilities made lengthy seated meditations too difficult at first, she found that our *one-minute meditation* was easy to fit regularly into her busy schedule. In addition to a *one-minute meditation* first thing in the morning and last thing at night, she also practiced at work. Whenever she sat down in front of a computer screen, even before she addressed the software problem, she closed her eyes and centered herself in a *one-minute meditation*. By simple arithmetic, we calculated that she was meditating a total of seven or eight minutes throughout the day.

When her blood pressure dropped to 100/70 after only days of *one-minute meditation* practice, the attending nurse asked if Julia had resumed her blood pressure medication. The answer, of course, was that meditation was her medication! But lowered blood pressure wasn't the only benefit Julia experienced. She began to feel a profound sense of calmness, gratitude and love—all of which enabled her to apply the teachings of yoga science more frequently in meeting the demands and needs of both work and family.

Part V

REVISITING OUR ROOTS

CHAPTER 20

The Foundation of Judaism, Christianity and Islam

A man asked his spiritual teacher, "Do you mean we should remember the Lord even in the give-and-take of business?" "Yes, of course," the rabbi replied. "If we can remember business matters in the hour of prayer, shouldn't we be able to remember God in the transactions of our business?

HASIDIC TALE

The regular, systematic practice of meditation helps you remember the Divine Reality within as you act in the world. Sustained mindfulness of your higher Self—moment by moment—frees you to skillfully serve the *shreya* and sacrifice the *preya* in mind, action and speech. The cumulative result of continuous *meditation in action* results in fulfilling and nurturing relationships. This is the essential truth of yoga science.

But the essential truth of yoga science is not found exclusively in the Eastern traditions. The very same philosophy and science is also found at the heart of the Judeo-Christian and Islamic traditions. As you earnestly practice *sadhana*, the similarities become more clear.

The *Shema*
The ancient Hebrew tradition gave birth to both

Christianity and Islam. The basic tenets are the same in all three. The essence of Judaism is expressed in a few verses from Deuteronomy called the *Shema* (pronounced *shem-ah'*). It is interesting to examine the truth it states and to discover that the spiritual core of these three traditions is virtually identical to those of yoga science and philosophy.

The first sacred pronouncement of the ancient Hebrew *Shema* represents an epiphany experienced by anonymous Hebrew sages and teachers. The statement is clearly the product of intense *sadhana* and deep *contemplation*. Through time and space these ancients lovingly proclaim:

Hear O Israel, the Lord our God, the Lord is One.

The Biblical origin of the word *Israel* is explained in the Old Testament story of Jacob, who was eventually to be known by the name Israel. In Genesis, Jacob wrestled through the night with an angel of the Lord. He was victorious in the struggle and transformed by it, but during the conflict he received an injury that caused a permanent limp.

Let's examine this story, looking for hidden levels of meaning. Like all individuals who seek to purify their body, mind and senses in order to find true Happiness, Jacob faced the demanding task of aligning every thought, word and act with his conscience. Jacob accepted the challenge and struggled to make conscious choices that served the Divine wisdom as reflected by the *buddhi*.

Wrestling with the angel can be understood as a metaphor for Jacob's determination to face and overcome the habits of his lower animal consciousness by renouncing attachments to the *preya*. Successfully wrestling with his individual, separate sense of I and mine, Jacob was able to overcome his limiting self-will. Through his conscious, willing effort, Jacob was reborn as an instrument of Divine Providence. Thus, Jacob's new name, Israel, represented an acknowledgement of the shift in his consciousness.

The new name did not describe a tribe, government or geographic location. Israel referred to the Inner Dweller, or Eternal Witness within—the true *land of milk and honey*. The name Israel honors Jacob's personal struggle with the ego (*ahamkara* or I-maker). It signifies that he was a human being who willingly, consciously and successfully wrestled with his alienating sense of separateness. Jacob was able to transcend the limitations of his mind, unite with the Divine Reality and realize a state of conscious equanimity. That peace, in turn, enabled him to experience Happiness.

Jacob's self-surrender also transfigured his body. His lameness is a symbol of the sacrifices he made in order to enter the kingdom of heaven within.

The essential proclamation of the *Shema* is very similar to the yogic concept of *sankalpa* or resolve. In effect, the declaration forms an unbreakable bond of love and dedication that is meant to inspire every Jew, Christian and Muslim to think, speak and act in harmony with the will of the ever-present Divine Reality.

Each recitation of the *Shema*: "Hear O Israel: The Lord is our God, the Lord is One," declares the absolute truth that there is only One Reality; that everything we can perceive through the senses—each name and form—has come forth as a unique manifestation of the One Divine Origin.

The *Shema* proclaims that the God of the entire Bible and the Quran is non-dualistic. Everything we perceive is a manifestation of the One—the physical and the spirit, the seen and the unseen. Nothing exists outside this One. There is no second.

Consider this most basic law, as recognized in the familiar workings of mathematics. Every number you can posit in mathematics is a manifestation of one. The number three, for example, is actually the number one, repeated three times. The number three hundred is actually the number one, repeated three hundred times. The very concept of numbers is dependent upon the One.

Yoga science does acknowledge the fact that there is a

multiplicity of names and forms. There is a multiplicity, but that multiplicity is transitory—subject to change, death, decay and decomposition. That which is eternal—pure consciousness—is the unity within the diversity. Having declared the profound paradigm shift from duality to non-duality, the *Shema* continues:

> *Blessed be his name,*
> *whose glorious kingdom is for ever and ever.*

This second verse of the *Shema* is an extrapolation of the first. If we accept that there is but one Absolute Reality—here, there and everywhere—it logically follows that everything with a name and form is Divine. Every gross and subtle object appearing in your awareness is a manifestation of the One.

Next, Deuteronomy presents the fundamental formula for the attainment of Happiness:

> *And thou shalt love the Lord thy God with all*
> *thine heart, and with all thy soul, and with all thy might.*

Through this verse, the Divine Reality issues an uncompromising commandment to the human race. "Love the Lord with all your heart, all your soul and all your might." Christianity and Islam, both children of the ancient Hebrew tradition, share the same teaching through the words of the New Testament and the Quran. In practical terms, what does it really mean? What is love, and how are we to exhibit that love toward the Lord?

Love songs must account for at least ninety percent of all recorded music, yet their lyrics give very little indication of what love is and less about how we might offer that love to God. But the sages do give us some guidance. Love, they teach, is attention. When you truly love someone, you can't stop giving him or her your attention. You are constantly thinking about the person—desiring to give your attention and to receive attention in return. Similarly, when you are able to maintain a continuous flow of attention—even toward a boring or tedious task—you slowly develop a fondness or love for it.

How, then, are we to give our attention, and therefore our love, to the Lord? The answer lies in our relationship with the *buddhi*. The *buddhi* is the mirrored reflection of the will of the Divine Reality. By continuously giving our attention to the *buddhi* and serving its wisdom in thought, word and deed, we are truly demonstrating our "love" for the Lord.

Deuteronomy continues:

> *And these words, which I command thee this day, shall be upon thine heart: and thou shalt teach them diligently unto thy children, and shalt talk of them when thou sittest in thine house, when thou walkest by the way, when thou liest down, and when thou risest up. And thou shalt bind them for a sign upon thine hand, and they shall be for frontlets between thine eyes. And thou shalt write them upon the doorposts of thy house, and upon thy gates.*

Through these verses of Deuteronomy, the Divine Reality is imploring each of us, "Give Me your attention!" In the midst of all your pleasure and in the midst of all your pain; while fulfilling all your duties and responsibilities; in the morning, afternoon and evening, "Remember Me always."

Rituals from every tradition are mechanisms for remembering the Divine Reality throughout the day—in every circumstance and relationship. To remember, Catholics pray with the rosary. Hindus use the *mala* beads or wear a *bindi*—a small dot between the two eyebrows. Muslims use prayer beads and religiously pray five times a day. Jews place a *mezuzah* on the doorposts of their homes, and some wear an undergarment called *tzi-tzit*. Yoga scientists listen to their *mantra*.

In every moment, we face a choice of how to direct our attention. In yoga science, the alternatives are described as the *preya* and the *shreya*—passing pleasure versus perennial joy. If we can remember the Divine Reality while making everyday choices, the sages promise that, in the process, we'll become detached enough from the charms and temptations of the world to serve the *shreya* freely and lovingly in thought, word and deed.

When you are earnest in your *sadhana*, the stored power of the *mantra* will come forward in the midst of your decision-making process in the form of love, fearlessness and strength. When you face an emotionally charged issue, the power of the *mantra* will remind you to ask the question, "Who am I? Who am I who is aware of this thought that evokes anger? Who has this thought that evokes fear? Who has this thought that evokes a selfish desire? Who am I?"

By giving your attention to the *mantra* throughout the day, you exhibit your love for the Divine Reality and create a healthy *samskara* in your unconscious mind. Then as you discharge your duties from the calm and bliss of your Essential Nature, you find the strength and creativity to make choices based on Divine wisdom rather than fear, anger or greed.

Early Christians experienced this stillness of the Eternal Witness as *Christ-consciousness*. But no matter what name you give it, that tranquility can become the center of your universe. Give your willing attention to your *mantra* throughout the day and all your thoughts, desires and emotions will flow into that sea of peacefulness. All your words and actions will flow outward from that Divine contentment, leading you for your highest and greatest good. This ancient practice is what the Jewish, Christian and Islamic sages referred to as loving the Lord with all their heart, all their soul and all their might.

Why Give Attention to the Divine Reality?

Why does the Divine Reality ask for your constant attention in every circumstance? The answer comes in the promises made in the very next verses:

> *And it shall come to pass, if ye shall hearken diligently unto my commandments which I command*

you this day, to love the Lord your God, and to serve him with all your heart and with all your soul, that I will give the rain of your land in its season, the former rain and the latter rain, that thou mayest gather in thy corn, and thy wine, and thine oil. And I will give grass in thy field for thy cattle, and thou shalt eat and be satisfied.

You are actually a citizen of two worlds. You are a citizen of this material world of changing forms, and you are a citizen of the subtle world of spirit, from which all Reality flows. The *real* you is essentially pure consciousness, or spirit, having a human experience. To pass beyond all sorrow, you need only to cherish and serve That which is eternal, as opposed to that which is transitory.

Live in the world, yoga science teaches, but be not of the world. Do not let yourself be defined or limited by that which decays and vanishes. In other words, do what is to be done, when it is to be done, moment by moment—based on the wise and good counsel of the *buddhi*—and the grace of the Divine Reality will bring you everything you need.

The habit of questioning if and when your needs will be met is the cause of much anxiety, alienation and depression. This verse promises that by remembering the Absolute Reality within and relying on Its intuitive wisdom, you can choose thoughts, words and actions that will result in consequences that fulfill your every need.

In the Old Testament, the Lord speaks of providing "wine, corn, oil and grass in the field for your cattle." Today, our needs are slightly different but the concept is the same. We need comfortable housing, nourishing food, serviceable clothing, a means of livelihood, reliable transportation, rejuvenating recreation and loving, nurturing relationships. The promise spoken of in the *Shema* is the same as in yoga science: all these things will come to us through grace if we let the wisdom of the Divine Reality guide our mind, action and speech in every circumstance.

Pain is the Consequence of Inattention

However, if we decide to serve selfish desires and choose not to become an instrument of Divine Providence by following the advice of the *buddhi*, Deuteronomy warns us that there is a price to be paid:

> *Take heed to yourselves, lest your heart be deceived, and ye turn aside, and serve other gods and worship them; and the anger of the Lord will be kindled against you, and He will shut up the heaven, and there be no rain, and that the land yield not her fruit; and ye perish quickly from off the good land which the Lord giveth you.*

In current terms, who are these "other gods" spoken of in Deuteronomy? In the twenty-first century, Americans don't pray to a golden calf. We are not idol worshippers. Or are we?

We may be far too sophisticated to succumb to pagan idolatry, but we easily fall prey to the seductive gods of fear, anger and greed. These motivate us to direct our attention— our love—away from the Divine Reality. Remember, two objects cannot occupy the same space at the same time. When we give our attention to our self-willed desires, we cannot give our attention and love to the Lord. As a result, we are certain to experience physical, mental and emotional dis-ease or pain. In other words, what Deuteronomy calls "the anger of the Lord" is understood in yoga science to be simply the natural consequence of cutting ourselves off from the flow of grace.

We have deep emotional attachments to the many gods that separate us from the One Absolute Reality. Trapped in the matrix of duality, we have a misplaced faith that relationships and material objects have the power to bring us happiness and eliminate our pain. Today, shopping centers have become our culture's most hallowed cathedrals and we allow Madison Avenue's commercials to erode our power to discriminate between what is needed and what is merely wanted.

Yoga science teaches that there is nothing intrinsically

wrong with consumption and enjoying sensory pleasures, but objects serve us well only when we use them with discrimination. Remember the *mantra*, *"namaha Shivaya"*: nothing is mine; everything is Thine. Everything is here for me to use and to enjoy, but not to possess, nor to be possessed by. When the allure of materialism beckons, yoga science suggests that before following it we ask this question: "Do I need the object I am attracted to, or am I merely habituated to want the object—thinking that it will bring me happiness or the eliminate my pain?" Then, let the *buddhi* guide your choice.

Ending Pain by Attention

A student of St. Teresa once asked her, "Do you love the Lord our God with all your heart, all your soul, and all your might as taught in the Bible?" St. Teresa answered humbly, "Yes, I do." Then the student asked, "And don't you hate the devil?" St. Teresa replied simply, "I don't have time."

Nisargadatta Maharaja, a twentieth century sage from Bombay, reminds us that "Evil is the shadow of inattention. When we forget our real nature, we become fearful, angry and selfish. Yet in the light of Self-awareness, evil withers and falls away."

Any form of pain is the shadow of the outstretched hand of the Divine Providence advising us that we need to change something in our lives. Pain is the only experience that consistently draws us inside our hearts to consider changing our course. Pleasure doesn't have that effect. If we were asked to vote on it, we'd all vote for pleasure, but the fulfillment of every desire for pleasure brings only another desire, not freedom or understanding. Desires are infinite in their expression.

Rather than shooting the messenger of pain, yoga science asks us to examine the communication and benefit from it. Pain is a superb teacher. The message of pain always offers us crucial information to contemplate so that we can make the changes in our lives that will free us to experience true Happiness.

CHAPTER 21

Where is God?

Late have I loved Thee, O Beauty so ancient and so new; late have I loved Thee! For behold, Thou wert within me and I outside; and I sought Thee outside and in my unloveliness fell upon these lovely things that Thou hast made. Thou wert with me and I was not with Thee. I was kept from Thee by those things, yet had they not been in Thee, they would not have been at all. Thou didst call and cry to me and break open my deafness; and Thou didst send forth thy beams and shine upon me and chase away my blindness; Thou didst breathe fragrance upon me, and I drew in my breath and do now pant for Thee. I tasted Thee, and now hunger and thirst for Thee; Thou didst touch me, and now I burn for Thy peace.

ST. AUGUSTINE

Every practice of yoga science has the same goal: to know the Divine Reality at all times—in every circumstance and relationship. Why? Because if you are aware of the Absolute Reality in the present moment and base your thoughts, words and actions on Its intuitive wisdom, you will always be led for your highest and greatest good.

Regardless of differences among religions, the basic concept of the Divine Reality, a.k.a. God, is universal. All traditions describe God as being omnipotent, omniscient and omnipresent. No matter what other religious, cultural or historical characteristics may be assigned to God, every tradition agrees that these three qualities always are true: God is all-powerful, all-knowing, and exists everywhere—simultaneously.

Omnipresence means that God is more than the traditional Judeo-Christian depiction of a wise, elderly, celestial being residing out in deep space—perhaps somewhere between Neptune and Pluto—even though God is, indeed, in deep space somewhere between Neptune and Pluto. Yoga science says it's equally true, however, that all the nine planets of our solar system, the Milky Way, all the galaxies and every other manifestation of the material universe, including you, are all manifestations of the One Absolute Reality.

Omnipresence means that the Divine Reality exists everywhere, including existence within each and every human being. The eternal capacity to be present in the moment to witness all gross and subtle objects as they appear *is* the Divine Reality. Although atheists and agnostics may exhibit an allergic reaction at the mention of a Divine Reality, this truth remains indisputable because even nonbelievers admit to believing in themselves—the thinkers of their thoughts, the experiencers of their experiences. The very Self of the atheist or agnostic also *is* the Divine Reality.

All gross and subtle objects in your awareness are, by definition, transitory: subject to change, death, decay and decomposition. For example: I am tall or I am short, I am happy or I am sad, I am stressed or I am calm, I am fearful or I am fearless. The physical, mental and emotional landscape is constantly changing. Any and all objects—gross or subtle—appearing in your awareness are not the real you. Nothing you can perceive is the real you. You are essentially consciousness Itself. Your awareness, the Eternal Witness, is the Divine Reality.

All the world's ancient scriptures, including the Old and New Testaments, have various levels of meaning. The level we're most familiar with is represented by the Sunday school stories we learned as children. But when our *sadhana* deepens, these elementary tales take on a richer, deeper tapestry of meaning. What we previously considered ancient historical texts are miraculously transformed into living, breathing, practical teachings on experiencing life more fully, freely and happily.

In the West, for instance, the most basic misconception concerning humanity's relationship with the Divine Reality starts with the first chapter and verse of Genesis: "In the beginning God created the heavens and the earth." The pronouncement implies that "in the beginning" there was God (an eternal, Divine force) and also a pre-existing supply of cosmic stuff (which was not God) that God used to fashion the heavens and the earth. This inherently dualistic concept of creation always leaves humanity isolated, estranged and fearful. Right from the beginning, mankind is taught that the individual is a separate entity, apart from God, and left alone to find happiness and to eliminate pain.

Yoga science would state it differently. Since nothing exists but God (consciousness), the process of creation is simply God manifesting into various forms—including our own human form. He, She or It (whichever personal pronoun you prefer) is the fullness from which fullness comes, yet His original fullness is never diminished by the multitude of the manifestation. God is, therefore, all things—while simultaneously remaining the One, without a second. We cannot possibly be separated from the Divine. Our very being is an aspect of the One Reality.

Listen to how Jesus the Christ explained this teaching in the *Gnostic Gospel of Thomas*:

> *I took my stand in the midst of the world, and in flesh I appeared to them. I found them all drunk, and I did not find any of them thirsty. My soul ached for the children of humanity, because they are blind in their hearts and do not see, for they came into the world empty, and they also seek to depart from the world empty. (Then) His disciples said to him: On what day*

will the kingdom come? Jesus said: It will not come by
expectation; they will not say: 'See, here,' or 'See,
there.' But the kingdom of the Father is spread upon
the earth, and men do not see it . . . I am the Light that
is above them all, I am the all, and all came forth from
Me and the all attained to Me. Cleave (a piece) of
wood, I am there; lift up the stone and you will find me
there.

Learning Numbers

To underscore the importance of Jesus's teaching, consider
the story of an earnest child who began to learn about
numbers. When his teacher finished explaining the number
one, she proceeded to explain the number two. This progress,
however, caused the youngster some consternation. He didn't
feel that he had comprehended the number one fully enough
to proceed to the number two. His endless questions about the
nature of one held the teacher back from her scheduled
curriculum. After persistent interruptions, the school teacher
suggested that the child go off on his own to learn more about
the number one while the the class was taught the higher
numbers. When the boy completely understood the number
one, the teacher said, he'd be welcome to rejoin the others.

After many years of study, the student did revisit his
teacher. Recognizing the grown boy, the teacher asked him
to share with her class all he had learned about the number
one. With steadfastness of purpose, the young man marched
up to the chalkboard. As he began to write the number one, the
board, wall, school, universe and every manifested distinction
disappeared—revealing only the awesome totality that is
One.

Consider the lives of the great sages from all traditions.
Logic tells us that if one human being has become one with the
"Father who is in heaven," then human beings possess that
potential. Nisargadatta Maharaj explained his enlightenment
this way: "When I realize I am nothing—that is wisdom. When

I realize I am everything—that is love. And between these two points I live my life."

Seeing God Everywhere

A very devout man lived on the banks of a river. It was springtime, and torrential rains brought threats of widespread flooding in his area. As he watched television, weather alerts warned those living in low-lying areas to evacuate their homes immediately. But the man wasn't worried. He had faith that the Lord would protect him.

As predicted, the rains continued, and soon his house was flooded. Under the circumstances, the man had no choice but to take refuge on his roof. A Red Cross rescue crew came by in a boat and offered assistance. "No thanks," the man replied. "The Lord will protect me. I have no fear." But as the water continued to rise, the man was forced to climb atop his chimney. As he held on, fighting the raging current, a helicopter appeared overhead and dropped a lifeline. Again, he waved them away proclaiming that the Lord would protect him.

The rains kept falling, the floodwaters raged and the man was swept away and drowned. When he entered heaven's gates, he angrily called out to the Lord in consternation, "I had perfect faith. Why didn't you save me?" Finally, the Lord spoke: "In your travail, I faithfully answered your prayers. I sent a weatherman and then a boat. When neither of those worked, I even sent a helicopter. What would it have taken for Me to get through to you?"

If an individual is earnest, the requisite will power and transformative insight will come—but not necessarily through the five cognitive senses and the ordinary intellect. Curiosity, openness and the willingness to experiment with our mind, action and speech introduce us to higher levels of understanding.

Sadhana acts as a transformative agent, helping any earnest seeker to unlock the mysteries of life both here and hereafter and to appreciate the richness and essence of all paths.

Although the road maps of various traditions may look different, the actual territory of the "promised land" is always one and the same.

The oceans surge, the rivers roll . . . in me, in me, in me.
The flowers smile, the zephyrs blow . . . in me, in me, in me.
Big fairs are held and battles raged . . . in me, in me, in me.
The mountains heave and Nature blooms . . . in me, in me, in me.
The comets fly, the meteors die,
Cold winds sigh and thunders cry . . . in me, in me, in me.
The foe contends, the friend defends,
The mother sleeps, the baby weeps . . . in me, in me, in me.

SWAMI RAMA TIRTHA[1]

[1]Reprinted from *"The Legacy of Rama,"* Published by Rama Tirtha Pratishtan, Lucknow, India.

Part VI

DEEPENING YOUR PRACTICE

CHAPTER 22

Romancing the Divine

Love your mantra and remember it slowly and gently and it will take you to the soundless state beyond body, breath and mind.

SWAMI RAMA OF THE HIMALAYAS

"Ask, and it shall be given you; seek, and ye shall find; knock, and it shall be opened unto you," the Bible instructs us. But for some new students of meditation, that door seems slow to open. They may sometimes forget to listen to their *mantra* through the day (*japa*) and then have difficulty directing their attention during meditation. The constant interruption of attractive and alluring thoughts and images can turn their meditation practice into a war of wills—a very frustrating experience. Consequently, they may lose sustained interest; their practice may become irregular or abandoned altogether, and that open door to the Divine remains an unfulfilled promise.

Novice meditators know from their limited experience that meditation is beneficial, but patience is not a common virtue in these hurried days. To sit and sustain concentration on the *mantra* becomes boring in the face of all those charms, attractions and temptations that unceasingly parade before the mind. Students want to see some progress and they want to see it now. They want to experience some immediate revelation, some profound spiritual breakthrough, or, at the very least, a sweet glimpse of the One, and they have doubts about how their practice can accomplish it.

The more we practice *japa* and seated meditation, the more the *mantra* establishes itself in the depths of our consciousness and begins to repeat itself—slowly opening a door to the Divine. As the *mantra* becomes our default thought throughout the day, old habits of fear, anger and greed become transformed into powerful reserves of energy, will power and creativity. Then, our power of concentration increases during daily meditations and the mind and *mantra* become one. In that union of mind and *mantra*, the *mantra* returns to its Origin, the Origin of all—and we experience the bliss-filled truth of our own Divinity. That truth, realized in silence, is the truth that sets us free. In that union, we know freedom from limitation and fear.

In practical terms, our challenge is to find a way to open the door to the Divine. We need to learn how to concentrate our attention without being distracted by all the competing and attractive thoughts, images and sounds.

We can draw inspiration from our everyday experience and desire for romance—the powerful attraction that draws one human being to another. When we are attracted to another person sexually, there are two forces at work: one is purely physical and the other is spiritual. The sense pleasure derived through sexual arousal invites and captures our attention easily because continuation of the species is Nature's highest priority. But beyond the physical attraction, a deeper, more meaningful and permanent desire for union exists. This spiritual affinity, or drawing power, is what Hindus refer to as *Krishna*—that aspect of the Divine Reality that beckons us into blissful union and our eventual *moksha* (liberation). When led to orgasm through the act of sex, a human being experiences a stillness in which the lover and beloved merge in the act of lovemaking, and each is swept away into a brief experience of peace, bliss and union. This momentary pleasure, however, is only a foreshadowing of the absolute bliss and fullness that awaits the meditator when sustained union with the Divine is experienced.

To attain an ongoing unity with the Divine, we need to follow a systematic procedure for meditation. We need to choose a convenient time and place for meditation, establish a steady, comfortable posture and attentively listen (as the Eternal Witness) to the sound of the *mantra*—the name of the Divine Reality.

When we begin to hear the *mantra* to the exclusion of all the mind's habitual chatter, we are entering into an intimate relationship. As we give even more attention to the *mantra*, it becomes obvious that this is a powerfully romantic liaison. Then, in the midst of our lovemaking we feel our love being returned, and extraneous thoughts, images and sounds have no more allure.

Focusing on the vibration of the name of the Divine, we begin to experience a genuine delight in the sound. Consequently, we give the *mantra* our attention with ease and without any intention, judgment or expectation. In the presence of such intimacy, the discipline of concentration effortlessly yields to love as we tenderly embrace the sacred sound. We humbly surrender all competing desires to the call of the *mantra*. Finally, through the act of surrender we experience the ultimate union of the *Atman* (individual soul) with the Universal Godhead (*Brahman*) in the climax known as *samadhi* (Self-realization).

Glimpses of such bliss are not so far from our own realm of experience as you might imagine. For instance, when you forget yourself while listening to a beautiful musical composition, it isn't the music that makes you happy, it is the union between the listener and the music that allows you to become aware of the bliss of your own true nature—the bliss of *Ananda*.

And it is the same in meditation. With one-pointed concentration on the *mantra*, you experience the bliss of *Ananda*, but when you begin to think and analyze, the energy field of the mind is no longer concentrated and the ego may conclude, "That was it! I experienced *nirvana*!" Of course, as soon as you think about the experience, you are no longer experiencing it. Still, that tiny peek at what awaits you in deep meditation serves to inspire your resolve the next time you sit for meditation.

The Gospel of John teaches that, "In the beginning was the word, and the word was with God and the word was God." In romancing the Divine, when the mind and the *mantra* become One, we understand that God *is* the *mantra* as well as everything and every one—including our very own Self. That realization transfigures our entire vision of life. We begin to see the world and all our individual relationships as a reflection of the unity of life. We break through the limitations imposed upon us by the old habits of the mind. Then, as we sustain our enthusiasm, attention and love, train our senses and coordinate the functions of the mind to reflect the Divine wisdom of a purified *buddhi*, we slowly and surely become the light of love we seek in the world by blossoming into That which we meditate upon.

CHAPTER 23

Meditation in Action

Under the sway of strong impulse the man who is devoid of self-control willfully commits deeds that he knows to be fraught with future misery. But the man of discrimination, even though moved by desires, at once becomes conscious of the evil that is in them, and does not yield to their influence but remains unattached.

SHRIMAD BHAGAVATAM

What is your most valuable asset? It's not your bank account, education, nor your good looks. The most powerful and valuable asset you possess is your thoughts, because your ability to focus your attention at will is a fundamental skill that determines how happy, creative and productive your life will be.

The techniques for training attention you've learned in seated meditation can be applied to every duty and responsibility throughout the day. The process is called *meditation in action*. Remember that every thought is only a suggestion of what to give your attention to, and that the *buddhi* will always identify the *shreya*, to be served by your mind, action and speech.

Every day is filled with many choices. What am I going to

think about? What will I say? How am I going to act? In every circumstance, learn to witness the mind's activity before taking action. Instead of giving attention to the debilitating energy of thoughts that evoke or reflect fear, anger or self-willed desire, you can choose to serve the intuitive wisdom that emanates from the center of consciousness.

Thoughts, desires and emotions are powerful reservoirs of potential energy. Just as gasoline fuels the automobile, fear, anger and self-willed desires—when they're transformed—can supply the power needed to fulfill the goal of life. The key to successful living lies in choosing not to let the potentially destructive and debilitating *preya* determine our actions.

Meditation in action instructs us to honor our powerful mental resources through the conscious control of our attention. By learning in seated meditation to withdraw our attention willingly from distracting thoughts and to surrender our attachments for them, we acquire a skill that can transform the inherent power of *preya*. Then, as *meditation in action* is practiced, we always have a fresh supply of energy available to help us meet every challenge. By skillfully surrendering the *preya* and serving the constructive and expansive *shreya*, we always have a full tank of gas.

Compassionately watch the mind. When a self-willed thought appears, recall your true nature as the Eternal Witness and consciously listen to the *mantra*. The power of the *mantra* will break the connection between the attractive *preya* thought and your attention. A compelling thought, emotion or sense craving has no power of its own. All the power any thought possesses comes from the attention you give it. When you consciously and willingly withdraw your attention from the *preya*, the *samskara* from which the thought originated is weakened. *Renunciation* of the *preya* stops the suggestion from propelling you into action and its raw power is transformed into strategic reserves.

When the energy of fear, anger or greed arises in your awareness and the *buddhi* advises that you're dealing with a seductive *preya*, you have at least three options:

Option No. 1: You can choose to give your attention to the *preya* thought; speak about the thought or do some physical action in service to it. This response initially gratifies the senses or ego, but ultimately leads to some form of physical, mental or emotional dis-ease or pain. Choosing this option indicates that your mind, action and speech are not in harmony with the *buddhi* and the Divine wisdom it reflects. Pain will inevitably result from such a choice. *For the yoga scientist this is not an acceptable option.*

Option No. 2: You can choose to repress the desire. You have good intentions and recognize that the *buddhi* is advising against giving your attention to the *preya*. Although you decide not to take overt actions that serve the *preya*, you cannot yet surrender your desire for it. On the surface it may appear that you are not serving the *preya*, but it still has your attention. In this case your mental energy still empowers the *preya*. This repression results in neither trustful surrender nor transformation. Like a steel spring held down forcibly, this repressed energy eventually manifests as neurosis, or erupts in sudden destructive behavior, pain and dis-ease. *For the yoga scientist this is not an acceptable option.*

Option No. 3: You can acknowledge the Divine Reality within—recognizing that thoughts are only suggestions and that your relationship with each of them is an integral part of your *sadhana*. Every *preya* thought represents an opportunity to move one step closer to fulfilling your deeply held desires for unbounded Life, Liberty and Happiness.

Because there is only One Absolute Reality (*Sat-Chit-Ananda*) into which all gross and subtle objects appear for a limited space and time, the *preya* thought—like all thoughts—is also a manifestation of the Divine Reality. The *preya* is energy, and it's *your* energy, but right now the *buddhi* is advising that this energy is presented in an unusable form. Recognizing its Divine nature and origin, simply welcome, acknowledge and honor the thought (a subtle object appearing in your awareness) and bathe it in the light of consciousness. When you are ready, offer the *preya* back to the Origin from which it has come.

To accomplish this sacrifice, fashion a prayer or internal dialogue in whatever form you find comfortable. For example:

> *"O, Inner Dweller (or any name for the Divine), right now I am so worried I can hardly focus on anything else, but I hear the buddhi telling me that this worry is a preya. O, Inner Dweller, I am earnestly and humbly offering this thought and its emotional turmoil back to you, the Origin of all. Please accept this offering as the loving gift of a dedicated heart. Consume it in the fire of your light and lead me toward my highest and greatest good."*

After you have offered back the *preya*, give your full attention to your *mantra*. By consciously and willingly withdrawing your attention from the *preya* thought in favor of the *mantra* (*shreya*), you can capture and transform the power of the *preya* into useable energy, will power and creativity, while increasing the *mantra*'s influence of love, fearlessness and strength.

If this process seems cumbersome and tedious, take comfort in knowing that in a very short time it will become effortless. To understand how that ease is accomplished, recall for a moment the first day you drove an automobile. You weren't sure how far to turn the steering wheel or how much pressure to apply to the gas and brake pedals. And who among us will ever forget the anxiety associated with learning how to parallel park? Now, however, once you've placed the key in the ignition, there's only driving. It's all second nature. You no longer consciously consider every component of the process, and driving has become a pleasure.

With the consistent practice of *meditation in action*, newly transformed resources will always be available—whenever you need to act in service to the *shreya*. That same energy, which formerly powered the *preya*, can now be used skillfully in any relationship that requires artistry, patience, forgiveness, detachment, compassion or understanding. The relationship might be with your family, lover or friend, work, pet or hobby. It might be a relationship with the food you eat, your body, breath, desires, the environment or even with the Divine Reality.

CHAPTER 24
Stillness: The Divine Physician

All human evil comes from this:
A man's being unable to sit still in a room.

BLAISE PASCAL

This will probably sound like a silly question, but after driving home from a busy day of work, would you leave the car running all night?

Of course not. You'd turn off the ignition. Otherwise, you'd waste gasoline, incur unnecessary wear and tear on moving parts and probably shorten the life-span of your automobile. It just makes good, common sense not to let the car run when you don't have somewhere to go.

Now here's a second question. If the answer to the first question was so easy to figure out, why do you let the mind run day and night without offering it some rest?

Just about everyone complains about the speed, stress and anxiety of modern life, about how the incessant demands of our spouse, children, aging parents, personal health, work and housekeeping drain us of the time and energy for the small pleasures we'd really like to enjoy. Sometimes things get so difficult that many of us feel as though our lives have been hijacked! So how do we respond? We further complicate the situation by trying to squeeze even more into our lives—

external experiences the ego or senses swear will be pleasant. Unfortunately, even if these experiences do turn out to be enjoyable, they are powerless to alter the basic controlling software of the mind that habituates us to unending desire and stress.

Yoga science, however, offers us an alternative to the habitual ways we live our lives—if we can simply learn to enjoy the therapeutic power of stillness.

The sages teach us that the mind moves first and the body follows. We can't even lift our hand without first entertaining a thought. The external movements of the body are consequences of what has already happened in the mind. This means that when the mind is racing at one hundred miles an hour in the passing lane of life, we simply don't have the option of making conscious choices. At such high speed, most of our actions will be based on our deepest *samskaras*, rather than the discriminative power of the *buddhi*. This continuous and unexamined stream of habitual thought and activity results in dis-ease, pain and limitation.

Just as the mind sends messages to the body, the body also sends messages to the mind—messages that we readily identify with. "A migraine exists in the head," the body complains. "A pain in the lower back is increasing. The breath is short and difficult. The heart is racing." When the already beleaguered mind receives an onslaught of such messages, it becomes even more agitated and unfocused as it attempts to integrate the data and ease the problems. The mind cannot remain calm under such pressure. As a result, the body—sooner or later—will reflect yet another level of dis-ease.

In order to experience the pleasures and benefits that a still mind brings, you must first calm the constant babble of the body. "Be still," the Psalms advise, "and know that I am God." This process begins when you learn the art of sitting for meditation in a quiet place, every day at the same time. Arrange your body so it is comfortable and steady, with your head, neck and trunk in straight alignment. Establish the *finger* and *root lock*s, and then with your full determination (*sankalpa*), pledge to yourself that no matter what charm, attraction or temptation appears in your awareness, the body will remain still, the mind will be calm and you will give your full and complete attention to the *mantra*. "I want to do it. I can do it. I have to do it. I am going to do it—no matter what!"

Once you establish a steady and comfortable posture, distractions of the body subside, and you will be able to develop a serene breath. A composed, diaphragmatic breath calms the mind and focuses creative energy. Then, as you sit regularly in meditation with complete concentration on the *mantra*, a quiet joy springs from the stillness. This bliss or fullness is what the sages refer to as *Ananda*—a facet of the Divine Reality within each of us. As you abide regularly in the joy of that stillness, a powerful purification and healing spontaneously take place in both the mind and body. In stillness, physical, mental and emotional dis-ease begin to melt away.

But the therapeutic quality of stillness is not associated only with seated meditation and the absence of movement. It can also be experienced while performing our duties and responsibilities in the world. The calmness, balance and focus of *meditation in action* allow us to make conscious, discriminating choices instead of being misled by the allure of *preya*. Real peace of mind and health of body come when we acquire the capacity to live free from all the conditioned responses of our fears, anger and selfish desires.

Without a sound philosophy of life, the leadership of our *mantra*, and first-hand experience of the profound benefits and joy of stillness, consciousness will continue to flow along our familiar, deep *samskaras*. This means that we will continue to think, speak and act according to old habits, day after day. We will scurry about in search of pleasant and comfortable objects and relationships we mistakingly believe will make us happy, and may exhaust ourselves chasing after rainbows—never attaining what we seek.

In contrast, meditation is a journey without movement that yields the highest blessings. In Sanskrit, the joy of stillness is referred to as *shanti*. The Bible calls it "the peace that passeth all understanding." This *shanti* is exactly what Christians call *Christ-consciousness*, Jews call the *land of milk and honey*, Hindus refer to as *Brahman*, Muslims refer to as *The Beloved* and Buddhists call *Nirvana*.

It doesn't matter what name is used to identify the blissful nature of stillness. The only question for each of us is, "How can we experience it?" As long as we avoid stillness in our lives, we are keeping ourselves apart from this great blessing.

Now, let's face it, most of our thoughts are not that useful. Worry, resentment, jealousy, dwelling in the past or future, never lead us for our highest and greatest good. So, why not employ practical Western know-how by exhibiting the same respect for our body and mind as we extend to our automobile? Just like turning off the car when we get home, stillness makes good, common sense. Stillness conserves our energy, enhances our creativity, heals the body and ultimately brings us what we are are all searching for—unbounded Life, Liberty and Happiness.

Meditators are Pleasure Seekers

Most people consider meditators to be disciplinarians, but many very pleasurable activities employ meditation techniques. For example, Olympic athletes receive greater joy from winning the gold medal than from indulging the variety of *preya*s they have willingly renounced along the training path to victory. The attainment of one-pointed attention and detachment (*vairagya*) is often the factor that empowers an athlete to win the gold. The athlete who has learned to focus attention down to that still-point, or *bindu*, is the one whose body can perform free of mental distractions. That calm competitor will win the Olympic gold.

The same holds true in the science of yoga and meditation. Each of us is aware of charms, attractions and temptations continually calling our attention. The senses are tirelessly venturing out into the material world to acquaint us with a host of tempting objects. These objects may be pleasant enough, but for the yoga scientist, like the Olympic athlete, there exists a greater perennial joy. By experiencing our own innate fullness in the stillness of focused attention, we become free of our limitations and can enjoy the objects and relationships of the world more completely.

Roar of the Ocean

Remember, all reality flows from the subtle to the gross. Every perceivable subtle and gross object—including sound—originates in silence. When you go to the shore and become aware of the roar of the ocean, do you ever wonder where this sound originates? To find out, follow the ocean back to the river from which it came, and then back even farther, to the mountain stream from which the river was born. Then, trace the stream back to its source, a spring in the highest mountains. There, all you will find is stillness.

Similarly, when you focus your undivided attention on the *mantra* in deep meditation, the mind and *mantra* become one and the *mantra* will lead you within to stillness at the Center of Consciousness. When you become aware of that ocean of bliss, you will know that the silent presence of pure consciousness is your own true Self and the Origin of all. In deep meditation you will realize that the blissful ocean of silence *is* the Divine Reality . . . within you. Through that revelation you will know what Jesus the Christ really meant when He spoke the words, "I and my Father are One."

CHAPTER 25

The Grand Charade

The two are really only one. It is the ignorant person who sees many where there is really only one.

BLACK ELK

If the sages are correct that our Essential Nature is eternal, bliss-filled consciousness (*Sat-Chit-Ananda*) and all gross and subtle objects appear in That—including our body, mind, thoughts, emotions and desires—why are we not aware of this Absolute Reality right from birth? The human being is a highly intelligent species. We have sent men to the moon, harnessed the power of the atom and cured polio. Why then are we blind to the most important question of all: "Who am I?" Why this grand charade? What keeps us unaware of the true nature of our being?

Part of the mystery can be explained through an acquaintance with the principle of illusion called *maya*. *Maya* is defined as the delusive power by which the One Reality, boundless and whole, is made to appear limited and divided. This potent illusion gives rise to our notion of bondage and separateness, self-willed desire and the mistaken conviction that there is something to be liberated from.

Preparing for the Birth Visualization

The power of *maya* operates at many levels of human perception, casting a veil of ignorance. However, by understanding how we have become so thoroughly identified with the limitations of body and mind, a spiritual seeker can begin to recognize and reverse this pervasive error. A short visualization will serve to initiate the process.

This visualization is not a meditation. While meditation requires the flow of attention to a single point, visualization asks you to allow your fertile imagination complete freedom to create detailed mental images.

Before you begin, remember that deep *samskaras* are created in your unconscious mind by the attention you habitually give to certain thoughts, and that consciousness flows through those most open and frequented channels in the mind. It follows that we, ourselves, are responsible for creating our own mental software, simply by repeatedly directing our attention according to habit.

In preparation for this visualization, assume your meditation posture. Gently close your eyes and mouth and establish the *finger lock*. The body should be motionless.

Now, imagine what it was like to be inside your mother's womb. To whatever extent your mind can visualize that experience, place yourself inside your mother's womb.

It's a perfect environment where everything you need is provided. It's warm, comforting, loving and nurturing. Mama's heartbeat is reassuring. Perhaps she's humming a sweet lullaby or lovingly caressing her belly. With complete one-pointed attention, continue to imagine what it was like to be in that perfect environment.

As you grow in the womb you might subtly perceive the need for more elbow room, but beyond that minor inconvenience, everything is perfect. Then, in the ninth month of gestation, you realize that dramatic changes are on the way. You're ready to be born. One day your whole environment begins to shift and squeeze. You experience a rush of adrenaline and expectancy as your body is pressed down through the birth canal. This is turning into a bit of a struggle, but you're ready for it. After all, you want to live!

Then, at last, you are born! Those first few moments after birth are momentous. Although your humanity has provided you with adequate physical and mental equipment for this new adventure, the intense onslaught of sensory information is overwhelming.

You have eyes, but they can't really focus yet, and the never-before seen light is painful and blinding. The mesmerizing and comforting sounds of Mama's heartbeat and internal organs suddenly disappear in a cacophony of loud, unidentifiable and even terrifying sounds.

For the first time you begin to smell and to experience the bodily functions of swallowing and tasting. So many new sensations! And the broad expanse of your naked skin is in pain. It's so cold! Everything the skin touches is rough and hard compared to Mama's womb. Then, if you're not already breathing, somebody might slap you on the behind. You have to breathe! You're on your own, baby.

Birth of the Ego and Installing the Software

So there you are, a newborn infant in a new world. In the midst of an overwhelming barrage of sensory stimulation, an innate desire for self-preservation propels you to search for comfort, safety and contentment. Above all else, you want to live! You must learn how to eliminate the pain! You must find happiness! But how? You have no frame of reference to remind you that this situation is merely temporary. You can certainly scream and thrash your arms and legs about, but beyond that, you can do little.

Then, as you try to comprehend and deal with this seemingly endless sensory assault, you begin to experience a very different kind of relationship. You are introduced to your mama, and Mama's breast. As Mama lovingly cuddles you in her arms and coos, you begin to nurse and all your mental and physical attention focuses down to a single point: Mama's nipple.

Because of your one-pointed attention, you are no longer aware of the stimulus of the senses and you begin to experience a cessation of pain and the establishment of pleasure. For the first time since the birth process began, you are aware of relative calm. You feel safe, secure, warm, nurtured, content and loved.

And, in the midst of this new, pleasant experience you reach your first profound, but ignorant, conclusion:

"I am a separate entity and Mama is a separate entity, and objects and relationships in the material world bring about contentment and happiness and cause the elimination of pain."

ॐ

Fueled by an intense desire for self-preservation, this memorable experience leads the newborn to conclude that I, the subject, perceive Mama, the object. The experience of nursing at Mama's breast is the dawning of the delusion of duality. It represents the birth of the *ahamkara*, the ego or I-maker—that function of the mind that effectively separates the baby from the One Absolute Reality. In fact, the ancient Sanskrit word *mama* means mine. The baby now believes, based on its own personal experience, that there is a me and there is also an "other."

Because survival depends on this new relationship, the baby mistakenly accepts duality as the true reality. Separation becomes the operative paradigm. Separation is now key to the newborn's self-preservation, and is stored in the unconscious memory bank of *chitta*. In fact, the attachment is so powerful that it strikes the virgin unconscious with a meteor-like force, creating a huge crater (*samskara*). Self-preservation is indispensable! The baby must survive!

As the newborn begins to experience, learn and make choices, he or she encounters continual reminders that reinforce the delusion that objects and relationships in the material world eliminate pain and establish relative calm and happiness. Remember, consciousness flows through the deepest, widest and most unobstructed channel in the unconscious. Only moments after birth, as soon as the baby nurses at Mama's breast, the baby's unconscious mind begins to spin a web of delusion because the only installed software program is based on the *samskara* of separateness and duality.

As the baby grows, the security of Mama's breast is replaced by a succession of different objects: new relationships with a bottle of formula, a pacifier, a stuffed animal, a suit of clothes, a shiny toy, a good grade on a spelling test, a high school diploma, a college degree, an automobile, a girlfriend, a boyfriend, a husband, a wife, or even a new baby. The human being continually substitutes one object and relationship for another, prodded and deluded by the notion that the next object or relationship is going to bring happiness and eliminate pain. Why? Because the mental operating system is based on habit patterns (*samskaras*) that define each human being and material object as an essentially separate entity.

The Lion and the Sheep

An orphaned lion cub was raised by a flock of sheep. Taught and nurtured by the adult sheep and frolicking with all the lambs, the cub never questioned his own identity. He always assumed he was a sheep.

One day as the flock was grazing near a small stream, they were chased by a pride of lions. In terror, the cub ran to escape. In a gallant attempt to elude the clutches of his pursuers, the young lion leaped across the stream. Once airborne, he happened to glance at the surface of the water, and, for the first time, he saw his reflection looking back at him. To his amazement, he did not see a white woolly sheep. Instead, he saw a leaping lion. When he reached a safe place, he bleated out his great relief and, to his amazement, his voice sounded exactly like the ferocious roar of a lion.

From birth, each of us grows up under a grand illusion. We innocently accept the suggestions of separateness that our own ego, family and culture present to us. Yet at a certain point in our lives, many of us begin in earnest the search for limitless Happiness. It is this inquiry that ultimately directs us inside ourselves to find the liberating truth of our Divine identity.

CHAPTER 26

Beyond Time, Space and Causation

The real voyage of discovery consists not in seeking new landscapes but in having new eyes.

MARCEL PROUST

The three principles of time, space and causation are the powerful forces that keep us enslaved to the dualistic paradigm. When the senses are engaged, a perceiving subject (me) becomes aware of some object and the concept of space is established in the mind. Space is the separation between subject and object. Time, the sages teach, is a mere construct of the human mind—a mechanism for comprehending and arranging the space between objects of awareness in a linear progression.

From this isolating perspective, most human beings see themselves as separate subjects viewing a procession of transitory objects. The space between subject and object—between *me* and *you*, or *me* and *it*—is a conditioned perception. It implies my separateness and engenders the fear that I might not get what I want or I might lose what I have. All fear inevitably invites danger. The mental software of dualism is the cause of pain and bondage.

The mind is your most powerful instrument and it can be your best friend. Yet, because of its capacity to separate you from the One Reality, the mind can also become your worst enemy. By your search for pleasing objects and your routine fixation on someone or something outside, you create a formidable obstacle to knowing your own Essential Nature. Consequently, many spiritual quests are frustrated by this limited "I" endlessly searching for an eternal "Thou." You remain an outsider in all your relationships. Not understanding your true Self, you put all your faith in the ever-changing external world.

The practices of yoga science help to purify the mind. By concentrating attention and by discriminating between the passing pleasure and perennial joy, the illusory space between the perceiver and the perceived disappears and the seamless Absolute Reality becomes apparent. By unifying the power of his or her aggregate desires through self-discipline, the spiritual seeker can experience the first great freedom: the freedom from fear. As the space between *me* and all *others* is annihilated, who or what is there to fear? Who is there to be angry at if there is only One Reality here, there and everywhere?

By refining your personality through detachment and *renunciation*, you free yourself from self-authored limitations and the inability to deal with the handicaps of others. Eknath Easwaran asks, "If a blind man knocks you down, are you angry with him?" No, because he cannot see you. "And if he doesn't react to the shock on your face as you sit on the pavement, do you think that he's insensitive?" No, he's simply blind.

The truth of the matter is that every one of us is blind! Each and every human being operates with physical, mental or emotional handicaps. Because our unconscious mental operating system is composed of huge *samskaras* of duality, we can see nothing else. We are constantly grabbing for that next brass ring that glistens with promise. Or, feeling that we have already gained something, we become fearful that we might lose what we have. This human condition is known as *samsara*—the unending cycle of birth and death, pain and sorrow.

Creating Waves of Desire

By operating under the delusion of duality—repeatedly directing your attention to an attractive thought, emotion or object—you create a wave of desire, rising in the lake of the mind. When you finally obtain the object of your desire, you experience a passing pleasure—a gratifying little thrill of satisfaction. You wanted the house. You wanted the house. You wanted the house. Now you have the house and you're happy . . . at least for the moment.

But, when you've obtained the object of desire, the *ahamkara* (ego or I-maker) muscles its way into your awareness—arm in arm with its constant companion, your belief in duality. The *ahamkara* is quick to attribute your happiness to the newly acquired object. "Aha!" ego concludes. "It's the object that made you happy." And why would you doubt such a conclusion? All of your experiences substantiate it: you believe you are a separate entity and that other entities in the material world have the power to eliminate your pain and make you happy. Consequently, this most recent experience is instantly stored in your unconscious mind—reconfirming and deepening an already cavernous *samskara* of ignorance.

Lesson of the Fountain Pen

The habit of anointing objects and relationships with the power to confer happiness is practically illustrated by my own relationship with a favorite fountain pen. Many years ago, a business acquaintance of mine had a beautiful fountain pen. The more attention I gave that pen, the more I wanted one just like it, and I imagined myself using it with an impressive flourish. One day I saw an advertisement for the pen in a prominent business magazine and my desire grew even stronger.

At last I received the pen as a gift and, as you can imagine, I was very happy. However, after only a few brief days with my new treasure, I lost the pen and could not find it—and I was miserable. I looked everywhere for the pen, retracing my movements from the time I realized it was gone. I looked in every conceivable place, but to no avail. The pen was lost and I grew increasingly depressed.

In the above illustration, I felt happy when I received the pen and depressed when I lost it. Was the pen the cause of my happiness or was it the cause of my depression? Neither, the sages emphatically teach. No object or relationship that is subject to change has any power to make us happy or depressed.

Metaphorically speaking, when I got the pen, the wave of desire for the pen crashed on the seawall of the mind—just as ocean waves crash at the shore. Watch the motion of the ocean and you will see waves endlessly rising, cresting and falling—one after another after another. But note that between two waves, there always comes a relative calm.

The same phenomenon occurs in the mind. When you give your attention to an object, a wave of desire begins to grow in your awareness. When the desire is fulfilled, the wave crashes and the mind is calm. For a brief time there is no desire calling your attention. In that stillness, the bliss that reflects into your awareness (*Chit*) is none other than the imperishable comfort of your own Divinity, *Ananda*—that aspect of your Essential Nature that is more full and rapturous than the passing pleasure experienced by fulfilling any desire.

Peek Experiences

When you obtain a desired object you get a rare glimpse into the nature of the One Reality. When the mind is still, the bliss of *Ananda* rises in your awareness, and for a brief time you can look deep into the placid, light-filled lake bed of the mind— into the Center of Consciousness from which thoughts themselves are generated.

The experience of bliss is brief, however, because the next wave of desire very quickly starts rolling in. Desires are endless. Every desire begets another desire. Now that I have the house, a desire for furniture grows. Yes, furniture! I want furniture. I want furniture. I want furniture. Now I've got some furniture and I feel happy. But without curtains, everybody will be able to see into my house, so a desire for curtains grows. I want some curtains. I want some curtains . . . It will never end.

Each desire gives rise to another. When a desire is fulfilled, the *ahamkara* attributes the passing pleasure to the object. The pen, the house and the curtains, the ego says, are the causes of your happiness. And you have no reason to doubt it.

As we have described, this ignorance can be traced all the way back to the moment you began nursing at Mama's breast. You experienced a passing pleasure and mistakenly attributed it to the object of your attention. This process gave rise to a sense of separate, limited self—the ego—which has continually concluded that "objects and relationships in the material world cause happiness and eliminate pain." Thoughts generated from deep *samskaras* habitually resubstantiate the correctness of this logic.

But the sages disagree. You are not separate. You are the formless, Eternal Witness (*Sat-Chit-Ananda*) having a human experience, and it is within that eternal, bliss-filled awareness and wisdom that all gross and subtle objects appear. You are aware of thoughts, desires and emotions, but you are *not* those thoughts, desires and emotions.

Yoga science calls for the conscious coordination of the suggestions of the ego, senses, unconscious mind and your discrimination—to allow the Divine Reality within to guide your actions. The effectiveness of this teaching is based on the power and skillful direction of your individual attention. It's so simple, Swami Rama always insisted. "Unplug there and plug in here."

Because the mental software of duality creates strong attachments, choosing to base your actions on the wisdom within is more easily said than done. But if you earnestly desire to be free from pain, misery and bondage, the sages promise that you can be. As you learn to cultivate one-pointed attention (*dharana*), you develop the facility to transform the old patterns of habit and personality into a newly expanded consciousness.

Understand that the term "expansion of consciousness" has nothing to do with tie-dyed shirts or the hooka-smoking caterpillars that symbolized the drug culture of the 1960s. Rather, it describes the scientific process for gaining increased access to an intuitive library of knowledge within—the super-conscious mind. To tune in to this practical wisdom, you simply need to pay attention to the *buddhi*. Be awake, as the Buddha advises, and you can gracefully align every thought, word and action with the *buddhi's* innate wisdom.

Thoughts, desires and emotions that limit you are continually generated from self-created *samskaras* (habit patterns). Breaking free of their powerful gravitational attraction requires strong resolve (*sankalpa*) and conscious effort. For that reason, our teaching offers a systematic program for purifying and re-engineering the software of the mind. Each practice presented in this book helps you focus attention, moment by moment. Within a very short time, your *sadhana* can rewrite the software of the mind—creating new habits that will lead you to realize your fullest potential.

Creating Healthy Habits

Have you ever noticed that the very same mechanism that formed your bad habits has also formed your good habits? In fact, the choice to form helpful or harmful habits is yours to make. We tend to dwell on our unhealthy habits, but we need to be more compassionate than condemning when we consider them. After all, the tide of our culture is constantly encouraging us to form habits in service to the *preya*. Choosing to go against that tide by regularly practicing meditation does require your courage, strength and will power.

The modern medical community already acknowledges that meditation can reduce hypertension and anxiety, as well as mitigate the harmful effects of fear, anger and depression. In addition, many spiritual traditions recognize that a consistent and regular meditation practice is a reliable path to Self-realization. Yet merely understanding the benefits does not supply an individual with the *sankalpa* to transform long-cultivated habits of the mind.

For many individuals, this is an area of considerable conflict. Although your intention is good, you may simply be unable to find time in an already crowded daily schedule. Or, you may not have been able to establish a minimal daily practice even though you have a strong desire to do so. Rest assured that these obstacles are commonplace and surmountable. All seasoned meditators remember the inevitable starts, stops and doubts involved in establishing a consistent and rewarding practice.

Like all animals, the human being has a tremendous capacity for conditioning. Just as dogs know when it's time for breakfast or a walk, human beings also anticipate a predictable event when we experience a certain circumstance. Most of our conditioning functions unconsciously. We're conditioned to work, play, snack, drink, talk, shop, smoke and sleep without making conscious decisions about behavior.

Should you decide, however, to dedicate yourself to a conscious and consistent *sadhana*, the sages promise that you can break free from the restraints imposed by time, space and causation. Instead of merely living in the world enslaved to desire and dis-ease, you will begin to experience the freedom of creativity and contentment. By aligning your mind, action and speech with the intuitive wisdom of the Divine Reality, you will come to know that you are not separate, but rather an integral part of the One.

CHAPTER 27

You are a Citizen of Two Worlds

When the mind soars in pursuit of the things conceived in space, it pursues emptiness. But when the man dives deep within himself, he experiences the fullness of existence.

MEHER BABA

Yoga science teaches that we are citizens of two worlds. Yes, we live in the material world. We have a body. We have a mind. We have thoughts, desires and emotions. We are constantly observing an endless array of names and forms. Furthermore, we have duties and responsibilities to perform and relationships to nurture in the world of names and forms. We perceive multiplicity through the senses, yet the sages remind us that there is only One Absolute truth . . . here, there and everywhere.

When the various forms and styles of gold jewelry are smelted in the crucible, only gold remains. For a limited time they appeared to be different—earrings, bracelets, rings and brooches—but they were always gold.

In its prescription for Happiness, yoga science does not demand the *renunciation* of all sense gratification—nor does it endorse the total annihilation of the ego. We are born with a body and senses that equip us to enjoy the pleasures of the world. Furthermore, human beings must accept, to a limited extent, the suggestion of separateness because a healthy ego is essential if we are to wisely perform our part in the Divine play of existence known as *lila*.

Nevertheless, while yoga science encourages us to live and actively participate in this world, it insists that we are not *of* this world. Our essential identity (*Sat-Chit-Ananda*) is of the realm of spirit—That from which all names and forms are manifested. Because of our ignorance, however, human beings identify with the limited and limiting body, mind and senses. We become attached to the transitory—believing that fleeting objects and relationships will somehow fulfill our desires.

The sages teach that we are also citizens of a second world, one that has neither beginning nor end, and where, in truth, nothing changes. *Sat-Chit-Ananda,* the eternal kingdom of bliss-filled consciousness and wisdom within each of us, is the other world spoken of by the sages. "Okay," the sages admit, "there is a multiplicity of forms with which we have relationships. But the multiplicity is ephemeral," they say, "subject to change just like the weather." Subtle and gross objects come, they're here for a brief period and then they're gone. It is foolhardy, the sages conclude, to give your deepest love and loyalty to that which will inevitably pass away. That is a prescription for pain. As Jesus the Christ taught, "Lay not up for yourselves treasures upon the earth, where moth and rust doth corrupt, and where thieves break through and steal: But lay up for yourselves treasures in heaven, where neither moth nor rust doth corrupt, and where thieves do not break through nor steal."

The sages of every tradition explain that we are on a journey. We have come from the formless sea of consciousness; we find ourselves in this human form for a brief time, and we are destined to return to the subtle. Yoga science insists that the journey should be meaningful and pleasant. We are meant to use and enjoy the objects and relationships of this material world, but not possess them nor be possessed by them. This becomes possible when we identify with the Eternal, rather than the transitory—when we are always aware of the Divine Reality and allow Its wisdom to guide our every action.

Evolution Versus Involution

There comes a certain point in our evolutionary trajectory when we begin to consider the possibility that true Happiness may not lie outside of us in the relative world. By grace, we may begin the involutionary process of seeking and finding Happiness within.

Our earnestness fuels this process of purification and Self-realization. As we learn to choose consciously which thoughts to think, words to speak and actions to take, we unencumber ourselves of crippling attachments to fear, anger and greed. In the process, we willingly renounce the contracting *preya* and discover our endless reserves of energy, will power and creativity.

Remember, Abraham was asked to sacrifice his greatest attachment in life—his son Isaac. He was able to make an offering (*yagna*) of his attachment, and through the process of *renunciation* Abraham attained the purification, inspiration, creativity and skill to become the patriarch of the Hebrew people.

As we willingly participate in the process of renouncing the *preya*, we unify the power of all our various desires. Our one-pointed attention yields creativity and genius as all our many small desires are consolidated in service to our deepest driving desire for unbounded Life, Liberty and Happiness. Just as the beam of a laser can penetrate steel, a concentrated mind can see beyond all illusion.

Yoga Ecology

If you resolve to practice the teachings presented in this book, you will be asked to give up some attachments in your life. In order to give your attention to any yoga practice, some other attractive object or relationship will have to be surrendered. It can be a seemingly insignificant attachment—a second cup of coffee, going back to sleep an extra ten minutes in the morning, listening to the car radio or the indulgence of an angry, fearful, selfish or self-deprecating thought.

For each of us, the offering will be different, but it will be perfect for our unique circumstance. Whatever *preya* presents itself in the moment is certain to be the ideal candidate for conscious and willing *renunciation*. Remember, it is impossible to serve the *shreya* and the *preya* at the same time. A choice will be made—either consciously or unconsciously. If you do not choose consciously, the choice will be made for you automatically, based on the deepest *samskara* in your unconscious mind. And *that* is slavery!

Each desire for the *preya* that comes into your awareness provides an opportunity for you to capture the intrinsic energy of that desire to increase reserves of will power and to expand your creativity. Instead of serving the *preya* and experiencing the pain of dis-ease; instead of repressing the *preya* and thereby cultivating the inevitable pain of neurosis, choose to experiment. Welcome and acknowledge the power of any thought that evokes fear, anger, greed, depression, resentment or jealousy. Its energy becomes available to you through your conscious act of surrender—the willing withdrawal of attention.

Inherent power resides in the *preya* that comes to you, and it belongs to you alone. If, through *renunciation*, you consciously inhibit that power from taking the form of an action, that power is automatically transformed into reserves of energy, will power and creativity—accessible whenever you need them.

This aspect of yoga science represents the most profound form of ecology. By consciously conserving and transforming the subtle thought power of *preya*, you are stewarding your most abundant natural resource. In effect, this practice unites your various human desires into an invincible force that can fulfill your deepest driving desire: the desire for freedom from pain, misery and bondage. As the Absolute Reality becomes the center of conscious awareness, the old cataracts of habit that previously obscured your vision begin to dissolve. This new consciousness frees you to blossom to your full capacity: creatively, artistically, productively and lovingly.

The entire process is based exclusively on the conscious use of your power of attention. It's an amazingly powerful tool. And it's free!

Part VII

POWER OF BREATH

CHAPTER 28

Pranayama: Science of Breath

Breath is the bridge that connects life to consciousness, which unites your body to your thoughts. Whenever your mind becomes scattered, use your breath as a means to take hold of your mind again.

THICH NHAT HANH

The Psalms inform us that "Each man's life is but a breath." Without breath, our lives would be impossible. The exchange of oxygen for carbon dioxide in the lungs is certainly essential for the human being to function, but yoga science suggests that it is not air that animates the city of life. Rather, our lives are sustained by an extremely powerful form of subtle energy known as *prana* that accompanies the air we breathe.

Traditional Western medicine defines humans as primarily physical beings. This approach logically evolved from a cultural attitude that continues to characterize each person as a separate, quantifiable entity. Reflecting the habits of the human mind, medical science has, until recently, limited its scientific inquiry to the perceivable and quantifiable.

Einstein Breaks the Mold

Albert Einstein wrote that "a problem cannot be solved on the same level at which it arose." This open-minded attitude helped him recognize that in the material universe an essential relationship exists between matter and energy. More specifically and scientifically, E=MC² (energy is equal to the mass of an object, times the speed of light, squared). In practical language, Einstein is telling us something profoundly important for our own health and well-being. He says that matter—the material stuff, like our physical bodies—can be transformed into energy, and that energy, conversely, can be turned into matter.

Einstein's mathematical equation serves as a bridge between metaphysics and physics. An obvious reality has now been explained in scientific terms. Our everyday experiences and observations have already taught us that energy and matter are one and the same. For instance, we count on the corn flakes we eat for breakfast to be turned into the energy with which we accomplish our work. With each bite of cereal, we are betting our lives that the energy of the sun will be reliably transformed into the carbohydrates and proteins our bodies and brains need to function. We accept without question that the calories (energy) we consume will become the physical bodies we inhabit and give the body strength to act. Such obvious and verifiable examples of the transformation of energy into matter, and matter into energy, did not become more true after Einstein's mathematical equation was stated, but his work has provided an interface between ancient assumptions about *prana* and modern physics.

Prana and the *Nadis*

In Sanskrit, the word *prana* refers to the first unit of life, a subtle energy emanating from the soul (*Sat-Chit-Ananda*) and flowing within the living human being. On the most subtle level, it is the vital *prana* that animates the body-mind-sense complex. If you were to force air into the lungs of a cadaver it would not get up and walk away. And why is that? Because it is the *prana* already present in a living body that invites, receives and distributes the life force of *prana* carried on the vehicle of breath. It is *prana* alone, not the mediums of air, food, or water, that enlivens the body.

The human body is maintained by an intricate network of subtle rivers of energy, through which the vital *prana* flows. These rivers are called *nadis*, and the aggregate complex of *nadis* and *prana* are known as *pranamaya kosha*. This body of energy is subtler than the physical body and serves as a link between the mind (*manomaya kosha*) and the physical body (*annamaya kosha*). Thus, the energy sheath of *prana* can influence both the mind and body, and is influenced by them as well.

Most ancient *pranayama* texts agree that there are some seventy-two thousand *nadis* within the body. Some texts contend that this number exceeds three million. The actual number need not concern us, however, since our interest is simply in maintaining the continuous, uninterrupted flow of *prana* through this complex network of *nadis*. Without *prana*, human life would cease.

Breath is the Vehicle for *Prana*

The breath is the body's primary delivery system for the vital *prana*. The relationship between the air we breathe and *prana* is analogous to the relationship that exists between a horse and its rider. Just as the horse is the vehicle for the rider, the air is the vehicle for the *prana*. According to the yogic science of *pranayama*, the air merely carries the *prana* to its destination in the physical body.

Pranayama (Control of *Prana*)

Prana means the first unit of subtle energy and *yama* means control. *Pranayama* is the science that controls the *prana*, primarily by breath regulation. Over thousands of years, the study of this vast and profound science has yielded a wide variety of effective practices. We will introduce a few that are safe, immediately helpful and require little preparation.

Breath awareness exercises help to normalize the motion of the lungs—thereby assuring the necessary flow of the vital force within the body. Regular *pranayama* helps direct and balance the flow of this subtle energy that sustains and coordinates all the body's physical and mental functions. Without such regulation, the intended flow of pranic energy may become blocked somewhere in the body. Trapped energy eventually manifests as pain (physical, mental and emotional dis-ease). Without a continuous delivery of vital *prana*, the respiratory system, the heart, the brain and autonomic nervous system do not function in a coordinated fashion. Disturbances in these physical processes can result in serious illness. For the *sadhaka* (spiritual seeker), such blockages may also limit progress in meditation.

In *pranayama*, the breath is considered to be the bridge between the body and the mind. Concentrated attention on the breath affects and directs the flow of the vital *prana* through the body. Every time we think about moving a part of the body, for example, vital *prana* rushes toward that site along the subtle network of *nadis* to make movement possible. Conversely, bodily movements also affect the flow of *prana*. A regular exercise program (including *Easy-Gentle Yoga* and *mantra* walks), therefore, is an essential element in maintaining and gently moving the vital *prana*.

Respiration is the body's primary mechanism for the strategic flow of energy. Proper inhalation and exhalation are like twin sentries guarding the city of life. The rate, rhythm and depth of breath directly impact the amount of energy available to the body and affect all the metabolic processes. The breath determines whether energy is delivered in irregular, short bursts or in longer, more sustained waves. With every breath we are redefining the patterns of energy that affect both the body and the mind—for better or worse.

Breathing air deeply into the lungs is a critical factor in maintaining good health. Diaphragmatic breathing calms the nervous system while massaging and stimulating the heart and all organs of digestion and elimination. In addition, it efficiently oxygenates the blood. Oxygen is inhaled into the lungs where it is transferred into the bloodstream for distribution to all the cells of the body. Because the human torso is carried in an upright position, gravity generally acts to keep greater quantities of blood in the lower portion of the lungs than the upper. With deep, diaphragmatic breathing, the lungs fill to their capacity, providing oxygen to the lower lungs where it can most readily be absorbed. Those who breathe shallowly, moving only the upper chest, often feel fatigued. Their improper breathing habits inhibit the process of oxygenation and deny vitality to the cells of the body.

Breath and Mind Connection

The breath is the physical manifestation of the mind. The ancients learned through direct observation that while they could not intellectually will the mind to calm down, they could create a serene, contented mind through conscious regulation of the breath. When their breath was full and even, without jerks, pauses or sounds, then their minds became calm.

The breath and the mind are inextricably linked—like two sides of the same coin. Through your own personal experience you may already know that your respiration always reflects the state of your mind. The rhythm, rate and capacity of your breathing changes instantly in reaction to your thoughts, desires and emotions. When emotional shock or strain is experienced in life, you can immediately observe its effects on the breathing process. When you are tense or surprised, you may hold your breath. When you are stressed, the breath may become rapid or shallow. When you are happy and content, the breath reflects that state of mind with its fullness and ease.

Five Breathing Irregularities

Most *pranayama* should be practiced in your regular seated meditation posture with your head, neck and trunk straight.

Once you have established a comfortable and steady posture, you may notice one or more of five possible irregularities in the breath.

1. Shallowness of breath
2. Interruptions in the flow of breath (jerks)
3. Noisy breathing
4. Extended pauses between inhalation and exhalation
5. Breathing through the mouth

To correct any irregularity, simply witness it with relaxed attention. This correction is the natural effect of your conscious attention to a formerly unconscious habit.

As you incorporate breath awareness into your *sadhana* and deepen your meditations, you will begin to recognize that most seemingly involuntary movements of the body are actually results of thought or emotion. When you observe your physical behavior, you will notice that no act or gesture occurs independently of the mind. The mind always moves first and then the body follows. The untrained mind often dissipates vital *prana* through nervous bodily movements and twitches—energy that could better serve the body-mind-sense complex in other ways.

Just being conscious of the breath helps you create an undisturbed and peaceful mind. When the breath begins to flow freely, smoothly and silently through the nostrils without any jerks, pauses or sounds, the mind experiences a state of joyful and calm stillness. This mental stillness allows the mind the freedom to consciously discriminate between the *preya* and the *shreya* and to know deeper states of consciousness through meditation.

Diaphragmatic Breathing

In properly regulating the breath, always remember *ahimsa*—

non-injury, non-harming. Never extend the breath beyond your comfortable capacity by inhaling or exhaling as much air as possible. With continued practice, your capacity will increase, but this should not be rushed. Rather, learn to turn your conscious attention toward establishing a gentle, full and even diaphragmatic breath.

Most of the time we are totally unconscious of the breathing process. Therefore, begin all your breath awareness exercises by observing the quality and rhythm of the breath before you attempt to alter it. As you breathe, investigate where in the body the breath seems to be moving, and then consciously visualize the desired movement and path of the breath. The goal of the science of breath is to re-establish the body's natural respiratory pattern—not by breathing from the upper chest, which is an unhealthy habit, but rather, by consciously employing the diaphragm, one of the body's strongest muscles, in your breathing process.

The Complete Yogic Breath

A full and smooth diaphragmatic breath is composed of three distinct, yet seamlessly integrated phases of inhalation: abdominal, thoracic and clavicular.

A newborn baby naturally uses the abdomen to breathe diaphragmatically. To feel the first phase of proper diaphragmatic breathing, imagine a balloon positioned just behind your navel. When you inhale, the balloon inflates and your belly gently swells outward. When you exhale, the imaginary balloon deflates and the belly contracts gently.

Physiologically, the diaphragm, in its resting state, resembles the dome of an open parachute. The abdominal phase of proper inhalation begins when the diaphragm contracts downward flattening into a disk, thereby expanding the thoracic cavity and causing the belly to protrude slightly. Exhalation then follows more or less automatically when the diaphragm relaxes and returns to its resting dome shape, compressing the lungs. Controlling the rate and duration of the exhalation becomes an important practice in *pranayama,* as is discussed in the instructions for *two-to-one breathing.*

A complete yogic breath, however, is more than the mere use of the abdomen and diaphragm. As the inhalation continues in its second (thoracic) phase, the belly expands outward and the lower ribs expand upward and forward, enlarging the thoracic cavity and increasing the circumference of the chest. The lungs fill this increased space, permitting oxygenation of blood in the lower lungs. In the final phase of the inhalation the clavicles (collar bones) rise slightly, allowing oxygen into the upper portions of the lungs.

When all three phases of diaphragmatic breathing are integrated into one continuous motion, the breath becomes the flywheel for a healthy mind and body. A full, smooth, quiet diaphragmatic breath should become your default breath.

In this ideal breath, all inhalations and exhalations flow through the nostrils rather than the mouth, and the entire process is without noise. If you are breathing rapidly and shallowly, or holding your breath between exhalation and inhalation, you are probably chest breathing. The inhalation and exhalation should gently yield to each other.

The fast pace and stress of modern life (and the constriction of tight pants, belts and pantyhose), have contributed to the unfortunate fact that most people experience nearly constant tension in the abdominal muscles. In addition, concerns about having a fashionably flat, hard abdomen keep many Americans pulling in their gut, military style. By not allowing the breath to be full and complete, you're utilizing only a fraction of your lung capacity.

Chest breathing is a dangerous habit. It tenses the body, disrupts the normal breathing rhythm, is said to be damaging to the heart and brain and does not allow for a complete exchange of gases through the lungs. Chest breathers never fully empty their lungs. Toxins that remain in the trough of the lungs are reassimilated through the semipermeable membrane of the lungs' lining, taxing the body and compromising the immune system.

Dangerous Breathing Patterns

Because the breath reflects our state of mind, a frenetic lifestyle is often accompanied by uneven breathing. Recent studies have found that a pause in the stream of breath, or holding the breath between inhalation and exhalation, is often associated with both coronary heart disease and dementia in the elderly.

Remember, consciousness (*Sat-Chit-Ananda*) is the background of all reality—into which all gross and subtle objects appear. This consciousness exists, in specialized ways, on every successive level of our being.

Imagine for a moment that you are your conscious heart and it's your responsibility to pump blood throughout the body. As the body breathes diaphragmatically, the heart muscle performs its duties with calm efficiency.

Now observe, from the perspective of the heart, what occurs when a human being reacts to thoughts that evoke fear or anger. Muscles immediately contract and the shoulders hunch forward, compressing the chest in a posture reflecting the dis-ease in the mind. Under stress, the body abandons its natural, diaphragmatic breath in favor of the shallow, uneven and often rapid inhalations of chest breathing, and the subsequent shortage of oxygen in the blood quickly becomes problematic.

The heart reacts immediately to this crisis. "Something's wrong," the heart concludes. "We're not getting enough oxygen. I'd better change the normal rhythm of my beat. Perhaps a faster beat will help move more blood through the lungs to access oxygen and bring this fellow back to a more composed state." But, of course, the elevated heart rate only makes matters worse, increasing stress on the heart muscle and vascular system and decreasing their efficiency while sparking further anxiety. Chest breathing accompanied by jerks and pauses in the breath may also be the beginning of a form of significant dis-ease—coronary heart disease.

You will note that we do not offer *pranayama* practices that involve breath retention (*kumbhaka*). We've observed with

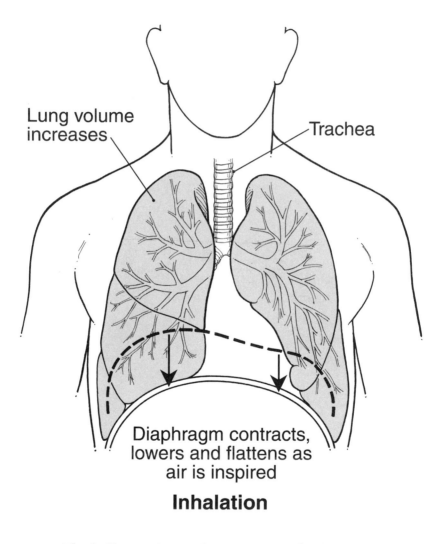

Lung volume increases

Trachea

Diaphragm contracts, lowers and flattens as air is inspired

Inhalation

The belly gently swells outward as the lungs fill.

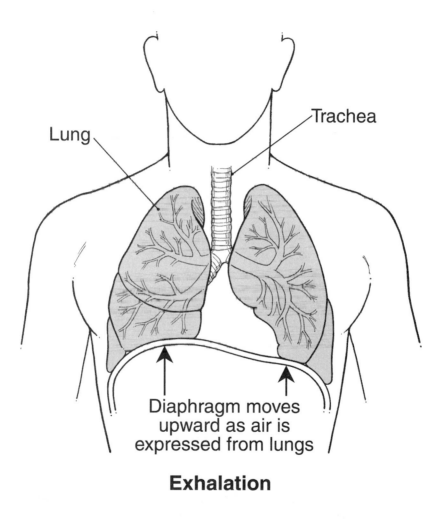

Exhalation

The belly contracts slightly inward as the lungs are emptied.

concern that most Western students are already suffering from the breath irregularities discussed here—especially the damaging habit of involuntary breath retention. Full recovery from this unhealthy condition is advisable before considering deliberate retention of the breath. Although others may offer such instruction in books, tapes and workshops, we strongly suggest that you first establish a smooth, continuous and healthy breath. Then, when you are prepared for *kumbhaka*, work only with a competent teacher who can gauge your individual capabilities.

Eliminating the pause between inhalation and exhalation, and between exhalation and inhalation is an important aspect of *sadhana* because it helps you keep a balanced mind and healthy body. The breath should become one continuous, unending stream in which the inhalation gently yields to the exhalation and the exhalation gently yields to the inhalation. It's like swimming laps in a pool. When the swimmer approaches the far end of the pool, he turns and kicks off with one fluid motion in preparation for the return lap. There is never a true pause.

Full and even diaphragmatic breathing constantly massages the internal organs. This rhythmic motion transmits beneficial messages to the entire autonomic nervous system, encouraging all systems within the body to operate optimally. A smooth diaphragmatic breath, not beyond your comfortable capacity, acts as a calming lullaby for the internal organs, while chest breathing invariably sends signals that some sort of crisis is at hand. Chest breathing is not only the result of anxiety, but can also be its cause.

Diaphragmatic breathing aids digestion, assimilation of essential nutrients and the elimination of waste products from the body. Whenever possible, cultivate the habit of loosening your belt and the waistband button of your pants at mealtimes to encourage deep, full breathing. By consciously incorporating the eating and breathing processes into your *sadhana*, you will enjoy your food more completely and the body will readily demonstrate its appreciation by exhibiting good health.

**Special Note for
Runners and Aerobic Exercisers**

Students often ask whether they should attempt to breathe diaphragmatically while running or engaging in other vigorous exercise. The answer must be practical. When you're exerting yourself by running or exercising, don't give any consideration to your diaphragmatic breath. Just allow the body to do whatever the body needs to do. However, once you complete your run or workout, and your breath returns to normal, consciously re-establish your diaphragmatic breath.

Are You Dancing?

In order to establish proper breathing, the head, neck and trunk must be correctly aligned. Therefore, be conscious of your posture—regardless of whether you are standing, walking, seated at a desk, in an easy chair or at the kitchen table.

Remember, "I have a body, but I am not the body." Because the body houses Eternity, every action is a sacrament. When you don't sit, stand and walk with your head, neck and trunk straight, you're not acting in harmony with *ahimsa*. Correct posture encourages the complete exchange of gases through the lungs, prepares the body to receive vital *prana* and allows the internal organs to rest unencumbered with an ease that permits them to carry out their normal functions efficiently.

Since the breath and mind are inextricably linked, proper diaphragmatic breathing and posture have the power to calm the mind. Only when the mind is calm can we hear and follow the encouragement of the *buddhi* to transform life into poetry and song.

Gently ask yourself this simple question, "Am I dancing?" Nearly everyone likes to dance or enjoys watching others dance. The question, "Are you dancing?" is a loving way of reminding yourself, or others, that the body is a shrine.

Why carry the body as if you have the weight of the world on your shoulders? Such posture is kind neither to yourself nor to others. It is not in harmony with *ahimsa*. Remember that *ahimsa*, non-injury, non-harming, begins with a loving relationship with your own body, breath, senses and mind. By learning to honor your true Self, you become an instrument that brings light to the world.

Body language is a reflection of the thoughts we entertain. If we give our attention to *preya*, contracting emotions will eventually be reflected in our posture, but a gentle reminder that Eternity dwells within is all we need to straighten up.

For example, like many seniors, my mother, who is now ninety years young, has mild osteoporosis. When we take her out for dinner and walk from the car to the restaurant, her body is often stooped. But invariably, when we ask her the question, "Are you dancing?" she smiles, and despite her medical problem, immediately stands up straighter. This is not to deny that for some people osteoporosis is a painful reality, but it does illustrate that poor posture—even in seniors—is often a reflection of the mind.

When you feel burdened by the weight of the world, simply ask yourself this question: "Are you dancing?" It's a thoroughly loving and non-intimidating question, in harmony with *ahimsa* and virtually guaranteed to bring a smile to your face.

Much lower back pain is caused by poor posture. If we trained ourselves to be mindful of proper posture throughout all daily activities, we would experience much less pain. I speak from personal experience. I suffered from debilitating lower back pain for many years. I visited general practitioners, neurologists, chiropractors and physical therapists, but none had an adequate remedy. Finally, through the practice of meditation, *pranayama* and *Easy-Gentle Yoga*, I began choosing new and different thoughts and activities—including a daily commitment to the stretching exercises described in Chapter 37. As habits of my mind changed, I became more flexible mentally and physically as a result. Within only a few weeks, I changed my body into a pain-free instrument of service, and you can do the same.

Crocodile Posture

The first breathing practice we recommend is the *crocodile posture*. Regardless of how long you've been a chest breather, you will automatically breathe diaphragmatically while you lie in the *crocodile posture*.

As with any breathing practice, always wear loose-fitting clothing—especially around the waist. Wear pants with a drawstring or a very soft elastic waist. If you normally wear eyeglasses, take them off and put them in a safe place during your breathing exercises. Without your glasses, and with your eyes closed, your concentration will deepen.

To practice the *crocodile posture*, lie face down on your stomach on the floor, positioning your feet a little wider than shoulder width apart. Your toes may turn either in or out, depending on your personal comfort. Crossing your arms in front of your body, clasp the right hand around the left bicep, just above the left elbow. Then clasp the left hand around the right bicep, just above the right elbow. Rest your forehead on your forearm, just above the wrist.

Don't position your arms too far out in front of you, which would bring the chest flush with the floor. Neither should you position the arms too close to the chest, which would put undue stress on the lower back and neck muscles. The ideal is to create a slight curve in the lower back, but without any strain.

Once you have established the *crocodile posture*, begin to focus your awareness on your breath at the navel region.

Your breath should be full, but not beyond your comfortable capacity. Remember *ahimsa* is the highest precept of all yoga science. Do not attempt to extend the breath beyond your present ability. With regular practice, your body's respiratory capacity will increase on its own.

If you have correctly established the *crocodile posture*, you will automatically breathe diaphragmatically. As you inhale, you will notice the belly swelling gently—pressing against the floor. As you exhale, you will notice the belly contracting slightly. When you inhale, the back will rise gently, and when

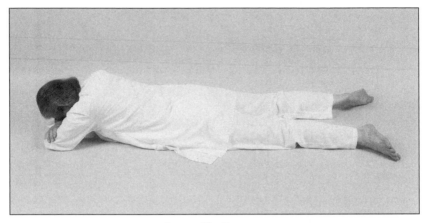

Crocodile Posture

you exhale, it gently falls. Both of these effects are produced by correct movement of the diaphragm. Keep your attention on your breath at the navel.

During all breath awareness exercises, only use the breath's natural *mantra*, *So-Hum*. With each inhalation, listen to the *SOOOO*, and with each exhalation, listen to the *HUMMMM*. Do not use your meditation and *japa mantra* in conjunction with any breath exercise. The vibrations of the personal *mantra* can produce subtle jerks and pauses in the breath.

The *crocodile posture* is not a preliminary practice for your meditation. Instead, perform diaphragmatic breathing in the *crocodile posture* four or five minutes every day at a time when other duties and responsibilities are not making demands on you. In addition to its benefits as a breathing exercise, this posture helps develop mental concentration. Avoid this posture when you are very tired so that you won't be tempted to drift off to sleep.

On Rising from the Floor

Before rising from any floor exercise, gently turn onto your right side and rest for a few seconds. Then, push off with your left hand and sit up for a moment before rising to a standing or seated position.

Guidelines for Diaphragmatic Breathing

Whether sitting at your desk, in your automobile, standing with friends at a party or lying on the couch watching television, diaphragmatic breathing enables you to feel your best, maintain emotional balance and reduce fatigue and stress. The following tips will help to evaluate your own breathing habits.

In relaxed, diaphragmatic breathing:
1. The breath flows smoothly—without any jerks.
2. There is no pause between inhalation and exhalation.
3. The breath flows silently.
4. Exhalation and inhalation are approximately equal.
5. The breath is full, with little movement of the upper chest.
6. All breathing is done through the nostrils, not the mouth.
7. As you inhale, the belly gently swells outward.
8. As you exhale, the belly gently contracts inward.
9. Never exceed your comfortable capacity.

Corpse Posture
With or Without a Breath Pillow[1]

Practice the *corpse posture* every day for five minutes with a weighted breath pillow and then five minutes without the breath pillow.

Conscious, diaphragmatic breathing while lying in the *corpse posture* (*shavasana*) is a very powerful exercise. When practiced with a weighted breath pillow, it reacquaints you with the natural movement of your diaphragm while it strengthens the diaphragm muscle itself.

Practiced with or without the breath pillow, the *corpse posture* helps establish diaphragmatic breathing, slows the heart rate, lowers blood pressure and, if done regularly, improves one-pointed attention and memory. In this position

[1]Breath pillows can be ordered directly from the American Meditation Institute Bookstore, 60 Garner Road, Averill Park, New York 12018. Tel. (800) 234-5115. Website: www.americanmeditation.org.

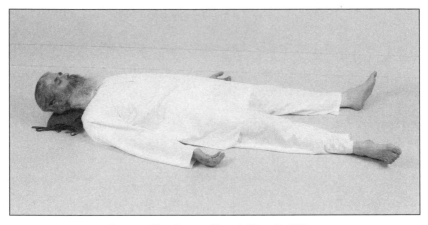

Corpse Posture without Breath Pillow

there should be no visible movement in any part of the body except for the slight rise and fall of the belly and chest with each breath.

Just as in your seated meditation practice, if a thought comes into your awareness, don't be upset with yourself or try to push the thought away. As the Eternal Witness, merely welcome and honor the thought and offer it back to the Origin from which it has come. Then redirect your attention to your diaphragm and breath. As with all breath exercises, use the *So-Hum mantra*. With each complete inhalation, listen to the *SOOOO* and with each complete exhalation, listen to the *HUMMMM*.

Begin by lying on your back on a firm surface. Depending on your personal comfort, place your feet a little wider than shoulder width apart. Position a small pillow or folded towel under your neck for support. Roll your head from side to side and adjust your back, shoulders and hips slightly until you've found a comfortable position with the head, neck and spine in a straight line. If the room is cool, cover yourself with a light blanket.

Place one hand directly on the navel region, and place the other hand on the upper chest. Pay attention to your breath and notice which hand is rising and falling with each

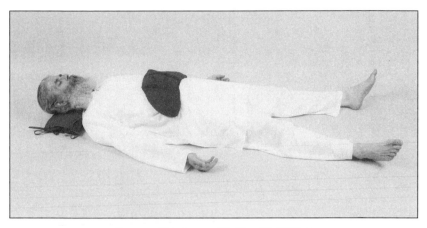

Corpse Posture with Breath Pillow

inhalation and exhalation. If the hand over your chest is moving more, you are chest-breathing. If the hand over the navel is rising and falling with each breath, you are definitely breathing diaphragmatically.

Now, place your arms on the floor, resting the hands eight to twelve inches away from the body, so the arms do not touch the torso. The palms face upward with the fingers slightly curled and relaxed. If you feel more comfortable with the palms facing downward, use that as an optional position. Your eyes and mouth should be gently closed.

Bring your attention to your breath. As mentioned in the previous section on diaphragmatic breathing, imagine a small balloon behind your navel. As you inhale, the balloon inflates gently, swelling the belly outward. As you exhale, the balloon contracts gently, flattening the belly. Your breath should be full, even and continuous. It becomes one unending stream. Concentrate on keeping the movement nice and smooth.

To derive benefit from this practice, it is essential that you do not exert beyond your comfortable breathing capacity. The regulation of your breath should be easy, kind and in harmony with *ahimsa*. Continue this exercise for five minutes.

After completing this first portion of the exercise, place a ten pound breath pillow directly on your diaphragm, just below the rib cage. Although the weight of the breath pillow may feel heavy in your hands, it will feel quite comforting when properly positioned. The weight will prove to be no real challenge since your diaphragm is one of the strongest muscles in the body. Practice this exercise with the breath pillow for five minutes every day.

At first, your breath may be irregular or jerky, but it will even out as you give your undivided attention to each inhalation and each exhalation. Remember, you're not trying to extend the inhalation and exhalation. The durations of your inhalation and exhalation should be approximately equal and the breath should be silent and deep. Never exceed your comfortable capacity. Minimize movement in the upper chest. All breathing should be done through the nostrils. The nose is uniquely constructed to warm, moisten and clean the air you breathe. The belly swells outward as you inhale and contracts gently as you exhale.

On Rising from the Floor

When you have completed this five-minute exercise with the breath pillow, carefully remove the weight from the diaphragm. Before rising from the floor, gently turn over onto your right side and rest for a few seconds. Rise to a seated position by pushing off with your left hand and rest again before standing.

CHAPTER 29

Alternate Nostril Breathing

And the Eternal God formed the man from the dust of the ground, and breathed into his nostrils the breath of life; and the man became a living soul.

GENESIS

The practice of alternate nostril breathing (*nadi shodhana*) is a powerful and practical tool for consciously working with *prana*. Before learning the mechanics, however, it's important that you understand the effects of alternate nostril breathing on both the physical body known as *annamaya kosha* and the energy body referred to as *pranamaya kosha*.

Structures within the physical body have counterparts in the energy sheath—a subtler, non-physical body composed of the rivers of *prana* known as *nadis*. In the practice of *nadi shodhana*, we will concern ourselves with three major *nadis*: *ida*, *pingala* and *sushumna*. The *ida nadi* controls all mental processes, the *pingala nadi* controls the body's vital (pranic) processes and the *sushumna nadi* awakens spiritual consciousness.

In the human body, the spinal column runs from the tailbone to the crown of the head. In the *pranamaya kosha* (the subtle energy body), the *sushumna nadi* (the central canal that is analogous to the spinal column) rises from the base of the spine to the crown of the head. The *sushumna* is part of a network of *nadis,* subtle rivers of energy (*prana*) that create and sustain the physical body.

The *ida, pingala* and *sushumna nadis* originate together at the *root chakra* (*muladhara*). From that shared point of origin the *ida* and *pingala* ascend toward the crown of the head in an undulating pattern along the vertical *sushumna.* Where the *ida* and *pingala* converge, swirling wheels of energy called *chakras* appear.[1]

From the *root chakra, sushumna* rises directly upward, while the *ida* flows to its left and *pingala* flows to its right. At each *chakra,* the three major *nadis* come together, as *sushumna* continues its upward flow toward the crown.[2] The *ida* and *pingala* continue their serpentine course until all three— *sushumna, ida* and *pingala*—merge at *ajna chakra,* the site of the pineal gland at the space between the two eyebrows. The *ida* accesses *ajna chakra* through the left nostril and the *pingala* through the right nostril.

The *pingala* flows with male energy. It is active, stimulates the left hemisphere of the brain, exemplifies the heat of solar power and is represented by the sun. The *ida* is a river of female energy. It is passive and intuitive, stimulates the right hemisphere of the brain, exemplifies the coolness of lunar power and is represented by the moon.

As the practice of *alternate nostril breathing* balances *ida* and *pingala,* their undulating paths straighten slightly, facilitating an opening of the *sushumna* channel.

The *Chakra* System

The *chakras* exist as subtle, non-physical patterns of energy (in the *pranamaya kosha)* that precede the formation of the body

[1]The modern emblem of the medical profession, the caduceus, is based on ancient illustrations of the *chakra* system and *nadis.*

[2]According to ancient yogic scriptures, the *sushumna* runs from the base of the spine (*muladhara chakra*) to the space between the two eyebrows (*ajna chakra*). From *ajna chakra,* the central canal flows to the crown of the head through *Brahma randra,* the channel named for *Brahma,* the creator.

and facilitate its creation. In the physical realm (*annamaya kosha*), muscles, nerves and glands form at these psycho-energetic centers. Consciousness, energy and structure function together at these points.

The organization of the seven major *chakras* corresponds roughly to the blueprint of the endocrine system. Because *chakras* serve as junction points for energy and consciousness, the vitality and balance of each *chakra* are reflected in a human being's physical, mental, emotional and spiritual well-being or dysfunction. The *chakra* system is an holistic entity; every part affects every other part.

Seven Major *Chakras*

Crown Chakra (Sahasrara)
Crown of the head; unification with the Divine

Eyebrow Chakra - Third Eye (Ajna)
Space between the two eyebrows; intuition

Throat Chakra (Vishuddha)
Throat; ether (space) element; communication and expression

Heart Chakra (Anahata)
Center of the chest; air element; unconditional love

Navel Chakra (Manipura)
The navel and solar plexus; fire element; metabolism; action

Genital Chakra (Svadhishthana)
Lower abdomen at the top of the pubic bone;
water element; procreation; fluidity

Root Chakra (Muladhara)
Base of the spine (coccyx);
earth element; self-preservation; fear

Shiva and *Shakti*: Male and Female Principles

The universe comes into being from the subtle to the gross, when the indivisible Absolute (*Sat-Chit-Ananda*) manifests as two interdependent aspects known as *Shiva* and *Shakti*. This is the first movement of "creation."

The apparently divided, yet inexorably united principles of *Shiva* and *Shakti* pervade all of creation. In the human body the apparent dichotomy manifests subtly at opposite ends of the spinal column. The male principle of transcendent consciousness known as *Shiva* is situated at the highest crown *chakra* (*sahasrara*), while the feminine force authoring all creation (*Shakti*) tends to lie dormant at the root *chakra* (*muladhara*).

Ancient yogic literature suggests that the second *chakra* (*svadhishthana*) is the true home of *Shakti*. From the second *chakra*, *Shakti* could more easily make her way through the higher *chakras* to provide the creative consciousness and energy for enlightened activity. But because of the stupefying downward force of sense attraction and pleasure, *Shakti* remains trapped within a triangular vessel (*kunda*) at the *root chakra*. Thus, the *Shakti* force, known as *kundalini*, can become a captive of her own creation—sometimes finding it difficult to do more than sustain the basic human functions. Consequently, the human being remains enslaved to the delusion of separateness and its progeny: fear, anger and greed, as well as the painful karmic consequences of actions dictated by such consciousness.

However, there is but One Absolute Reality. Because *Shiva* and *Shakti* remain essentially One—even in their separation—it is their proclivity and destiny to unite. When Divine grace offers the perennial sacred knowledge to an individual, the spiritual seeker (*sadhaka*) begins to undertake various practices that require a sacrifice of the downward gravitational force of *preya*. Through sacrificial human effort, the dormant creative energy of *Shakti* slowly rises to her true abode at *svadhishthana*. Once appropriately situated, the *Shakti* force of inspiration, creativity and energy is free to flow through any *chakra*, unencumbered, to lead the human being for his or her highest and greatest good.

Anatomical View of the
Chakras, Ida, Pingala and *Sushumna Nadis*

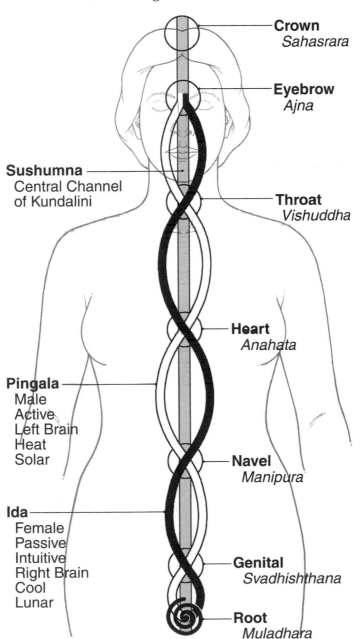

Crown
Sahasrara

Eyebrow
Ajna

Sushumna
Central Channel
of Kundalini

Throat
Vishuddha

Heart
Anahata

Pingala
Male
Active
Left Brain
Heat
Solar

Navel
Manipura

Ida
Female
Passive
Intuitive
Right Brain
Cool
Lunar

Genital
Svadhishthana

Root
Muladhara

Wedding of the Sun and Moon
The Rise of Creative Energy (*Kundalini*)

If you pay attention to your breath at various times throughout the day you will find that you're usually inhaling a greater volume of air through one nostril than the other. This is normal. One nostril becomes active (while the other remains passive) for about two and one-half hours, and then they switch. For example, if the right nostril has been active for that period, it then becomes passive, and the left nostril, which was passive, becomes active.

In preparation for your meditation practice, *nadi shodhana* balances the breath so that the same volume of air is carried by each nostril simultaneously. Through the practice of *nadi shodhana*, the *pingala* (right nostril: male, active, left brain, solar energy) and the *ida* (left nostril: female, intuitive, right brain, lunar energy) become equally active at the same time. This phenomenon is referred to as the *wedding of the sun and moon*.

Through the practice of *nadi shodhana*, the *ida* and *pingala* become balanced and their undulating pathways become straighter. This facilitates the widening of *sushumna* (known as *sushumna application*) and allows *kundalini* (creative energy) to rise to the higher *chakras*. Following *nadi shodhana*, you will meditate at the sixth *chakra—ajna chakra*.

For most human beings the creative energy of *kundalini* resides primarily in the lowest *chakra—muladhara*. This *chakra* manifests the consciousness of duality, or separateness. Consciousness at this *chakra* is concerned with self-preservation and reflects the belief that "I am a separate entity in search of whatever will make me happy or eliminate my pain." When too much of our consciousness resides here, an individual exhibits fear, self-centeredness, insecurity, greed, anger and even violence.

The general practice of yoga science and the specific practice of *nadi shodhana* facilitate the rise of creative energy to the higher *chakras*. As *kundalini* activates the consciousness of higher *chakras*, we expand our sense of *I-ness* by understanding and manifesting such universal ideals as unconditional love, selfless service, forgiveness, compassion, intuition, insight and Self-realization.

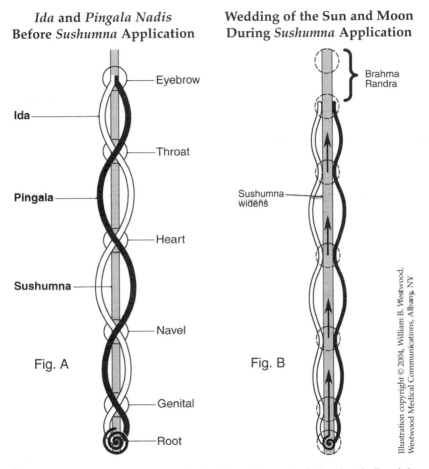

Ida and Pingala Nadis Before Sushumna Application

Eyebrow
Ida
Throat
Pingala
Heart
Sushumna
Navel
Fig. A
Genital
Root

Wedding of the Sun and Moon During Sushumna Application

Brahma Randra
Sushumna widens
Fig. B

Illustration copyright © 2004, William B. Westwood, Westwood Medical Communications, Albany, NY

Fig. A. The *ida* and *pingala nadis* rise from the root *chakra* (*muladhara*) in serpentine pathways. At their points of confluence, swirling wheels of energy appear.

Fig. B. After three complete cycles of *nadi shodhana* (alternate nostril breathing), both the right and left nostrils carry an equal volume of air. This is referred to as *sushumna* application, or the "wedding of the sun and the moon." When the *nadis* are cleared and the male and female, the active and passive aspects of the human being are in balance, the *ida* and *pingala* straighten their pathways slightly and *sushumna* swells—allowing *kundalini* (consciousness) to rise to the higher *chakras*.

Mechanics of
Alternate Nostril Breathing (*Nadi Shodhana*)

First, relax in your comfortable meditation posture and observe your breath. Allow your breath to become deep, even and diaphragmatic.

Before beginning the practice of *nadi shodhana*, determine whether you will inhale first through the right or left nostril.

If the sun is rising or in the sky, or if you must be mentally or physically active in the evening, inhale first through the right nostril. By breathing through the right nostril first, you flood the entire body with the energy of the sun (*pingala*).

Generally, if you're doing this practice prior to your evening meditation after sunset, or in preparation for sleep, inhale through the left nostril first (*ida*) to access the cool, calming energy of the moon.

Regardless of which nostril you inhale through first, close off that nostril and exhale fully through the opposite nostril before your first inhalation. This empties the lungs of toxins and, in the subtle body, clears the energy channels or *nadis*. The inhalation and exhalation together should form a full and complete yogic breath.

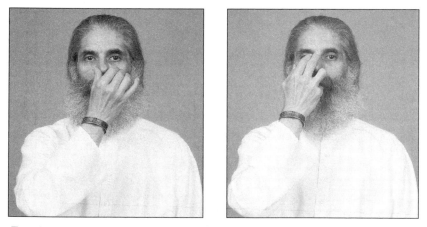

For the practice of *nadi shodhana* (alternate nostril breathing), apply a modest amount of gentle pressure with the thumb and fourth finger to open and close the appropriate nostril.

To close and open your nostrils, use your thumb and fourth finger (ring finger) and exert very little pressure. If you are right-handed, use your right hand. If you are left-handed, use your left. Practice the motion by placing your hand in front of your face with fingers pointed upward and fluidly turning the wrist first in one direction and then the other.

Using the *So-Hum Mantra*

If you are inhaling through the right nostril, visualize the breath rising along the right side of the spine (*pingala*) from the base of the spine to the crown of the head. If you are inhaling through the left nostril, visualize the breath rising along the left side of the spine (*ida*) from the base of the spine to the crown of the head.

If you are exhaling through the right nostril, visualize the breath descending along the right side of the spine (*pingala*) from the crown of the head to the base of the spine. If you are exhaling through the left nostril, visualize the breath descending along the left side of the spine (*ida*) from the crown of the head to the base of the spine.

For example, as you inhale through the right nostril, visualize the breath rising from the tailbone along the right side of the spine to the crown of the head.

As you exhale through the left nostril, visualize the breath descending along the left side of the spine from the crown of the head to the tailbone. With each inhalation, follow the breath and silently listen to the *mantra SOOOO*. As you exhale, follow the breath and silently listen to the *mantra HUMMMM*.

Methodically continue giving your attention to each inhalation and exhalation while listening to the *So-Hum mantra*. As previously stated, *So-Hum* means "I am That." The word "That" refers to *Sat-Chit-Ananda*, the Divine Reality within.

As you visualize your inhalations and exhalations while listening to the *So-Hum mantra*, the vital *pranas* carried on each breath are directed through either the *ida* or *pingala nadi*. Just as the pattern of the invisible force field around a magnet is made visible by iron filings on paper placed over the magnet, so this visualization makes us aware of the movement of *prana* through the subtle body. But the objective is not only to perceive, but to direct this energy by our attention. The resultant organizing effect resembles the synchronizing of light energy in laser technology.

As you practice *alternate nostril breathing*, your exhalation with the *mantra Hum* will excite the fire of creative energy at *muladhara chakra*. This flame consumes and transforms your *samskaras*, and prevents the dust of ignorance from covering and cooling the embers.

The "fire" ablaze at *muladhara chakra* has two transformative qualities: heat and light. When you inhale, listening to the *mantra SO*, the heat (of determination) and the light (of wisdom) from the "fire" of an awakening *kundalini* are allowed to rise through the central *sushumna* channel, activating the spiritually liberating and creative consciousness of the higher *chakras*. Through this process, the personality is gradually purified as your mind, action and speech increasingly reflect the unerring wisdom and limitless power of the Divine.

With each breath, the visualization and *mantra* vibration aspects of *nadi shodhana* are coordinated and vital *pranas* flood the *nadis*, which, in turn flow into the *chakras*. This transfusion of subtle energy into the *chakras* awakens and balances the consciousness within these centers and, on the physical level, purifies and revitalizes the muscles, nerves, glands and internal organs within the domains of the individual *chakras*.

Procedure for
Alternate Nostril Breathing (*Nadi Shodhana*)

To practice one entire cycle of *nadi shodhana*, complete three inhalations through one nostril and then three inhalations through the opposite nostril. The total practice consists of three cycles (rounds)—a total of nine inhalations through each nostril.

To prepare for this practice, sit in your chosen meditation posture. Initially, inhalation and exhalation should be of equal duration (see *Two to One Breathing*, at the end of this chapter). Do not force the breath. Keep it slow, controlled, continuous and free from jerks, pauses or sounds.

During this practice, you should never exceed your comfortable capacity. With each inhalation, visualize the breath (along either the right or left side of the spine) from the base of the spine to the crown of the head, and mentally hear the *mantra SOOOO*. With each exhalation, visualize the breath (along the opposite side of the spine) from the crown of the head to the base of the spine and silently listen to the *mantra HUMMMM*. As you inhale allow the belly to swell gently, and as you exhale allow the belly to contract gently.

Bring the right hand to the nose and gently fold the second and third fingers in toward the palm so that the right thumb can be used to close the right nostril and the fourth (ring) finger can be used to close the left nostril.

Morning and Afternoon *Nadi Shodhana*
When the sun is active or you need extra energy
REPEAT STEPS 1 - 5 THREE COMPLETE TIMES

1. In the morning and afternoon, close the right nostril. Exhale completely through the left nostril, visualizing the path of the breath, and silently listen to the *mantra HUM*. At the end of each exhalation, close the left nostril and inhale through the right nostril slowly and completely—visualizing the path of the breath and mentally listening to the *mantra SO*. Inhalation and exhalation should be of equal duration.

2. Repeat this cycle of exhalation and inhalation two more times.

3. At the end the the third inhalation with the right nostril, exhale completely through the same (right) nostril, keeping the left nostril closed with the fourth (ring) finger.

4. At the end of the exhalation of the right nostril, close the right nostril and inhale through the left nostril.

5. Repeat the cycle of exhalation through the right nostril and inhalation through the left nostril twice.

Morning and Afternoon Nadi Shodhana

Exhale Left (*Hum*)—— Inhale Right (*So*)
Exhale Left (*Hum*)—— Inhale Right (*So*)
Exhale Left (*Hum*)—— Inhale Right (*So*)
Exhale Right (*Hum*)
Inhale Left (*So*)—— Exhale Right (*Hum*)
Inhale Left (*So*)—— Exhale Right (*Hum*)
Inhale Left (*So*)
Continue two more cycles, as above.

Evening *Nadi Shodhana*
**At night, or when you need the calm,
centered, intuitive energy of the moon**

1. In the evening, close the left nostril. Exhale completely through the right nostril to begin the cycle, listening to the *mantra* HUM. Then, as you inhale through the left nostril, continue visualizing the path of the breath and silently listening to the *So-Hum mantra* as the instructions indicate.

Before Sleep Nadi Shodhana

Exhale Right (*Hum*)
To begin the practice, exhale completely on right, then:

Inhale Left (*So*)—— Exhale Right (*Hum*)
Inhale Left (*So*)—— Exhale Right (*Hum*)
Inhale Left (*So*)

Exhale Left (*Hum*)—— Inhale Right (*So*)
Exhale Left (*Hum*)—— Inhale Right (*So*)
Exhale Left (*Hum*)—— Inhale Right (*So*)
Exhale Right (*Hum*)
Continue two more cycles, as above—beginning with Inhale Left (So).

Practical Benefits of *Nadi Shodhana*

Nadi shodhana is a very powerful practice. Complete it before morning and evening meditation and again at noontime if your schedule permits. During times of great emotional stress, it's recommended that *nadi shodhana* be practiced five times a day. The practice is both centering and extremely energizing—a more effective pick-me-up than two cups of black coffee. It cultivates one-pointed attention, enhances memory, calms your nerves and oxygenates the blood. The entire practice takes only a few minutes and is free of the harmful side effects of sugar and caffeine.

Two-to-One Breathing

After you have practiced *nadi shodhana* for at least six months, gradually lengthen the duration of your exhalation until you can exhale twice the length of the inhalation. This *two-to-one breathing* will enhance physical well-being by oxygenating the blood as it fortifies physical, mental and emotional strength.

When practicing *two-to-one breathing*, do not mentally count. Counting creates subtle jerks in the breath and sends unhealthy messages to your heart and autonomic nervous system.

To lengthen your exhalation without counting, mentally follow your controlled exhalation from the crown of the head through the entire body to the toes. Then begin your inhalation, at the same rate, from the base of the spine and proceed upward through the body to the crown of the head. Continue listening to the SO-HUM *mantra* and allow the belly to swell gently as you inhale and contract gently as you exhale.

Part VIII

POWER OF THE MIND

CHAPTER 30

Four Major Functions of the Mind

One must first discipline and control one's own mind. If a man can control his own mind he will find the way to enlightenment, and all wisdom and virtue will naturally come to him.

THE COMPASSIONATE BUDDHA

The Anatomy of Your Real Being

Yoga science defines the human being as three separate selves: the *mortal self*, the *semi-immortal self* and the *immortal Self*.

Emanating from the eternal ocean of consciousness, wisdom and bliss (*Sat-Chit-Ananda*), a bubble—having exactly the same intrinsic qualities as the ocean—rises from the deep. This is the *immortal Self*, or soul.

The soul issues forth an energy called *adi prana* (literally, the first unit of life) that is essential to the creation and maintenance of the mind and physical body.[1]

The mind in its totality, consisting of both the conscious

---

[1] *Adi prana* is analogous to the Christian concept of a "silver cord" that facilitates human life. Researchers into near-death experiences document accounts of people leaving the physical body and observing a "silver cord" connecting the physical body to their soul. Biblical reference to a silver cord is found in Ecclesiastes: "Remember Him, before the silver cord is severed . . . and the dust returns to the ground it came from, and the spirit returns to God who gave it."

and unconscious portions, evolves from the *adi prana*. The mind then projects the body, breath and senses as a vehicle for action. The breath is the bridge between mind and body, and facilitates the ongoing infusion of new *prana* required to maintain the city of life.

According to yoga science, death is not annihilation. It is merely the separation of the *mortal self* from the *semi-immortal self* and the *immortal Self*. At death, the body, breath, senses and conscious mind separate from the unconscious mind (*chitta*) and soul (*Sat-Chit-Ananda*).

Following physical death, as in sleep, the unconscious mind and individual soul remain linked in a resting state. Eventually, as latent impressions in the *chitta* begin to activate, a vehicle, or body, becomes necessary to resolve and fulfill remaining *karmas* stored in the unconscious mind, and the process begins again with a new birth.

In Eastern traditions, to be human is considered the greatest of gifts. Right now you have a body, breath, senses and a mind blessed with the discriminative faculty of *buddhi*. You already have available all the equipment necessary to dissolve your attachments, exhaust your *karmas* and free yourself from pain and bondage. By *sadhana*, the animal nature can evolve—through your humanity—to unite with the Divine.

Acquaintance with the relationship between the *mortal self*, *semi-immortal self* and *immortal Self* helps clarify how decisions are to be made in this lifetime. Every time we take an action, a consequence follows. Each consequence leads us closer to fulfillment or farther away. Once we appreciate the mechanics of the *law of karma* (that thought precedes action and action precedes consequence), the nature of our decision-making emerges as a critical factor in determining our condition in this life. To examine the decision-making process, it is essential that we understand the functioning of the human mind.

The *Yoga Sutras* teach that true yoga begins with "*chitta vritti narodha*," coordination of the modifications of the mind-field. This does not mean suppression of the thought process, but rather, regulation and mastery of the mind.

The Anatomy of Your Real Being

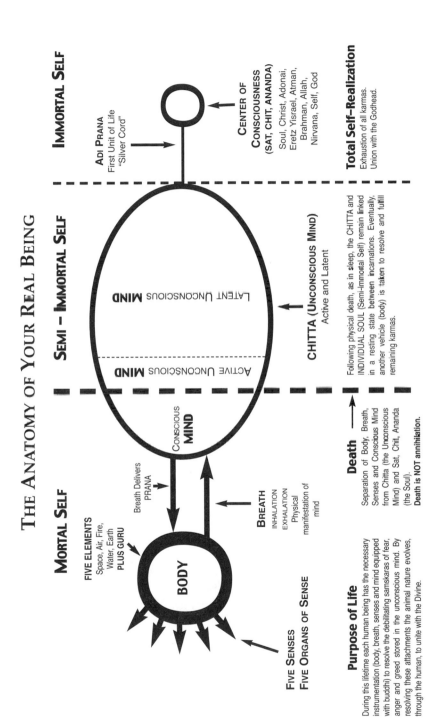

Mortal Self

Semi – Immortal Self

Immortal Self

FIVE ELEMENTS
Space, Air, Fire, Water, Earth
PLUS GURU

FIVE SENSES
FIVE ORGANS OF SENSE

BODY

Breath Delivers PRANA

Conscious **MIND**

BREATH
INHALATION
EXHALATION
Physical manifestation of mind

Active Unconscious **MIND**

Latent Unconscious **MIND**

CHITTA (UNCONSCIOUS MIND)
Active and Latent

ADI PRANA
First Unit of Life
"Silver Cord"

**CENTER OF CONSCIOUSNESS
(SAT, CHIT, ANANDA)**
Soul, Christ, Adonai, Eretz Yisrael, Atman, Brahman, Allah, Nirvana, Self, God

Total Self–Realization
Exhaustion of all karmas.
Union with the Godhead.

Purpose of Life

During this lifetime each human being has the necessary instrumentation (body, breath, senses and mind equipped with buddhi) to resolve the debilitating samskaras of fear, anger and greed stored in the unconscious mind. By resolving these attachments the animal nature evolves, through the human, to unite with the Divine.

Death

Separation of Body, Breath, Senses and Conscious Mind from Chitta (the Unconscious Mind) and Sat, Chit, Ananda (the Soul).
Death is NOT annihilation.

Following physical death, as in sleep, the CHITTA and INDIVIDUAL SOUL (Semi-Immortal Self) remain linked in a resting state between incarnations. Eventually, another vehicle (body) is taken to resolve and fulfill remaining karmas.

The mind is our most powerful instrument. Through it we perceive and consciously participate in this Divine dance of creation. The human mind has the capacity to transform desires into the realities of this world we experience. A disciplined mind, therefore, can be our best friend and strongest ally in that endeavor, and conversely, an undisciplined mind can be our fiercest adversary.

To explore the deepest aspects of our internal being or to deal successfully with the countless objects and relationships of the external world, we must understand the four major faculties of the mind. Understanding the total mind prepares us to establish inner coordination of these faculties. Without inner coordination, serious conflicts eventually arise in the mind, and since all reality flows from the subtle to the gross, conflict within the mind inevitably manifests as conflict and dis-ease in the external world.

Learning to become free of interior conflict, therefore, is one of the major challenges facing the human being. The practice of seated meditation and a practical understanding of the mind help us transform the latent power of thoughts, desires and emotions, and establish a relative calmness in the mind. When the mind becomes still, there is no longer separation between the individual and the Divine Reality. In that still awareness of our Essential Nature, we realize freedom from conflict and pain.

In the daily practice of *meditation in action*, a yoga scientist consciously evaluates the character and merit of thoughts as they appear. Probing questions emerge. What is the purpose of this thought? What will be its consequence? To whom is this thought appearing? Who am I? Who is the thinker of the thought? All these questions cultivate identification with the Inner Witness: *Sat-Chit-Ananda*. Only from this perspective can we evaluate fairly the worthiness of each thought.

Remember, the word responsibility is a compound of two words: response and ability. This teaching helps you train the mind to utilize its capacity to respond creatively, rather than to react habitually. This is the key to freedom.

To begin this study, we draw upon the teachings of the Himalayan masters. The following diagram illustrates a wheel comprised of three basic components: the rim of the wheel, the spokes and the hub. The spokes move, and then the rim of the wheel rolls forward. The hub facilitates the turning of the spokes and the wheel rotates as a result of that movement.

In this analogy, the wheel represents the human body. No movement can occur in the body unless and until there is movement in the four modifications (functions) of the mind. These faculties of the mind are like the spokes of the wheel. The mind always moves first and the body follows.

The hub is the Eternal Witness or soul (*Sat-Chit-Ananda*). This core itself never moves, but it is the cause and the power of the mind, and the mind ultimately animates the body. Without the existence of the hub there could be neither mind nor body.

The four spokes in our analogy represent the four major functions of the mind: *manas* (active mind), *ahamkara* (ego or I-maker), *chitta* (the unconscious, storehouse of impressions or *samskaras*) and *buddhi* (intellect, discrimination).

The Four Functions of the Mind

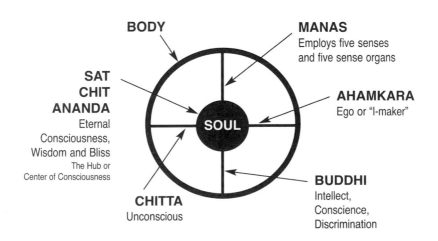

Manas

The word *manas* comes from the Sanskrit root *man*, which means mind. *Manas* operates both internally and externally; it is an importer and exporter of information. In relating to each thought, desire and emotion, we constantly face the decision of whether or not to take an action. Toward that end, the *manas* collects the various bits of pertinent information from the external world and from the various other functions of the mind, organizes the data and presents it to our awareness (*Chit*).

In order to collect information from the external world, the *manas* employs five senses and sense organs: sight (eyes), smell (nose), hearing (ears), taste (mouth) and touch (hands, feet and skin). These employees are constantly going out into the material world and bringing back information about the multitude of objects with which there exists potential for a relationship.

Ahamkara (Ego, or I-Maker)

The *manas* also collects and organizes data from the *ahamkara*. Information from the *ahamkara* can be valid and useful, but its inherent bias must be taken into account. As is explained in Chapter 25, the individual consciousness of ego is born when an infant begins to view existence exclusively in terms of subject and object. This limited "I" perceives every object or relationship as either pleasant or unpleasant. Left undisciplined, the unruly *ahamkara* continually reinforces a human being's alienation from the One Absolute Reality.

Chitta: The Unconscious Human Hard Drive

As the *manas* debates whether or not to take an action, information retrieved from the unconscious portion of the mind (*chitta*) is added to the various suggestions of the *ahamkara* and senses. The *chitta* is analogous to a computer's hard drive—a reservoir of all your *samskaras* and the storehouse of information defined as useful in fulfilling your desires.

Manas **Presents its Findings**

When the *manas* has concluded its preliminary fact-finding, it presents two possible choices for consideration. Addressing our awareness, the *manas* begins by saying, "You have two basic alternatives. There is *alternative A*, which will probably result in consequences one, two, three and four, and there is *alternative B*, which will probably result in other consequences one, two, three and four. What is your decision? In support of which alternative will you take an action?"

After the *manas* concludes its monologue on alternatives and consequences, it waits a bit for our decision. If none is forthcoming, it automatically begins again. "You have two basic choices: *alternative A* with certain consequences and *alternative B* with these different consequences. Have you made a decision yet?"

Without a decision, *manas* repeats again and again, "You have two choices: A or B. Will you do it or will you not do it? A or B? A or B? A or B?

The relentless repetition becomes first annoying, then frustrating, and eventually, exhausting. The doubt and indecision play on like a broken record, and our inability or unwillingness to make a decision based on the available information is a major cause of stress in our lives.

The functioning of *manas* is analogous to the performance of the computer. No matter how sophisticated and swift its operation, the computer is always dealing with the solitary question: yes or no? (one or zero?). The function of the *manas* is vital, but like the computer, the *manas* has no capacity to discriminate nor to judge responsibly the information it collects and presents.

Buddhi **(Discrimination)**

The *buddhi* is the only function of the mind that has the competence to discriminate and decide. It has the potential for great wisdom. However, without sufficient exercise and purification through *sadhana*, the *buddhi* may reflect the limited perspective of the senses, *ahamkara* and *chitta* instead of the wisdom of the superconscious mind. This is a perfect example of the "squeaky wheel" theory. Sometimes the loud insistence of the ego, senses, memories, imagination, fear, anger and selfish desires can become the sole basis upon which *buddhi* makes a decision.

When employed regularly, however, the purified *buddhi* has the reflective quality of a well-polished mirror. It is the instrument through which the conscious mind can know the will of the Divine Reality. With the regular practice of seated meditation, the *buddhi* increasingly reflects the intuitive library of knowledge of the superconscious mind. The purified *buddhi* can always discriminate between the *preya* and the *shreya*. When the *manas* presents us with choices that echo the calls of the senses, *ahamkara* (ego), and *chitta* (unconscious mind), the purified *buddhi* will unerringly define and endorse the *shreya*—that choice that will lead us for our highest and greatest good.

In many respects, the *buddhi* is similar to the Western concept of conscience, but the powers of the *buddhi* are potentially far greater than what we usually attribute to the conscience. The *buddhi* honors, but also goes beyond, situational ethics and conditioned morality. The purified *buddhi* can instantaneously access the infinite creativity and wisdom of the Divine intelligence at the center of consciousness.

This knowledge requires no verification. When knowledge from the superconscious mind comes into your awareness through a purified *buddhi*, you don't need a Ph.D.—or any other special qualification—to know that the advice is correct. You intuitively know that it's true. You know that you know. This is the knowledge that sets you free—if you can muster the will power to act on it.

Purifying the *buddhi* is essential. The more you cleanse and clarify the *buddhi*—by the practice of seated meditation and all forms of *meditation in action*—the greater will be your access to the superconscious mind.

Your Soul is the Hub of the Wheel

The four major functions of the mind animate the body. But as illustrated in the wheel analogy, it is, in truth, the hub that empowers the wheel to turn. The hub of the human being is our essential, eternal identity: *Sat-Chit-Ananda*. Just as awareness is the Essential Nature of the human being, awareness is also the Essential Nature of all animals, plants and minerals. In fact, consciousness is all that really exists. It is both the cause and the substance of the material universe. Every transitory object that appears does so within that Awareness—including the mind, with its thoughts, desires and emotions, and the human body.

Listening to the Signal Despite the Noise

If the *buddhi* is always directing us, why is it so difficult to hear the message?

The science of engineering is often faced with problems concerning signal and noise. To maximize the audibility of a signal that cannot be enhanced, an engineer finds a way to lessen or eliminate the interfering noise. When the noise level is lowered, the signal becomes relatively more audible.

During the Cold War, the United States Information Agency broadcast news and rock 'n roll to Eastern European countries twenty-four hours a day. Although the signal of Radio Free Europe was transmitted every day, many of the people of Hungary, Czechoslovakia, Poland and East Germany rarely heard it. Why? Because the Soviet Union employed sophisticated electronics to jam the signal.

Yoga science recognizes a parallel in human life. The collective noise of the senses, the opinions of the ego and the power of *chitta's* memories and imaginations are so loud that they often drown out the quiet but resolute signal of the *buddhi*. In order to hear the signal and to heed its message, the yoga scientist must first be able to turn down the noise of the *manas* (and senses), ego and *chitta*. Controlling and directing attention accomplishes this.

Coordinating the Four Functions of the Mind

Recognizing how the mind functions and training it properly constitute the prime spiritual discipline of the yoga scientist. When all the four major faculties of the mind are coordinated in service to the wisdom of the soul, the human being can transcend the limitations of the animal body and live in union with the Supreme Reality. Conscious coordination of the functions of the mind makes it possible for us to know the Divine within.

To a great extent, the effectiveness of yoga science depends on your remembrance of the Divine Reality in every circumstance. I have a body. I have a mind. I have thoughts, desires and emotions. I have an ego and unconscious mind. But I am not defined by these. Then, who am I? The body, mind, senses and ego have manifested to serve our true identity, the Eternal Witness. When a human being knows and serves this Witness, the small, separate self becomes an instrument of Divine Providence. When we do not follow the light of intuitive wisdom, however, we condemn ourselves to living in the darkness of ignorance and pain.

An Ancient View of the Mind

More than five thousand years ago, the wisdom of yoga philosophy was revealed to ancient seers through meditation. It was recorded in scriptures that became known as the *Upanishads*. The word *Upanishad* literally means "to sit down near;" that is, to sit in front of a *guru* to receive some important teaching.

One of the principal *Upanishads*, the *Katha Upanishad*, presents the story of a teenager named Nachiketa who sought enlightenment by asking life's most perplexing questions: Who am I? From where have I come? Why am I here? What is to be done? Where will I go?

Nachiketa's spiritual inquiry was no mere intellectual or philosophical exercise. Rather, it was meant to challenge and inspire each of us to put an end to the suffering and alienation wrought by our doubts and fears. According to the scripture, this liberation is accomplished by experimenting with yoga science in order to experience the eternal, bliss-filled Divine Reality for ourselves, in this lifetime. This realization, the sages tell us, is the only freedom worth attaining—the very purpose of our lives.

Know the Self as Lord of the chariot, the body as the chariot itself, the discriminating intellect (buddhi) as the charioteer, and the mind as the reins. The senses, say the wise, are the horses, selfish desires are the roads they travel.

KATHA UPANISHAD[1]

In the *Katha Upanishad* a vivid metaphor is used to help us understand the importance of coordinating the various functions of the mind in service to our Essential Identity. Our body, we're told, is like a chariot drawn by five powerful horses, the five senses. These horses gallop from birth toward death along the roads of desire, pursuing objects and relationships in hope of finding happiness and eliminating pain. The *buddhi* (discriminative faculty or conscience) is the charioteer, whose job it is to ensure that we're not pulled over a cliff by unrestrained horses. The reins held by the charioteer represent the mind, with its many thoughts, desires and emotions. And you, the Eternal Witness, the Divine Self, are the ever-present passenger—the true Master of the chariot.

This image has many important implications. First, it's the role of the *buddhi* to keep you headed in the best direction. The mind serves as reins to steer you for your highest and greatest good. When all the major functions of the mind are coordinated

[1]Translation of the *Katha Upanishad* from *Dialogue with Death*, by Eknath Easwaran, Part I, Canto 2. © 1981, 1992, The Blue Mountain Center of Meditation. Reprinted by permission of Nilgiri Press, P. O. Box 256, Tomales, Ca 94971, www.nilgiri.org.

to work in harmony, the real Self makes all the decisions. The *buddhi*, reflecting the will of the Divine Reality, communicates this wisdom to the mind, and the senses and body obey. But when the senses are uncontrolled, they immediately take to the road of desire that promises pleasure. Then we are not determining our destiny. We are enslaved to the whim of our horses.

In practical terms, a yoga scientist can always identify which modification of the mind is presenting information into his or her awareness. These four faculties of the mind must be coordinated and placed in service to the Self, the hub of the wheel (*Sat-Chit-Ananda*). *Manas*, ego and *chitta* must each do their job, but not more. Recognizing that the purified *buddhi* reflects the will of the Divine Reality, we can be at ease as we serve the *shreya* and willingly surrender the *preya* in thought, word and deed. This ongoing practice ensures the blessings of a joyful and creative life.

CHAPTER 31

Managing Your Thoughts

When a sage is angry, he is no longer a sage.
THE TALMUD

Every kingdom divided against itself is brought to desolation; and every city or house divided against itself shall not stand.
JESUS THE CHRIST

The Importance of NOW

When a yoga scientist understands that all reality flows from the subtle to the gross, individual thoughts can be viewed as embryos, and attention as an incubator employed in the process of creation. When you give attention to a thought, that subtle embryo is incubated. When sufficient attention has been given, a concrete form of the thought-object is born into the material world. The more you think a thought, the more likely you are to speak about that thought. With sustained attention to the same thought, you're likely to undertake some physical action in the material world that can successively create ever more complex relationships—all in service to that original embryo called thought. Both the words and the actions are concrete manifestations of that subtle thought-embryo you nurtured with your attention.

Let's assume that a specific thought comes into your

awareness. No one else is aware of this particular thought, just you. Others, of course, get their own thoughts that you are not aware of. You have received this specific thought *now*, in the present moment. At this point in space and time you are in a unique relationship with a certain constellation of relationships throughout the universe, and your body-mind-sense complex is the one perfectly qualified to take some action in response to this subtle thought-object appearing in your awareness. So it has come to you.

If, in the present moment, your *buddhi* advises that the thought, desire or emotion in your awareness is a *shreya*, give it your complete attention. This message from the *buddhi* means that you have been chosen, from among the billions of people in the world, to incubate this thought-embryo that the Divine Reality is bringing forth from the subtle world. Your capacity to focus attention on that thought, in the present moment—*now*—is the Divine mechanism for transforming the subtle thought-object into manifest form. This progression from the subtle thought to the more concrete forms of speech, action and consequence is the process of creation. By aligning every thought, word and action with the *buddhi*, you become an instrument of the Divine Reality in the process of creation.

In Hindu literature, *Krishna* is the personification of the longing a spiritual seeker feels in his or her heart—the yearning that draws one into a deeper relationship with the Divine. *Krishna*, strong, beautiful and charismatic, is often depicted playing a hollow reed flute. The seeker who can purify the body, mind and senses by renouncing attachments to fear, anger and self-willed desire becomes the instrument through which the Divine melody is played.

St. Francis taught, "It is in dying (to the separate sense of self), that we are born to eternal life." Many writers have defined yoga science and meditation as the "art of dying"—learning how to die to our attachments before we have to die physically. As we learn to unencumber ourselves of our limitations, we can "become One with the Father who is in heaven" and experience *turiya*—the fourth state of consciousness beyond waking, dreaming and deep sleep. This is the state of tranquility and equanimity that sages of various traditions have called *moksha* (liberation), *Christ-consciousness*, *nirvana* or the *land of milk and honey*.

Considering Your Options

When the *buddhi* suggests that the thought, desire or emotion in your awareness is a *preya*, you have three basic choices of what to do with your attention.

You can continue to give your attention to the attractively familiar *preya*, but if you do, the *preya* will eventually manifest as some form of physical, mental or emotional dis-ease or pain.

Or, you may repress the *preya*. However, this repressed energy will eventually manifest as destructive neurosis, bringing pain and dis-ease.

The only desirable choice for a yoga scientist is to surrender the *preya*. As your practice of *japa* and seated meditation becomes more consistent, the power of the *mantra* will naturally come forward when you're faced with the allure of the *preya*. The *mantra* will help center you in the awareness of the Eternal Witness. Then, secure in the fullness of your true Self, you are free to surrender the *preya* back to the Origin from which it has come. This act of *renunciation*, in complete harmony with the will of the Divine Reality as communicated through the purified *buddhi*, transforms the power of the *preya* into energy, will power and creativity. These reserves can be accessed at another time to perform any demanding duty or responsibility the *buddhi* suggests. By offering your mind, action and speech in service to your Inner Wisdom, you are no longer the author of the action, and therefore have no claim to its outcome. The act of *renunciation* is not a *quid pro quo*—you do not make this offering expecting a specific result. Your willing sacrifice of the *preya* is an act of trustful surrender. Regardless of the consequence, the earnest seeker always knows she is being led for her highest and greatest good. For the yoga scientist, this option is the only acceptable choice.

Danger in Serving the *Preya*

If you are ignoring your Divine Nature at the moment a thought, desire or emotion appears in your awareness, you're likely to disregard or overlook the wise and good counsel of the *buddhi* and fall sway to the siren call of the senses, *ahamkara* and *chitta*. You may even be fooled temporarily into believing that you're choosing the *preya* through your own free will, but actions chosen on the basis of fear, anger and greed will always result in dis-ease.

A purified *buddhi* encourages you to serve the *shreya*. Disregarding the *buddhi*, however, and serving the *preya* in thought, word or deed amounts to a miscarriage, or abortion—subtle violence against the unique thought-embryo that the Absolute Reality has suggested you bring forth into the material world.

In this sense, each of us is guilty of "murder." Many times a day we betray our conscience (*buddhi*) and abort potential manifestations of *shreya*. The physical, mental and emotional pain rampant in our society, and our futile reliance on pharmacological, consumptive, penal and military remedies to ameliorate the dis-ease, can be viewed yogically as direct consequences of the violence we inflict individually and collectively on the *buddhi*. All Reality flows from the subtle to the gross. When the precept of *ahimsa* is disregarded, the resulting injurious action inevitably has an injurious effect.

Analogy of Abortion

Imagine that a woman becomes pregnant and that the fetus is aborted sometime during the gestation period. This does not mean that the woman cannot give birth to a child at some future time. In all likelihood she will be able to have another child. However, she will never give birth to the child she lost.

Similar rules apply to our thoughts. If, in the present moment, we receive a thought that the *buddhi* defines as *shreya*, the Divine Reality is asking us to give this particular thought our attention in order to facilitate the birth of its more concrete form. But we have free will. We can choose not to participate further in developing the form of this subtle embryo. We can ignore or forget it.

We can receive another thought, or even the very same thought, at some future time. At that point in space and time, however, a new constellation of relationships will exist—one entirely different from that which existed at the time of the first thought. Living in the present moment is essential to our health and well-being. If our conscious attention is not focused in the *now*, we will miss the message of the *buddhi* and remain enslaved to a whirlpool of painful consequences (*karmas*).

This is not to suggest, in any way, that meditators must deny themselves the enjoyments of the world. Quite the contrary. Through *sadhana* the yoga scientist becomes even more free and prepared to experience the world joyously and completely.

We have a body and senses, and life is to be enjoyed, but it is only through discrimination that the world can be fully appreciated. Only with an exercised and purified *buddhi* can the human being become truly happy, healthy, creative, productive, artistic, loving and nurtured to the fullest extent. Therefore, the sages teach, if what you had hoped and planned for is fulfilled, be grateful. If what you had hoped and planned for is not fulfilled, be equally grateful. Through your own experience, and despite the protests of the ego, senses and habit, you come to know that you are indeed being led for your highest and greatest good.

The Shell Game

You've probably seen some version of the old shell game. In this carnival trick you're asked to follow the pea under one of three moving walnut shells. A skillful operator can move the pea in the blink of an eye from one shell to another, and unless you're present in the moment and totally focused, you're likely to make the wrong choice. Of course, in real life situations our errors are not the fault of a deceitful operator, but rather the result of our own inattention. Unless you are present in the *now,* know your true Self and can identify which function of the mind is presenting information, you may miss the Divine counsel of the *buddhi.*

An important point to remember is this: what is clearly the *shreya* on one occasion might become the *preya* the next. What is *preya* in one particular circumstance may well become the *shreya* in another. Consider your desire for a slice of apple pie, for example. Let's say that apple pie represents one of your strongest food desires. If you've enjoyed a special dinner at a friend's home and you're offered a slice of apple pie for dessert, the *buddhi* might appropriately suggest that it is the *shreya.* After all, life is to be enjoyed. Besides, if your host has lovingly prepared apple pie especially for you, it would not be kind to refuse the thoughtful gesture. However, if you're offered a *second* piece of apple pie ten minutes later, the *buddhi* will probably advise that this slice is a *preya.*

How to Deal with Thoughts

In yoga science, the only way to determine if a thought, desire or emotion is *preya* or *shreya* is to:

1. Be focused in the moment.

2. Center yourself in the fullness of your Essential Nature (*Sat-Chit-Ananda*).

3. Recognize which function of the mind is speaking to your awareness.

4. Listen to the subtle voice of the *buddhi.* As you concentrate on the *buddhi* with one-pointed attention, the noise of the *manas,* ego and *chitta* will become relatively quiet.

5. Upon hearing the Divine counsel of *buddhi,* face the challenge: surrender attachment to the *preya* and, with all the will power you can summon, align every thought, word and action with the *buddhi.*

It takes strength, courage and will power to harmonize mind, action and speech with the *buddhi.* You may have to go against the tide of our culture and the habits of a lifetime.

While the *buddhi* is always defining the *shreya*, the senses, ego and *chitta* may very well be attempting to jam that signal. Meanwhile, Madison Avenue is relentlessly generating new mantras that sing the praises of the *preya*, reinforcing the notion that you are a separate entity in search of other separate entities that can make you happy and eliminate your pain.

Without conscientiously serving the wisdom of the *buddhi*, we are all susceptible to the pitch. When conflict exists in the mind, it can be difficult to maintain the focused attention needed to evaluate each suggestion in the moment. But if we fail to make the effort, our deepest *samskaras* determine our actions, and we unconsciously deny ourselves the unbounded Life, Liberty and Happiness we seek.

CHAPTER 32

Four Primitive Urges

Nothing is more important than being able to choose the way we think—our feelings, aspirations, and desires; the way we view our world and ourselves. Mastery of the mind means that we can begin to reshape our life and character, rebuild relationships, thrive in the stress of daily living and become the kind of person we really want to be.

EKNATH EASWARAN

Four basic urges power our thoughts and emotions. In all animals, including the human being, these sources of mental energy arise from great fountains deep in the unconscious mind. These four primitive fountains, or channels of energy, are our desires for food, sex, sleep and self-preservation. Like Old Faithful at Yosemite, these individual geysers are not always active. However, when one of them is operating, a certain thought may be absolutely overwhelming—almost as if the thought had the strength of a freight train pulling you in the direction of its own fancy. At other times, that primitive fountain may be dormant. If a thought that previously was so compelling recurs when the fountain is not active, it may do so with little or no power to make you act.

Virtually all animal activity is motivated by an urge for food, sex, sleep or self-preservation. Human beings, however, can master these urges by coordinating the major functions of the mind: *manas*, ego, *chitta* and *buddhi*. If these mental faculties are not coordinated and do not function in service to Intuitive Wisdom, the intensity of power emanating from the primitive fountains can manifest as unhealthy habits, such as food or sleep disorders, addictions, sexual excesses or dysfunction, excessive worry or a crippling fear of death.

In truth, this unbridled power is manifested by Divine Providence to fulfill your life's purpose. To begin working with this titanic force, it's important to recognize which primitive fountain is the point of origin for a particular thought, desire or emotion. While it is true that we cannot control the thoughts that come into our awareness from the four primitive fountains, we do have the capacity to decide what to do with the energy each thought represents. Often, the simple recognition of the source of a compulsive thought is enough to begin the harnessing of its power and the diminishment of its control over us.

Through the various practices of yoga science, an earnest seeker can gain the perspective to see what changes to make and, at the same time, cultivate the will power and skill to institute these changes in daily life. In order to begin this process we must become better acquainted with the four primitive urges.

Food

Dietary habits play an enormous role in determining how we feel physically, mentally and emotionally. Many people today eat more often for entertainment, companionship, convenience and emotional comfort than for sustenance. With most adult household members in the workforce, there's little time for anyone to prepare well-planned, nutritious meals with love every day. Instead, the need for convenience rules. If it's quick and tasty, even though its nutritional value may be questionable, the pace of our culture encourages us to go for it. This sounds like choosing the *preya*, and in many cases it is.

Serving the *shreya* in our food choices provides us excellent opportunities to undo our enslavement to unhealthy habits. Each time we choose to eat something, we should remember that the body is a shrine that houses Eternity. Eating, therefore, is a sacrament. As a yoga scientist, take care that each food consumed is in harmony with *ahimsa*—non-injurious and non-harming to you. Try to choose a diet that does not pollute the body or agitate the nervous system. Reduce sugar, salt, fat and caffeine, and eat healthy, first-generation foods (see Chapters 34-36). The mind will become more calm, you'll be attracted to fewer junk foods and you'll feel more satisfied physically, mentally and emotionally. But remember, it's neither necessary nor advisable to change everything at once. Small changes add up.

Sex

It's interesting to note that while the desire for food begins in the body, the desire for sex usually emanates from the mind. Food goes through the body and affects the mind, but sex originates in the mind and then is expressed through the body. If our mind maintains its balance through reliance on the *buddhi* in thought, word and action, we can enjoy sex in a healthy, loving and discriminative manner.

Many people are consumed with thoughts of sex, but when the opportunity comes, they can't enjoy it. To experience this enjoyment fully, as it is intended, a person needs inner strength and consistent awareness of the Divine Reality within. Without these, we may view our sexual partners as mere objects for our own personal satisfaction, or we may remain fearful of sexual exploitation and manipulation.

Sleep

The enjoyment and satisfaction provided by sleep are higher than those provided by any other pleasures, even food or sex. In sleep the body rests and repairs itself. We are more likely to have a deep, restful sleep if we resolve every choice during the day by following the advice of the *buddhi*. Such diverse choices could include: attention to *ahimsa* in all our relationships, eating our biggest meal at midday, relaxing the body and mind through *Easy-Gentle Yoga*, practicing *pranayama* exercises like *nadi shodhana*, and sitting for meditation. When it is difficult to sleep, or when we awake in the morning feeling tired, it's often because we have many anxieties about issues left unresolved. Learn to wake up before sunrise. Sloth and inertia are the greatest detriments to progress.

Self-Preservation (Fear)

Among these four primal forces, self-preservation is the strongest in both human beings and animals. Self-preservation, however, relates to more than the preservation of a living body. It also concerns honor, social status, position, being right, physical attractiveness and proficiency. Self-preservation is about the fear of losing love, nurturing and income, just as much as it is about the fear of illness or death. If we believe our life is threatened, we try to run away or seek to protect ourselves with all our strength and skill. Because our deepest *samskaras* enslave us to the notion that we are a separate entity in the universe, we are bound to experience an inherent fear of losing our body. Fear is the consequence of believing that objects and relationships in the material world have some magical power to make us happy or to eliminate our pain. Therefore, we fear losing what we have, or not gaining what we want.

The fear of annihilation (the central concern of self-preservation) leads to a variety of symptoms, including anxiety or panic disorders, possessiveness in relationships, irritable bowel syndrome, the fear of losing belongings and the fear of heights or flying, as well as other debilitating phobias.

When we know the Absolute Reality within, however, and understand our four primitive urges, it becomes easier, moment by moment, to make enlightened choices.

Harnessing Your Power

Through *sadhana*, the yoga scientist learns how to harness and direct the energy flowing through the four primitive fountains. If, when one of these primitive fountains is activated, we can align every thought, word and action with the Divine counsel of the *buddhi*, we will be able to transform enormous amounts of raw power into reserves of energy, will power and creativity.

Without a coordinated and discriminating mind, we may develop habits, cravings and even compulsions related to the energy of one or more of these primitive fountains. Without a purified and fully employed *buddhi*, we may eat too much or too little, engage in too much or too little sex or in compulsive thoughts of sex, sleep too much or too little, or be constantly plagued by fears of loss or failure. In other words, our energy will be wasted or turned against our best interests.

Until the mind is coordinated in service to the true Self and unless conflict within is resolved, the external world will appear to be filled with pain and dis-ease. When, on the other hand, the internal world is coordinated in service to the Eternal, Bliss-filled Witness (*Sat-Chit-Ananda*), we are in harmony with the universe and free to choose the thoughts, words and actions that will always lead us for our highest and greatest good.

CHAPTER 33

Relationships:
The Essence of Living

Most of us never really see the people we live with. Our boyfriend may be right before our eyes, but we do not see him. We see our idea of him, a little model we have made in chitta, and on that we pronounce our judgments. To me it seems quite unfair. The mind takes some exaggerated impressions, memories, hopes, and insecurities, draws a quick caricature like one of those sidewalk cartoonists, and then turns up its nose. The person in question should retort, "That's not me; that's your caricature of me. If you don't like it, you don't like your own mind."

EKNATH EASWARAN

Do you truly desire to experience loving, meaningful and richly rewarding relationships? Is it important for you to be happy and content? Do you want to reduce or eliminate the various forms of dis-ease in your life? If so, you can achieve everything you earnestly desire by honestly examining the ways you deal with relationships.

Building, Healing and Spiritualizing Relationships
Just for a moment, stop and think about the wide variety of relationships you have every day. Think of your spouse or lover, your child, parents, siblings, friends, extended family,

people you work for or with, and those you do business with (like the banker, supermarket cashier, auto mechanic or plumber). Now, consider your more remote relationships with your local, state and national government officials, all the celebrity types you know through television, radio, films and recordings. You have relationships with the house or apartment you live in, your work, tools, car, computer, clothes, pets and the environment. Then add the thousands of other, more intimate relationships you have—with your body, the food you eat, your breath, your senses, as well as your mind and its many thoughts, desires, memories, imaginations and emotions. Let's face it, you have a lot of relationships!

Every single relationship requires you to take some kind of action. Essentially, that's what having a relationship means. When you have a relationship, it means that a thought, desire or emotion is commanding your attention and requiring you to respond. Relationships imply action just as action implies a relationship, and your choice of which thoughts to think, which words to speak and which actions to take will determine whether your relationships bring you happiness or sorrow.

We experience pain and dis-ease in our relationships because most of us merely adopt the goals, fashions and ideals of our society, without really knowing ourselves first, within and without. This leaves us ignorant of our Divinity and Its wisdom, and dependent on the suggestions of others. As each new generation takes on the handicaps of the previous generations, humanity continues to look outside itself for new objects and relationships that—it is hoped, or expected—will bring the desired happiness and contentment. Unfortunately, what we often wind up with is stress, anxiety, frustration, anger or even depression.

This beleaguered state is not new. More than six thousand years ago, certain wise people had already understood that our ignorance is the root cause of the pain experienced in dealing with life's constant and inevitable change. In response to their dis-ease, these women and men began to experiment with knowledge received intuitively in meditation and came to know that although change is indeed constant and inevitable, responding to that change with pain and bondage is not.

In Sanskrit the word *lila* is used to describe the vast, joyful and spontaneous play of creation. The word "play" implies fun, and *lila* is the Divine Reality's game that we are well equipped to enjoy. Whether we understand the word play to mean a theatrical production or the everyday events of an infinite cosmic game with defined rules and regulations makes little difference—we are the players.

As skilled actors we're required to play a variety of roles as perfectly as we can, but no truly accomplished performer identifies so completely with the role that she forgets who she is. Likewise, the skilled athlete is never so consumed by the winning or losing that he forgets how to play the game. As Shakespeare says, "The play's the thing!" We merely need to know how to play well and enjoy it.

The foundation of the ancient wisdom of yoga, known as the *yamas* and *niyamas*, was formulated to guide human beings through every relationship and circumstance—to transform life's "play" from a dreary noun into an exhilarating and rewarding verb. By employing the *yamas* and *niyamas*, the ancients found their lives became the engrossing and fulfilling kind of play that children long for and revel in.

Essentially, the *yamas* and *niyamas* reflect the understanding that in every relationship action must be taken, and for relationships to become loving and rewarding, every thought, word and deed must be guided by the discriminative faculty of *buddhi*. The sages teach us that the secret to establishing meaningful relationships—whether they are external or internal—is the recognition that when you consistently serve the *shreya* and surrender the *preya*, you will naturally experience happy, creative, productive and loving relationships.

The science of yoga rests upon precepts designed to inspire spiritual seekers in the creation of meaningful and rewarding lives. The first of these building blocks are the *yamas* and *niyamas*. (For a complete overview of the eight steps of traditional yoga science, see Chapter 1.)

YAMAS:
DISCIPLINES AND RESTRAINTS

1. Non-violence (*Ahimsa*)

Non-injuring, non-harming is the highest precept of yoga science and is to be applied to every thought, word and deed in every relationship—including the relationship you have with yourself. Charity must always begin at home. Unless you serve *ahimsa* in all your relationships, they will inevitably bring you varying forms of physical, mental, emotional or spiritual dis-ease.

2. Truthfulness (*Satya*)

Satya is the avoidance of all falsehood, exaggeration and pretense. But *satya* is more than mere conventional honesty. First and foremost, a fact, in order to be the truth, must be in harmony with *ahimsa*. If a thought, word or deed is injurious, it is considered to be only a fact, but not the truth. When your every action, subtle and gross, serves truth, the body and mind will experience health. When your actions are not in service to truth, the body and mind will experience dis-ease. Truthfulness is required for the unfoldment of your intuitive, discriminating faculties. (See *Truth Versus Fact*, pages 307-308.)

3. Non-stealing (*Asteya*)

Asteya means not stealing physical objects, but also refers to not taking credit for anything that is not rightfully ours. *Asteya* is an expression of the freedom from craving that dawns with the realization of our innate fullness.

4. Chastity (*Brahmacharya*)

Brahmacharya is usually translated as chastity or celibacy. However, it also implies an ongoing awareness of the Absolute Reality within and a reverence for our sacred energy in every form it may take. Learning to steward this energy is an important step in realizing our life purpose: the attainment of freedom from the pains and bondages of human existence.

Regulating sexual desires—and the desires for sense gratifications in general—frees our resources. We lose nothing. In fact we find ourselves newly equipped to act in ways that were formerly beyond our means. In intimate relationships, for example, this means replacing the selfish desire for pleasure with the desires to give, to serve and to understand. If we see ourselves, our partner, and the world as manifestations of the One Absolute Reality, we experience both giving and receiving as selfless acts of love in our relationship with the Divine. This attitude helps free us from enslavement to the senses and transforms us into spiritual ecologists.

Practicing *brahmacharya* allows the energy of the senses to be used for higher purposes. Instead of permitting the senses to dissipate energy in pursuit of *preya*, the purified *buddhi* is employed to discern which actions will lead us for our highest and greatest good, which is the good of all. Each time we align mind, action and speech with the *buddhi*, that action adds to our storehouse of will—the power to choose the long-term good consistently.

5. Non-possessiveness (*Aparigraha*)

Aparigraha literally means non-holding. It means seeing every relationship as an opportunity for spiritual unfoldment, with no sense that we own the person, creature or object, or that we are owned by them. Everything is here for us to use and to enjoy, but not to possess nor to be possessed by. In our search for Happiness, attempts to possess any thing or anyone will only block our access to our creative energy.

Every action gives rise to an equal reaction, or fruit of that action. So states the *law of karma*. When we recognize the One Reality in all manifestation, every relationship becomes a relationship with our Divine Self. Therefore, when we think, speak and act selflessly—giving away the fruit of our action—some benefit accrues to us, and our energy becomes an expansive and loving force in all our relationships.

NIYAMAS:
CONSTRUCTIVE OBSERVANCES

1. Purity and Cleanliness (*Saucha*)

We purify the mind and body by surrendering undesirable thoughts, desires and emotions through the practice of *renunciation*. The importance of this purification cannot be overstated, since all that occurs in the manifest world is preceded by events in the subtle world of our past thoughts and intentions. As it relates to the physical body, *saucha* means more than keeping our skin and hair clean. *Saucha* is achieved by loving attention to the condition of the entire body-mind-sense complex. This means eating pure, healthy, first-genera-tion foods, regulating the breath (*pranayama*) and getting appropriate exercise. Adhering to the the common sense principles of *Ayurveda* that are outlined in Chapter 34 can also contribute greatly to purification of the body.

2. Contentment (*Santosha*)

Contentment should not be confused with satisfaction. Continually give your best effort. If the result of your action is other than what you had planned or expected, you are free to act again, but always with the contentment (*santosha*) of know-ing that when mind, action and speech have served the *buddhi*'s discrimination, you are being led for your highest and greatest good.

3. Austerities and Ascetic Practices (*Tapas*)

Tapas refers to acts of surrender or *renunciation* that generate the heat and fire necessary to facilitate transformation. These offerings purify the mind and body and increase the resolve (*sankalpa*) to expand consciousness and realize greater freedom. *Tapas* does not mean the repression of every pleasurable desire and emotion. However, it is helpful to remember that self-discipline is a necessary ingredient in the transformation and storage of potential energy—energy that can be used for the attainment of a higher and greater good. Throughout the day you are called upon to make thousands of decisions. Make them mindfully. Consistently making conscious, discriminating choices is what the sages call freedom (*moksha*).

4. Self-Study (*Svadhyaya*)

Self-study is the process of looking within, seeking within and finding the Absolute Reality within. *Svadhyaya* helps an individual act skillfully and lovingly in the world and leads to Self-realization. It includes the study of the scriptures and of our internal states of consciousness, as well as the practices of contemplation, repentance and prayer (see Chapter 39).

5. Surrender to God (*Ishvara Pranidhana*)

When we unite our individual will with the greater intelligence existing beyond the mind, our egotism, pettiness and selfishness evaporate. Living in this state of equanimity and tranquility, we no longer perceive the world through the dualistic paradigm of subject and object. By seeing the unity in the diversity, "I" and "mine" give way to "Thou" and "Thine." When the space between subject and object is annihilated, then I and my Father truly become One.

To experience the best from every relationship, experiment with these yogic guidelines for successful living. Starting today, evaluate whether the thoughts, words and actions in your daily life are in harmony with the *buddhi* and the principles of the *yamas* and *niyamas*. Rely on yoga philosophy in all your decision-making and you'll begin to experience less stress and anxiety. You'll find creative answers to dilemmas that have plagued you for a long time. As your *sadhana* deepens, contentment (*santosha*) will dawn as you realize that a new ease of being has become your constant companion.

A Contemplation on Oneness

The following contemplation has proven helpful in our *sadhana*, and we offer it to help you achieve the final *niyama*: surrender to the Absolute Reality.

In the Hindu tradition the individual soul within each of us is called *Atman*. The collective soul, of which we are all a part, is known as *Brahman*.

As you sit comfortably, ponder the words of this contemplation. Using your intellect, consider how the meaning of these words apply to you. If it is more meaningful to you, feel free to substitute the name of the Divine Reality from whatever tradition you call your own.

The universe is unreal.
***Brahman* is real.**

There is only one *Brahman* without second.
Realize the unity in the diversity.

I am *Brahman*.
Realize the Absolute Reality within.

All is *Brahman*.
There is only one absolute truth . . .
Self-existent, all pervading, within and without.

ॐ

Truth versus Fact

A brief story set in Nazi Germany during World War II illustrates and clarifies the concept of truthfulness (*satya*). A Jewish man, seeking refuge from an uncertain future, went to the farmhouse of a neighbor. The two had grown up together as best friends, so he had no reservations about asking the German, "May I stay in your house? Will you hide me?"

"Of course," the German replied without hesitation.

The brave farmer made a small apartment for his Jewish friend in the basement of the house and provided food, water and clothing.

Days later an SS officer knocked at the door. When the farmer opened the door, a Nazi officer briskly asked, "Are there any Jews in this house?" As a yoga scientist, the farmer knew intuitively that if he answered "Yes," he would be violating the precept of *ahimsa*. By declaring the presence of a Jew, he would be committing an act of violence, not only against the Jew, but against himself and the SS officer as well, because they would both become implicated in the injury that would surely befall his friend.

Remembering the wisdom of the *yamas* and *niyamas*, the farmer knew that truth must always be in harmony with *ahimsa* in thought, word and deed. Therefore, his impeccable response was "No, there are no Jews in this house."

In twenty-first century America it seems that almost everyone believes he or she has a corner on what is the truth. Ask the person on the opposite end of an argument, listen to talk radio or watch any number of television news commentators. All claim to know the truth. Decisiveness in our culture is clearly more highly prized than thoughtfulness. Often wrong, but never in doubt, seems to have become the signature of our modern age.

Truth, however, in order to merit the support of our thoughts, words and actions, must be in harmony with *ahimsa*. Without meeting this criterion of non-harming, a so-called truth can only be considered a relatively true fact, and, therefore, a *preya*—to be willingly sacrificed.

Yoga science asks us to think, speak and act in service to the truth at all times, in all places and in all circumstances—regardless of the suggestions or protestations of the ego, *chitta*, *manas* and senses. In practical terms, *satya* demands that a yoga scientist must always be willing to experiment—to surrender his or her *raga/dveshas* (likes and dislikes) and attachments in favor of *ahimsa*.

Remember, if it's not in harmony with the Divine counsel of the *buddhi* and the *yamas* and *niyamas*, then it's to be considered *preya*—an opportunity for *renunciation*. In the story of Abraham and Isaac, Abraham renounced his greatest attachment and he became the patriarch of the Hebrew people. But the cause and effect described in this story was not a business deal between Abraham and God. Abraham became newly fit for his ultimate life's calling only because of the purification his sacrifice accomplished.

In order for each of us to make this kind of choice in our lives, we first must be awake—conscious of our Divinity and aware that we have choices every moment. This is why *japa*, or repetition of the *mantra*, is so important. The sacred vibrations of the name of the Divine Reality have the capacity to lead us to the wisdom and contentment at the Center of Consciousness.

All power lies in the realm of the subtle, not the gross. The gross comes from the subtle. By the time a thought has become manifest, its power is a mere shadow of the power residing in the subtle form. Therefore, the more we remain centered in the Eternal Witness and the more we are in harmony with the Divine Reality the safer we are, the more protected we are and the more our needs are met by the sacred energies that are allowed to flow through us.

Don't just Believe—Experiment!

Remember that yoga, as a science, is verifiable or refutable, based on your own personal experience. Do not accept any suggestion presented in this book or elsewhere without verifying its truthfulness through your personal practice. Once you have begun assimilating the knowledge of yoga science, start actively experimenting with these concepts.

While respecting your personal duties, responsibilities and limitations, begin to work with those practices that initially are most comfortable for you. Don't take on too much too soon. Remember, this book reflects many years of study and experimentation. Neither Jenness nor I read any one book nor attended any one lecture that changed our lives radically overnight. Yoga science is a process, not a quick fix.

Living free from stress and worry is not a distant goal, but rather the path upon which you are presently traveling. Learn to enjoy the journey, for the present moment is all you ever have. Before you commit to any action, turn yesterday and tomorrow into today, and turn today into *now*. Centered in your true Self, in the present moment, *now*, you will find the wisdom and the truth that sets you free.

However, you can never know this truth if you merely believe what you've read in a book, or what's been suggested to you by your parents, clergy, meditation teacher, or Madison Avenue gurus. Dependence on external resources, suggestions and habits will only prolong the bondage. No one other than your own true Self can bring you this liberating wisdom.

You must light your own lamp. To fulfill this great purpose, you first need a burning desire for unbounded Happiness. Then, metaphorically, you must gather together a wick, oil and lamp by working with practices that help you build a philosophy of life. You can know the truth only by *experiencing* the truth, and you can experience the truth only by renouncing the ground of *preya* upon which you stand. You must practice. Prepare yourself and make your life an embodiment of this teaching, and you can achieve the ultimate goal of real freedom. Remember, the truth is self-evident and empowering. It unerringly applies in *every* relationship in *every* circumstance.

The Blind Man and the Lame Man

Two men walking in the forest approached a swift-flowing

stream. For each, the stream's rapid current and uncertain footing proved insurmountable obstacles to the continuation of their journey. One man was blind, and the other was lame.

After much consternation, the blind man had an idea. "Look here, my friend. You are lame and cannot walk well, but have excellent sight. I am blind, but have strong and steady legs. If you sit on my shoulders, you can guide my sure-footed steps with your keen vision. Together we can cross the stream." And so the lame man climbed onto the shoulders of the blind man and they crossed the river. By sharing unique resources, their desired goal was accomplished.

If your intention is pure and you dedicate yourself to your *sadhana*, what you may lack personally will become available to you through the grace of Divine Providence. Despite seemingly insurmountable physical, mental or emotional handicaps, as you follow the Divine wisdom of *buddhi* confidently and fearlessly—knowing yourSelf to be none other than the One eternal, universal and compassionate intelligence—difficult relationships will either heal or wither away. New relationships will appear to lead you beyond your personal limitations and you will find that life can indeed be lived in peace and joy.

Part IX
AYURVEDA

CHAPTER 34
Ayurveda—The Science of Life

Humility and relentless industry should characterize your approach to knowledge. The entire world consists of teachers for the wise and enemies for the fools. Therefore, knowledge—conducive to health, longevity, fame, and excellence, coming from even an unknown source—should be received, assimilated, and utilized with earnestness.

CHARAKA SAMHITA

In grade school science class we learned that two objects cannot occupy the same space at the same time. Similarly, when we hold on to the familiar and comfortable, we continue to think, speak and act in our habitual manner because there's no room for change. If we always do what we've always done, we'll always get what we always got. But when we freely follow the Divine wisdom reflected by the *buddhi*—renouncing our habits of fear, anger and self-willed desire—we begin to see creative solutions to problems that have perennially plagued us.

By this same mechanism the ancients discovered *Ayurveda*. When human beings with unique proclivities and abilities began to meditate and practice yoga science, certain truths, including *Ayurveda*, were revealed to them from the superconscious mind. This same revelatory process brought the Ten Commandments to Moses through deep meditation at Mt. Sinai.

Widely practiced in India for more than five thousand years, *Ayurveda* is a holistic system of medicine. The Sanskrit word *Ayurveda* means "the science of life." *Ayur* is life, and *veda* is knowledge or science. It is a complex science, yet its basic principles are easily employed in making everyday decisions about our health and well-being. It also offers us a profound understanding of our bodies, personalities and relationships.

Process of Manifestation

All reality flows from the subtle to the gross. Every object is a manifestation of the One, eternal, unmanifested, bliss-filled consciousness (*Sat-Chit-Ananda*). In order to truly know and be all, the Divine Reality must experience the infinite variety of potentialities. In Hindu cosmology, this process of the Divine manifesting and experiencing Itself is represented by a Holy Trinity. Though depicted as three separate deities, this Trinity is essentially monotheistic. The differing characters of the three gods express the three essential aspects of the One Absolute on which the existence of the entire phenomenal universe depends.

The first aspect of this ongoing creation process is represented by *Brahma* (the Creator)—that aspect of the One that brings forth a form from the subtle world into the material world. *Vishnu* (the Sustainer), the second aspect of the One, maintains the manifestation for a limited period of time, and *Shiva* (the Destroyer), the third aspect of the Eternal One, causes a dissolution back into the unmanifest Origin through the mechanisms of death and decomposition. This endless cycle of creation, sustenance and dissolution has been called the eternal breath of the Lord in ancient literature. This causeless "breath" of God is without beginning and without end. It is the very nature of Being.

The process of manifestation begins with formless consciousness (*Sat-Chit-Ananda*), existing in its potential state. The Essential Nature of this consciousness is to manifest Itself, and Its first, most subtle expression came forth as an unstruck vibration—the primal sound of the universe itself. According to the science of yoga and *Ayurveda*, that first sound was, and is, the *mantra AUM* (also written and pronounced as *OM*). *AUM* is considered the "mother of all mantras" because everything—past, present and future—is contained in the *AUM*. The very first verse of the *Gospel According to John* echoes this understanding. "In the beginning was the word and the word was with God, and the word *was* God." To say that *AUM*[1] is the sum of manifestation containing an infinite number of possibilities is simply another way of understanding God.

Verifying the Truth of *AUM*

The ancients teach us that all creation—every gross and subtle object, all the seeds and the possibilities of life—is contained in the *AUM*. To comprehend this more completely, remember that modern physics has proven no object to be truly solid. Each object exists as a unique, shimmering vibration of particles. Certainly, in everyday life we act as though objects are solid. No one would claim, for instance, that the chair you are sitting in is not supporting your body. Physics, however, tells us that gross objects actually contain much more space than they do solid material. It is their distinctive vibration, as perceived by the human mind and senses, that makes them appear as they do.

To verify the claim that every gross and subtle object is contained in the *AUM*, you would have to visit the past, present and future and collect every gross and subtle object

---

[1]The mantra *AUM* is the origin of the Western liturgical word amen. In fact, the Hebrew word shalom also has its genesis in *AUM*. In modern usage, shalom has three meanings: hello, goodbye and peace. However, from a yogic perspective, the ancient derivation of shalom is best understood as a compound of the Hebrew word *shel*, which means of, and the Sanskrit word *AUM* (*OM*), meaning the One Divine Reality—the Origin of all manifestation. Spoken as one compound word, shel-om, or shalom, it confers a spiritual blessing upon its recipient: "May you always be aware of *Om*." If an individual experiences the truth of *Om*—the One Divine Reality without second, referred to as God—then, whether she is coming in or going out, she will always be at peace for she is centered in her Essential Nature and living in the true *land of milk and honey*.

that ever existed, that exists now, and that will exist some time in the future. Then, you'd need to record the unique vibration of each individual object (including every human being, thought, desire and emotion), mix the separate sound tracks together and play them back simultaneously. Yoga science says that the resulting sound would be OMMMM. Everything with a name and form is contained in the *mantra AUM*.

MANIFESTATION BEGINS WITH THE *MANTRA AUM*

Creation begins with pure, undifferentiated consciousness (*Sat-Chit-Ananda*). From that Divinity emanates *AUM*, the first vibration, containing the seeds of all potential manifestation. Out of the *AUM* are birthed a progressive sequence of elements or *tattvas*: space (ether), air, fire, water and earth.

The Five Basic Elements

The sacred vibration *AUM* gives rise to the first element: ether or space. Inherent in space is the concept of the presence of a subtle framework—the basis of all that will be manifest. In the analogous Chinese system of elements, wood is the corollary to ether/space. This apparent incongruity can be explained by considering that in Eastern countries bamboo scaffolding is still used today in the construction of buildings made of concrete, stone and steel.

Also, prior to the advent of the computer, graphic designers created the pages of newspapers and magazines by laying down black type and photographs on a grid printed in blue ink. When the page design was photographed, the blue grid, unrecognized by the camera, disappeared and only the black type was visible in the final printing. Similarly, the grid— upon which all the successive elements are organized in the material world—exists invisibly in the ether.

With the manifestation of space, a movement or vibration occurs that subsequently gives rise to the second element: air (ether in motion). As the movement of the space and air continues, friction is produced, and that friction generates heat. As heat grows in intensity, it gives rise to the third basic element: fire. In the presence of fire, certain ethereal particles liquefy, manifesting the water element. Finally, the liquid state of matter/energy (the water element) cools and solidifies, forming the physical element: earth. From earth, all organic and inorganic substances are born, including the kingdoms of minerals, plants and animals.

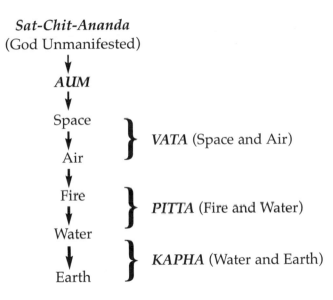

Man as Microcosm of the Cosmos

As they learned to focus their attention, meditate and practice yoga science, ancient practitioners of *Ayurveda* realized that every perceivable object in the universe—including the human being—is both a microcosm and macrocosm of everything else. Seeing that the five basic elements of space, air, fire, water and earth appear in nature as they do in each human being, *Ayurveda* considers man's individual existence, health and dis-ease in holistic terms—inseparable from the intrinsic cosmic unity of consciousness, energy and matter. Therefore, in order to determine what makes an individual body healthy, the first practitioners of *Ayurveda* studied the laws and interrelatedness of the cosmos. In order to understand the functioning of the universe, they examined the operations of the human body.

THE ELEMENTS (*TATTVAS*) AND THE HUMAN BODY

Ether/Space

Within the human body lie many cavities comprised of the ether element. For example, space exists in the mouth, nose, respiratory and gastrointestinal tracts, capillaries, lymphatics and in all the tissues and cells. All functions of the body take place within space. All relationships and responses of the physical body require space as an element of their operation.

Air

Space in motion is air, and in the human body the air element manifests in the movement of the muscles, stomach and intestines, the beating of the heart and the expansion and contraction of the lungs. On the molecular level also, constant motion within the human body is governed by the air element. These movements include the motility of individual cells, sensory and motor activity of nerve impulses and the wide-ranging operations of the central nervous system.

Fire

The fire element is responsible for digestion, metabolism and the maintenance of body temperature. In the brain, fire facilitates the thinking process. In the functioning of sight, fire makes it possible for the retina to perceive light.

Water

Three quarters of the human body is composed of water.

Water manifests in all bodily secretions, and is vital to the workings of the body's mucous membranes, tissues, organs, plasma and cytoplasm. Water cools and cleans all vital systems.

Earth

Every solid structure of the human body is a manifestation of the earth element. Bones, cartilage, muscles, tendons, skin, hair and nails are all constructed of the earth element present in the food we have ingested.

THE ELEMENTS AND THE FIVE SENSES

Ayurveda teaches that in addition to constituting the body, each of the five basic elements (*tattvas*) of space, air, fire, water and earth also relate to one of the five senses of hearing, touch, vision, taste and smell.

Hearing - Ether/Space

Space is the medium through which sound is transmitted, and the ear, the organ of hearing, expresses action through the mouth and throat, the organs of speech (sound).

Touch - Air

The air element is related to the sense of touch, and the sensory organ of touch is the skin. The organ of action for the sense of touch is the hand. Therefore, the skin of the hand is especially sensitive since the hand is responsible for actions of holding, giving and receiving.

Vision - Fire

The fire element manifests as light, heat and color, and is

related to the sense of vision. The eye, the organ of sight, governs the action of walking and is related, therefore, to the feet. An individual without the sense of sight has difficulty walking. The eyes give direction to the action of walking.

Taste - Water

The water element is related to the organ of taste. Without water, the tongue cannot taste. In *Ayurveda*, the function of the tongue is closely related to the performance of the genitals; therefore the penis or clitoris is considered the "lower tongue," while the tongue in the mouth is termed the "upper tongue." The individual who controls the "upper tongue" naturally controls the "lower tongue."

Smell - Earth

The earth element is related to the sense of smell. The nose, the sensory organ of smell, is related in function to the excretory function of the anus. This relationship is demonstrated in the person who has constipation or an unclean colon; he generally has bad breath and his sense of smell is diminished.

THE THREE *DOSHAS*

Vata, Pitta and Kapha

The science of *Ayurveda* states that each human being is born with a certain unique and perfect individual balance of the five elements: ether, air, fire, water and earth. In each manifested form, including the human being, the five basic elements combine into three categories called *doshas*.

The three *doshas* of *Ayurveda* are *vata*, *pitta* and *kapha*. When balanced, the *doshas* maintain a healthy physiological and psychological condition; and when imbalanced, they contribute to the process of physical, mental and/or emotional dis-ease.

These *doshas* govern the everyday activities of both the body and mind. The balance of *vata*, *pitta* and *kapha* is responsible for the rise of natural urges and for individual preferences in such qualities as the flavor, temperature and degree of spiciness of foods. The *doshas* influence the creation, maintenance and destruction of bodily tissue and the elimination of waste products from the body. Imbalanced *doshas* contribute to the arousal of emotions like fear, anger and greed, while balanced *doshas* facilitate human understanding, compassion and love.

Vata dosha, the combination of space and air, is present wherever there is movement in the body. *Vata* regulates such processes as breathing, blinking of the eyelids, beating of the heart, as well as the expansion and contraction in muscles, tissues, cell membranes and nerves. It is the cause of pain, tremors and spasms. The large intestine, pelvic cavity, bones, skin, ears and thighs are all sites where excess *vata* tends to accumulate. Excess *vata* is responsible for such emotions as worry, fear and anxiety. *Vata* is also expressed as cheerfulness, flexibility and creativity.

Pitta dosha represents the combination of fire and water elements. *Pitta* governs the processes of digestion, absorption, assimilation, nutrition, metabolism, temperature, skin coloration, eyesight and intelligence. The small intestine, stomach, sweat glands, blood, fat, eyes and skin are the sites in the body where excess *pitta* tends to accumulate. Excess *pitta* incites anger, hatred and aggression. Pitta is also expressed as efficiency, leadership and focus.

Kapha dosha is formed by the combination of the elements of earth and water. The bonding quality and heaviness of *kapha* provides the material for the body's physical structure. *Kapha* lubricates the joints, provides moisture to the skin, helps heal wounds, gives strength, vigor and stability, supports memory retention, gives energy to the heart and lungs and maintains the immune system. Excess *kapha* manifests as symptoms in the chest, throat, head, sinuses, nose, mouth, stomach, joints, cytoplasm, plasma and such liquid secretions as mucus. *Kapha* is responsible for emotions of attachment, greed and jealousy. It is also expressed as calmness, forgiveness and compassion.

A variety of factors combine at the time of human conception to determine an individual's basic and unique constitution—their perfect balance of *vata*, *pitta* and *kapha*. For example, both the time of day and seasons of the year have a certain balance of *vata*, *pitta* and *kapha*.

Time of Day

Each twelve-hour segment of the day is divided into three periods, each lasting approximately four hours. When a particular *dosha* dominates one of these time periods, it also influences our individual *dosha* balance and, therefore, our capacities for physical, mental and emotional activity. Remember, according to *Ayurveda*, everything is either a microcosm or macrocosm of everything else. As above, so below.

Vata, Pitta and *Kapha* Time

Through their meditation and personal experience, the ancients learned that just as the greatest heat of the day accompanies the noontime sun, so also, the fire element in our body (digestion and metabolism) is most efficient at that same time. *Ayurveda* observes that the fire of our human digestive furnace works at maximum efficiency from 10 A.M. to 2 P.M. This period is known as *pitta* time—when the fire element predominates. Therefore, *Ayurveda* instructs that for optimal digestion and nutrient assimilation, we should eat our biggest meal of the day at noon or 1 P.M.—just as rural Americans did when our culture was more in harmony with the natural rhythms of life.

Kapha rules the hours between six and ten o'clock, in both the morning and evening, when the heavier elements of earth and water predominate in the body. The science of *Ayurveda* tells us that when it's difficult to awake from sleep at 7 A.M., we are under the weighty influence of *kapha dosha*. Similarly, at the end of the day, after extensive physical and mental activity, and after the dinner meal is eaten, we may feel a little lethargic and tired. This is *kapha* time, when the heavier elements of earth and water predominate in the body.

Applying this knowledge, *Ayurveda* advises that we eat a light dinner at the end of the day so our digestion will be complete before the evening meditation and sleep. In addition, it is most beneficial for the human being to fall asleep before 10 P.M. Just as a lead-weighted sinker on the end of a fishing line carries the hook far beneath the surface of the water, the heavy elements of earth and water draw us down into a deep, restful sleep—if we get to bed in *kapha* time. *Vata* constitutions, especially, benefit from this effect of entering sleep before 10 P.M.

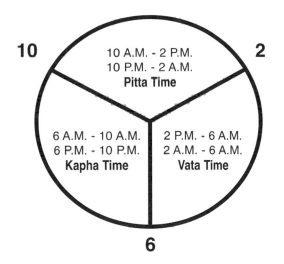

Most of us don't fall asleep in *kapha* time. Around 9:30 or 10 P.M., we experience a burst of renewed energy. Instead of meditating and retiring for the night by ten o'clock, we may expend our newfound energy in outward activity. Influenced by our twenty-four hour culture, we might go to a movie, watch television, have a snack, write a letter, surf the internet, call a friend or read a book. This "second wind" is actually the onset of evening *pitta* time—when the fire of our metabolic furnace becomes more active again. When we fall asleep in *kapha* time, the extra heat and energy of evening *pitta* can fulfill its intended purpose: the repair and restoration of body cells—correcting damage that routinely occurs during the normal wear and tear of daily life.

Vata dosha (air and space) predominates from two to six o'clock, both in the afternoon and early morning. Because the *vata* elements of air and space facilitate movement, *Ayurveda* encourages us to rise before 6 A.M., within *vata* time. This enables us to start our meditation practice under the activating influence of *vata* rather than the sedative influence of *kapha*.

Many *vata* types suffer from insomnia around 2 A.M. when the morning *vata* time begins. For those who are prone to sleepless nights, a cup of lightly boiled milk with an added teaspoon of ghee (clarified butter), taken just prior to bedtime, is suggested. The boiling helps to pre-digest the milk proteins, and the hot liquid has a very calming effect. The heavy earth and water elements of milk promote deep, prolonged sleep.

Seasons of the Year

Ayurveda divides the year into three main seasons. Each season reflects the general character of *vata, pitta* or *kapha,* although specific days within each season may exhibit characteristics from any of the three *doshas.*

Kapha Season (mid-March to mid-June)
Pitta Season (mid-June to mid-October)
Vata Season (mid-October to mid-March)

Summer is considered the *pitta* season, combining the fire and water elements—it is hot and humid. Spring is a *kapha* season, the time of year when the water and earth elements predominate. It is a time of rain, floods, mud, new growth and allergies. Late fall and winter is considered *vata* season, when the cold and drying elements of air and space manifest in freezing temperatures and wind.

Throughout our daily lives, ceaseless interaction takes place between the internal and external environments. The *vata, pitta* and *kapha* of the external macrocosm, such as the seasons and the time of day, constantly intermingle with and influence the *vata, pitta* and *kapha* of the internal microcosm of the human mind and body. For example, during the spring *kapha* season, individuals with allergies benefit from reducing their intake of such *kapha*-producing foods as dairy and wheat products and citrus fruits. During *pitta* season, it is prudent to honor the fact that the fire element of summertime heat can often inflame a physical, mental or emotional symptom. During *vata* season, individuals who are especially susceptible to the drying effects of increased air and space elements should take appropriate precautions by dressing warmly and increasing their intake of warm, moist foods.

Everyday activities also affect the doshic balance within the human body-mind-sense complex. When *vata* types (predominantly space and air) fly in an airplane or take a long automobile trip, they can counterbalance the inevitable increase of *vata* by consuming oatmeal for breakfast. Oatmeal, a *kapha* food, increases the water and earth elements and tends to stabilize the movement of *vata*. This conscious *dosha* balancing provides a *vata* constitution sustained energy while decreasing susceptibility to the exhaustion associated with travel. By understanding and applying such practical principles of *Ayurveda*, we can foster balance in the body and mind by altering our diet and habits in response to our changing external environment.

Forming the Individual Constitution

The basic *vata-pitta-kapha* constitution of each individual is determined by a combination of doshic factors. The unique *vata-pitta-kapha* of the father, mother, time of day and season of the year all merge together into the unique *vata-pitta-kapha* of the egg and sperm to form the *vata-pitta-kapha* of the embryo at the moment of conception.

Although each person's doshic balance is unique and specific, for the sake of practicality, *Ayurveda* recognizes seven constitutional types: (1) *vata*; (2) *pitta*; (3) *kapha*; (4) *vata-pitta* or *pitta-vata*; (5) *pitta-kapha* or *kapha-pitta*; (6) *vata-kapha* or *kapha-vata*; and (7)*vata-pitta-kapha* (also referred to as *tri-doshic*).

The constitution, or nature, of an individual is called *prakriti*. *Prakriti* includes not only the physical form, but temperament as well. It is the unique and perfect balance of the five elements present at birth, and it should remain virtually unaltered throughout one's lifetime. However, this balance is subject to continuous influence by the *vata*, *pitta* and *kapha* of the external environment. The balance of space, air, fire, water and earth found in the food we eat, the seasons of the year, the time of day and the activities we engage in all interact and modify the internal balance of elements present in the human body. However, *Ayurveda* maintains that healing can take place only when an individual's internal *vata-pitta-kapha* returns to the unique balance present at birth.

Balancing the Elements for Health

This natural balance can be re-established by working with diet, habits and attachments, as well as by making changes in the external environment. By consciously making discriminating choices, the knowledge of *Ayurveda* becomes an integral part of *sadhana*. Working with this wisdom helps purify the discriminating *buddhi* so that conscious choices are made in service to the *shreya* and not the *preya*.

The body is designed to operate in health, but habit patterns stored in the unconscious mind can motivate debilitating human actions that contribute to physical, mental and emotional dis-ease. Because the vast majority of diseases start in the mind, most are preventable—and many existing diseases are completely reversible—if individuals can adopt an enlightened holistic approach to maintaining good health.

The practice of *Ayurveda* promotes human contentment, health and creative growth. A sister science to yoga, *Ayurveda* is considered the mother of all intuitive healing arts. It helps the healthy person maintain health, and the diseased person regain health. Unlike some other medical systems, *Ayurveda* is not merely a band-aid applied to ameliorate a distressing symptom. By earnestly integrating the principles of *Ayurveda* into *sadhana*, an individual can actually retard the processes of physical deterioration and disease, develop skills that access superconscious knowledge and even accelerate the process of spiritual transformation.

During national healthcare debates in our country only two questions are generally considered: "What is my coverage?" and "How much is it going to cost me?" Media experts don't raise the specter of personal responsibility or ask the basic questions like, "What can I do right now, today and tomorrow, to enhance the odds that five, ten or twenty years from now my body is going to be healthy—not in need of any expensive medical procedure or confusing pharmacological regimen?" These questions aren't asked because our medical culture accepts disease as inevitable, and in most cases, unpreventable.

Yoga science and *Ayurveda*, however, assure us that there is much we can do proactively to improve and maintain our health. The key to good health is to be awake in the moment and to align every thought, word and action with the Divine wisdom reflected by the *buddhi*. By incorporating the knowledge of *Ayurveda* into our *sadhana*, we will find abundant opportunities to increase our reserves of energy, will power and creativity. Many of these opportunities involve food choices, which are discussed in Chapter 36.

Understanding the Disease Process

Ayurveda asserts that if we maintain the original balance with which we were born, the body will naturally function at its optimal level of health. However, for a number of reasons, this personal balance may not be easily maintained. A different balance of space, air, fire, water and earth forms the character of each food we consume. The specific hour of each day, the various seasons of the year and our own physical and mental processes all contribute *doshic* influences.

When we do not consider these factors, our natural *doshic* balance can become altered. This imbalance of the *doshas* retards the complete digestion of the food we eat and sets the disease process in motion. Incompletely digested food generates a poison called *ama*, which begins to accumulate in different receptive sites in the body. The most hospitable locations for *ama* are determined by our genetic weak links.

According to *Ayurveda*, all disease begins in the gut. When our imbalanced *doshas* cause food to be incompletely digested, the resulting *ama* is deposited in much the same way road crews fill springtime potholes in city streets. When sufficient *ama* is produced, the accumulating site can become so aggravated that it is effectively sealed off from the nourishing life force of vital *pranas* provided through the air and food. At that point, the seeds of dis-ease begin to sprout. Remember, the seeds of disease were always present in the potential state. The sages remind us that everything is contained in the *mantra AUM*. All of the seeds and the possibilities of life—past, present and future—exist at creation. Even the seeds of potential disease appear at the moment of conception. But in order for illness to manifest, the right conditions must arise, and in most cases, those right conditions mean an aggravation by *ama*.

Reversing the Disease Process:
The Role of Allopathic Medicine and Pharmacology

Neither *Ayurveda* nor yoga science advises, "Do not see a doctor; do not have an operation; do not take medicine." If the disease process has advanced to a critical stage, the best remedy at that point may indeed be an allopathic medicine or even surgery.

It's generally prudent to work in partnership with your

allopathic physician (M.D.). After all, yoga science proclaims that every thing and every one is a manifestation of the Divine Reality. That includes your medical doctor, surgeon and appropriate drugs, should any of these become necessary to restore your health.

In preventing or reversing disease, we can benefit our health simply by conscientiously filtering all thoughts, desires and emotions through the *buddhi*. Since we eat so often and have developed many attachments to foods we like and aversions to those we dislike, Swami Rama of the Himalayas taught that: "If we control the palate, we control our destiny."

The implications are profound. If the disease process has not advanced too far, we can initiate and accelerate the healing process by restoring our natural balance of *vata*, *pitta* and *kapha*. With a basic understanding of *Ayurvedic* principles we can retard the production of *ama*, enhance receptivity to healing *pranas* and encourage the body to fully manifest its inherent potential for good health.

CHAPTER 35
Understanding the Doshas

This food is Brahman; offered by Brahman; taken by Brahman; all is Brahman. May the fire of this food unite in yoga with the fire of our body and lead us for our highest and greatest good. May we convert this food into selfless acts of love.

PRAYER BEFORE EATING

The *doshas* provide a blueprint for understanding innate human tendencies. Each person's constitution can be understood as a combination of *doshic* characteristics, with one *dosha* typically predominating. Although one *dosha* may dominate, all three exist in varying proportions in each individual and in every cell, tissue and organ of the body. Once you understand the qualities of your particular body type, you can improve your health by making food and lifestyle choices according to *Ayurvedic* principles. These conscious choices become an integral part of your *sadhana*.

Vata Dosha

People in whom *vata* is predominant are generally the thinnest of the three *dosha* types, with narrow shoulders and / or hips. Some *vatas* have difficulty maintaining enough weight, others effortlessly stay slender and flexible, and some *vatas* who are willowy in their youth do become overweight in middle age. *Vatas*, ruled by movement, are creative, enthusiastic and adaptable in their work and relationships.

Vata Characteristics

Vata types generally perform activities quickly and have an aversion to cold weather. They are often animated, imaginative and quick to learn new information. Because most *vata* types tire easily from overexertion and have changeable energy levels, they need sustained nutrition throughout the day and imposed rest periods. *Vatas* can exhibit outbursts of emotion that are quickly forgotten. They are often worriers and may suffer from various symptoms of anxiety. *Vata* types are disposed toward constant change and irregular habits. They commonly walk quickly, speak with animated body language and often have a vocation that requires movement.

Vata constitutions may exhibit physical irregularities. Hands or feet may be too large or too small for the body, and teeth may be unusually small, large, unevenly spaced or protruding. An overbite is a fairly common *vata* characteristic. High *vata* types may have bowlegs, pigeon-toes, spinal curvature (scoliosis), a deviated septum or eyes that are close together or far apart. Their bones may be unusually light or heavy, short or very long. Joints, tendons and veins are visible on many *vata* bodies because the layer of fat beneath the skin is thin. Cracking joints are common.

Vata dosha is responsible for all motion. *Vata* regulates breathing, muscle movement, digestion and the workings of the central nervous system. When imbalanced, *vata* types experience such nervous disorders as depression, insomnia and many psychosomatic symptoms. Therefore, rebalancing the *vata* often ameliorates symptoms that do not respond to other forms of treatment.

An excess of *vata* can motivate a person to begin new projects without the desire or sustained energy to complete them. Such people may shop compulsively without buying anything, talk incessantly without making a point, and become chronically fatigued and dissatisfied. In the excitement of the moment, *vata* types may expend their resources imprudently, wasting money, energy and words.

Vata's inclination toward movement translates into short sleep cycles. Six hours or less is characteristic, growing shorter as *vata* types age. Common digestive complaints are chronic constipation, painful gas, cramping and bloating. Menstrual pain and arthritic conditions are also generally attributed to this *dosha*.

A balanced *vata* person is cheerful, enthusiastic and energetic. The *vata* mind is clear and alert, but extremely sensitive to change. *Vata* types have quick, acute responses to sound and touch, and dislike loud noise. Personalities that are vivacious, vibrant, excitable, unpredictable and imaginative typify *vata*.

Perhaps the most important quality of *vata* is that it portends change—movement. *Vata dosha* is considered the leading *dosha*, because when it is properly balanced, *pitta* and *kapha* are usually balanced as well. Because *vata* tends to go out of balance before *pitta* or *kapha*, *vata* is the *dosha* most responsible for the onset of the dis-ease process. *Vata* can mimic both *pitta* and *kapha doshas*, which sometimes makes it difficult to determine the precise cause of a specific problem or symptom.

Cautions for *Vata*

Vata types need sufficient rest and must not overburden their everyday routine. Movement is the predominant characteristic of this *dosha*, so *vata* types are inclined to overextend themselves and then to experience a sudden depletion of energy. However, by conscientious discipline, careful conservation of energy and making conscious choices between the *preya* and the *shreya*, *vata* types experience healthy, creative and joyful relationships.

Pitta Dosha

Fire is the predominant element of the *pitta dosha*. An

individual with red hair exhibits *pitta dosha*, as do those who are diligent, industrious, ambitious, sarcastic, opinionated, clever, contentious, resentful or sharp-tongued. The quarrelsome tendency of *pitta* is not uncommon, but it does not have to be indulged. When *pitta dosha* is balanced, *pittas* are amorous and enthusiastic in physical, mental and emotional relationships.

Pitta Characteristics

Pitta types have a moderate body build, vitality and stamina. They generally possess a fair or red-toned complexion, often with freckles or moles. The fire element causes most *pitta* types to be uncomfortable in hot, sunny weather, but it is also responsible for a powerful digestive system, intense hunger and thirst, and irritability when meals are late. *Pitta* types prefer cold foods and drinks and may awaken feeling hot and thirsty in the middle of the night. *Pittas* have enterprising personalities and like to be challenged. They have a keen intellect, and are generally astute, resourceful and shrewd. *Pittas* are good public speakers, have a strong memory and perform activity at a moderate rate of speed. They tend to become angry or impatient under stress. *Pitta* types feel comfortable controlling situations and often display a tendency to be abrupt, demanding or critical. They walk and move with determination and purpose.

Pittas usually maintain their body weight without drastic change—not finding it too difficult to gain or lose weight as they desire. Facial features are well-proportioned; eyes are of medium size, often with a penetrating glance. Hands and feet are also of medium size and joints are normal.

Pitta hair is usually straight and fine, red, blond or sandy colored, and may gray prematurely. Baldness, thinning hair or a receding hairline are all signs of a strong *pitta*.

Pittas generally have above-average powers of concentration. They are methodical and steward their resources, such as energy and money, with efficiency. Spending on luxuries is one notable exception—*pittas* love to be surrounded by the finer things of life. They are generally more visually observant than the other *doshas*.

Because of the predominance of the fire element, *pitta* types may experience warm hands and feet and burning sensations in the eyes, skin, stomach or intestines.

The fire element of *pitta* can be expressed in widely diverse behavior. Unbalanced *pitta* types can become short-tempered or argumentative in their search for perfection, but they often become precise, articulate speakers and leaders.

For all body types, *pitta dosha* is the controller of metabolism. *Pitta* types tend to have a strong digestive fire (*agni*), but eating too much *pitta* food (defined in the next chapter) can cause them to experience heartburn and may eventually lead to stomach ulcers and hemorrhoids.

Other areas of the human body are similarly affected by the fire of *pitta dosha*. The skin, for example, can easily become irritated with rashes and acne. The white portion of the eyes often turns red, causing an uncomfortable burning sensation. *Pittas* generally sleep for eight hours a night, but when their fire *dosha* is out of balance, they may experience insomnia—very often as a consequence of their all-consuming desire to work.

Cautions for *Pitta*

The best advice for *Pitta* types is to take the path of moderation. As with the other *doshas*, physical, mental and emotional well-being is dependent on the conscious choices we make. Since every cell in the body depends on the element of fire to maintain its healthy function, conscious decisions about what and when to eat quickly impact the experiences of *pitta* types. Remembering to respond with patience and tolerance in everyday situations is especially valuable to *pitta* types in improving their relationships.

Kapha Dosha

Kapha dosha expresses the attributes of earth and water.

Therefore, *kapha* types are often relaxed, balanced, steady and poised, with great physical strength and endurance. As a rule, they enjoy good health, while expressing a serene, joyful and tranquil view of the world.

Kapha Characteristics

Kapha types have solid, heavily built bodies with great physical strength and resilience. Slow and methodical, they possess consistent levels of energy. *Kapha* hair is plentiful, thick and wavy, and the skin is oily and smooth.

Because *kaphas* possess only a moderate supply of the fire element, they may experience slow digestion, mild hunger and frequent weight gains. They often use food for emotional comfort. *Kapha* types generally have an easy-going personality, but have difficulty with change. Though *kapha* types are caring people—often showing concern and empathy for others—they also have a tendency to be possessive, jealous and complacent. *Kaphas* are generally slow learners, but they do have good retentive memories. Their sleep is often heavy and prolonged.

Kapha types exhibit reliable, natural strength, resistance to disease and a sense of inner security. They tend to have wide hips and/or shoulders. They generally have large, attractive eyes and thick eyebrows and eyelashes.

Kapha dosha is expressed by slow, deliberate eating, digestion and speaking. Composed and self-contained, *kapha* types are slow to anger and try to reconcile differences. It is very *kapha* to be affectionate, tolerant, forgiving and nurturing. To be motherly is to express *kapha*.

Kaphas are not easily jangled in a crisis, and they support others around them. Expressing the elements of earth and water, their natural response to the world is through taste and smell. *Kaphas*, therefore, tend to place a great deal of importance on food. *Kapha's* accumulate money, possessions, energy, food and fat. The fat is usually stored in the thighs and buttocks.

Cautions for *Kapha*

Because this *dosha* controls the moist tissues of the body, a *kapha* imbalance will tend to be expressed in the mucous membranes. In the *kapha* seasons of late winter and spring, *kapha* types are prone to experience sinus congestion, chest colds, allergies, asthma and painful joints. The prevalent negative emotion for *kapha* is covetousness or over-attachment. Anyone who finds it difficult to throw out old clothes or other possessions is expressing an excess of *kapha*.

Kapha types need movement and stimulation. Any inactive situation turns *kapha* stability into grogginess or lethargy. *Kapha* types need to be vigilant concerning their attachment to memories, people, possessions and circumstances, and must consciously strive to be more open to new possibilities.

Ayurveda's Hidden Benefit

On a beautiful Sunday afternoon during a Christmas visit to California, we were driving across the Golden Gate Bridge from San Francisco to Marin County. Because schools were on recess, the walkways were filled with hundreds of students, families, friends and lots of tourists.

As we proceeded across the bridge, we began to make some mental observations based on our knowledge of *Ayurveda*. We informally calculated that 80 percent of the people on the bridge that afternoon were *vata*. Most of them were smiling and very happy. We estimated that another 15 percent were *pitta*. The *pitta* types were not quite as ebullient as the *vatas*, but they were having a good time. Then there were the five percent we viewed as *kapha*. They were easy to spot. Their unmistakable body language was broadcasting to the world that they'd rather be somewhere with plenty of comforting earth under their feet.

This story illustrates an important point: *Ayurveda* not only teaches us about ourselves—it also provides a virtual encyclopedia of information about the physical, mental and emotional propensities of other people. Because each one of us is a unique mixture of *vata, pitta* and *kapha,* this kind of casual application of *Ayurveda* cannot be 100 percent accurate. Still, it does provide an experienced observer valuable information in the first minutes of a new acquaintance, and increased sensitivity in established relationships. Its practical wisdom allows us to be more understanding and compassionate with our own limitations and more skillful in the ways we meet the daily challenges of all our personal interactions.

Ayurveda Body Type Test

The following quiz will help you determine your Ayurvedic body type. The analysis is divided into three sections. For each of the 28 questions, choose the *dosha* that best describes you (*vata, pitta* or *kapha*) and mark, on a numerical scale from zero to six, the extent to which it applies to you.

0 = Doesn't apply to me
3 = Applies to me somewhat (or some of the time)
6 = Applies to me very much (or nearly all of the time)

At the bottom of the *vata* column, write down your total *vata* score. For example, if you mark a 6 for the first question, a 3 for the second, and a 1 for the third, your total at that point would be 6 + 3 + 1 = 10. Total the entire section in this way until you arrive at your final *vata* score. Proceed in the same way to find your totals for *pitta* and for *kapha*. When you are finished, you will have three separate scores. Comparing these will determine your body type. Your highest score indicates your leading *dosha*. (See page 326 for more information about dual or *tri-doshic* types.)

Our bodies and attitudes may change slightly over time. Answer according to how you have been, have felt and have acted most of your life, or at least for the last few years.

Once you've completed the *Ayurveda* Body-Type Test and

are familiar with the characteristics and influences of your primary *dosha*, identify any physical, mental or emotional issues you are presently dealing with. If there are none, it probably means that your *doshas* are in balance and your food choices are serving you well. However, if you do note symptoms, begin to experiment with changes in your diet that can rebalance your *doshas* and ameliorate your discomforts. Learning to base your food choices on the *buddhi*'s discrimination will yield profound results. This process will be explained in the next chapter.

	VATA	PITTA	KAPHA
Body	Small Frame	Medium Frame	Large Frame
Weight	Thin, Hard to Gain	Medium Weight	Heavy, Easy to Gain
Skin	Dry, Rough	Soft, Medium Oily	Oily, Moist
Complexion	Dark	Pink to Red	Pale, White
Amount of Hair	Average	Thinning	Thick
Type of Hair	Dry	Medium	Oily
Endurance	Poor	Good	Excellent
Strength	Poor	Good	Excellent
Size of Teeth	Very Large or Small	Small to Medium	Medium to Large
Mental Activity	Quick Mind, Restless	Sharp Intellect, Aggressive	Calm, Steady, Stable
Memory	Short Term is Best	Good Memory	Long Term is Best
Dreams	Fearful, Flying, Running	Angry, Fiery, Violent	Water, Clouds, Romance
Weather	Aversion to Cold	Aversion to Heat	Aversion to Damp & Cold
Sleep	Interrupted, Light	Sound, Medium Length	Sound, Heavy, Long
React to Stress	Excites Quickly	Angers Easily, Quick Temper	Slow to Irritate

	VATA	PITTA	KAPHA
Resting Pulse Rate, (Beats/Minute)			
Women	—— 80-100	—— 70-80	—— 60-70
Men	—— 70-90	—— 60-70	—— 50-60
Hunger	—— Irregular	—— Sharp, Needs Food	—— Easily Misses Meals
Food & Drink	—— Prefers Warm	—— Prefers Cold	—— Prefers Dry & Warm
Eat	—— Quickly	—— Medium Speed	—— Slowly
Financial	—— Doesn't Save	—— Saver & Big Spender	—— Saver, Accumulates Wealth
Sex Drive	—— Variable, Irregular	—— Moderate	—— Strong
Elimination	—— Dry, Hard, Constipation	—— Frequent, Soft to Normal	—— Heavy, Slow, Thick, Regular
Walk	—— Fast, Quick Steps	—— Average	—— Slow & Steady
Voice	—— High Pitch, Fast Speech	—— Medium Pitch, Clear	—— Low Pitch, Resonating
Moods	—— Change Quickly	—— Change Slowly	—— Steady, Slow to Change
Totals	—— **Vata**	—— **Pitta**	—— **Kapha**

CHAPTER 36

Food Sadhana

The seed of God is in us. Given an intelligent and hard-working farmer, it will thrive and grow up to God, whose seed it is; and accordingly its fruits will be God-nature. Pear seeds grow into pear trees, nut seeds into nut trees, and God seed into God.

MEISTER ECKHART

Would you be pleased if each new day brought you plenty of energy for all of life's duties and responsibilities? Would you be relieved if you never again experienced pangs of guilt for not having sufficient will power to do what your conscience suggests? Would you be happy personally and successful professionally if you could become the creative person you always wanted to be? Yoga science professes that you can experience the changes you seek. One practical mechanism that is always available for accomplishing these changes is *food sadhana*—the spiritual practice of transforming your everyday desires for certain foods into ready supplies of energy, will power and creativity.

The ancient *Mundaka Upanishad* describes two golden birds who are constant companions, perched in the same tree. One bird is the separate, individual self, ignorantly living in the world of duality and believing that objects and relationships bring happiness. The second bird is the immortal *Atman* (*Sat-Chit-Ananda*). The former tastes the sweet and bitter fruits of the tree, seeking the pleasant but experiencing the pain as well. The latter remains still, calmly watching with *vairagya* (non-attachment), and eternally enjoying its own perfect fullness and the abundance of all it sees. The limited self, having forgotten its own true identity, experiences various forms of dis-ease until it recognizes that the same Divine Reality within its companion is also within him. It is through this Self-realization that the separate self unites with the One Absolute Reality, *Brahman*, and becomes free of pain.

The image of the two birds illustrates the ultimate truth about man's real and apparent natures. Our suffering, the story explains, is a function of being ignorant of our Essential Nature—the bliss-filled *Atman*. But suffering need not be the norm. As we practice and experience the truth of yoga science, we recognize the innate power hidden within all of our desires—including our desire for food.

Our bodies are made up of food and water, a delicate balance of the five elements. The body itself is transitory—subject to change, death and decomposition—yet it houses the Eternal. When we begin to understand and incorporate this knowledge into our daily practice of yoga science, the act of eating becomes a sacrament. When we begin to make conscious choices about which foods to eat and what to give attention to during the eating process, our *food sadhana* can become a powerful and practical mechanism to increase our inner reserves of energy, boost our will power and expand our capacity for creativity.

Desire, in and of itself, is not bad. It's like gasoline in a combustion engine: it's the fuel for action. Without desire, nothing is ever accomplished. But not all desires, including desires for certain foods, will lead us for our highest and greatest good. Only when every thought, word and action is in harmony with the *buddhi* can the transformational power of yoga science manifest the energy, will power and creativity we need.

When a thought about what to eat comes into your awareness, remember that the food you consume builds, repairs and maintains the instrument of action that the Divine Reality uses to unfold the continuing story of creation. When the desire for a certain food begins to grow, ask immediately, "Who is the thinker of this thought? Who am I? Who is aware of a desire for this particular food?" This process of self-inquiry breaks your identification with the body and helps you to analyze which function of the mind is suggesting that a particular food be consumed. Ask yourself if the *manas* is merely transmitting messages it has received from the non-discriminating senses. Ask yourself if the *ahamkara* is trying to steer you toward the pleasant or away from the unpleasant. Ask yourself if the suggestion is being fueled by some comforting memory or desire from the *chitta*.

Then, become proactive. Step out of old habit patterns. Ask the *chitta* to bring forward information you've learned about *Ayurveda*. Ask the *chitta* to list foods that will help balance your *doshas*. Ask the *buddhi*, your discriminative faculty, if your choice of food is in harmony with *ahimsa*. Will consumption of the food be an act of kindness toward the body? Will the food assist the body in serving the Divine Reality, without causing illness or discomfort?

Armed with that information, consult the *buddhi* again and listen as it defines the prospective food choice as either *preya* or *shreya*. If the answer comes back "*shreya*," consume the food and enjoy it. It will lead you for your highest and greatest good. If the *buddhi* defines the food choice as *preya*, exercise the muscles of your will power by lovingly and willingly surrendering the desire back to the Origin from which it has come. In simple terms, consciously decide that for the attainment of your deepest driving desire for unbounded Life, Liberty and Happiness—you are willing to give up the *preya*.

The result of this kind of spiritual practice is remarkable. When you willingly and consciously surrender the desire for a specific food, the power residing in the *preya* is transformed into strategic reserves of energy, will power and consciousness. Because we eat so frequently, many opportunities come our way every day to increase our personal bank accounts of energy, will and creativity. These resources are not produced magically. They result from our own choices—the conscious use of our own inherent energy.

Medieval city-states were protected by high, impenetrable walls. To gain access, a visitor was required to announce himself at the main gate, credibly identify himself, state his intended purpose and justify the duration of his stay. Only after such thorough examination was right of entry granted.

When a thought or desire for a specific food seeks entrance into our city of life, most of us wave it in with hardly a second glance. Our habitual food choices are based on our likes and dislikes (raga/dveshas), and these have generally been formed by the boisterous clamor of the senses, ego and chitta. By remaining under the sway of this committee, we are actually choosing to satisfy our likes and dislikes in preference to attaining our supreme Happiness. Food sadhana changes the priorities. It acknowledges the information of the senses, ego and chitta, but employs the discrimination and Divine wisdom of a purified buddhi before a decision is made.

A spiritual seeker once asked his master to teach him the truth that would bring him Happiness and end his sorrow. The master agreed. "You will know the truth," he said, "when you go to the nearby well, draw three buckets full of water, and fill a large tub for bathing." With great eagerness the student lowered the bucket, filled it with water and raised it, only to find that the bucket was empty. He lowered the bucket to the bottom of the well a second time, filled it with water, raised it up and again found it to be empty. Then, before he lowered the bucket for the third time, he carefully examined the bottom of the bucket and discovered that it was riddled with tiny holes.

The mind is our most powerful instrument for realizing our ultimate Happiness, but we unconsciously allow more energy to pour out of the mind in service to our habits than we can harness to attain our highest and greatest good.

Food sadhana is not intended to deprive us of the small, sensory pleasures that life offers. Though we are not the body, yoga science acknowledges that we certainly do have a body.

We have senses, and life is to be enjoyed. Therefore, if you have a persistent desire for chocolate, order chocolate mousse or a slice of chocolate cake every couple of months at your favorite restaurant and thoroughly enjoy the pleasure without any guilt. However, do not constantly deplete your reserves of energy, will power and creativity by bringing these items into the home every week. This only further enslaves you to your habitual likes and dislikes (raga/dveshas) while increasing your physical, mental and emotional dis-ease.

Remember, every desire is made up of three basic components: energy, will power and creativity. If you feel tired, stressed and anxious because of the demands life is making, if you wish you had more will power to successfully fulfill your responsibilities, and if you could use more creative ideas in dealing with all that comes to you, then expand your practice of yoga science and *Ayurveda* by consciously examining your relationship with food. As you begin to choose those foods endorsed by the *buddhi* as *shreya,* and are able to surrender your desires for foods the *buddhi* defines as *preya,* you will gain access to a limitless store of strength, will and creativity. Your body will become less taxed and more healthy, and new-found wisdom from the superconscious mind can lead you to the summum bonum of life.

General Suggestions for all *Doshas*

The following suggestions are garnered from *Ayurvedic* authorities, common sense wisdom and our own personal experiences. As with all practices of yoga science, honor *ahimsa* in your experimentation. After you've worked with each suggestion, its beneficial effects will increase your openness to making further constructive changes in your life. The most important step is simply to begin.

Avoid taking a meal until the previous meal has been digested, allowing three to five hours between meals. Always sit down to eat in a settled and quiet atmosphere at roughly the same time each day. Do not work, read or watch television during meals. Don't eat too quickly or too slowly. Consume about three quarters of your stomach's capacity, and chew your food twenty to thirty times before swallowing. Never eat during a serious emotional upset. Do not leave the table feeling very hungry or feeling very full. Take a few minutes to sit quietly after eating before returning to your activity.

A desire for food may be your physiology's means of expressing what it needs to achieve a balance of the *vata*, *pitta* and *kapha doshas*. However, when the *buddhi* advises that your desire for a certain food arises from some habitual pattern (*samskara*) or is the expression of an existing doshic imbalance, it is an indication that the desire may be *preya*. If so, the attachment to the desire is to be welcomed and surrendered.

Eat first-generation foods whenever possible—reducing your reliance on frozen foods and prepared mixes. Food should be freshly cooked. Vital *prana* begins to disappear from food soon after it is prepared, so minimize your consumption of leftovers. Food is best eaten warm and well-cooked. Your meals should be pleasing to the eye—providing a balanced variety of colors, textures and tastes (sweet, sour, salty, bitter, pungent and astringent). Yogurt, cheese, cottage cheese and cultured buttermilk should be avoided at night. Do not bake or cook with honey. When heated to high temperatures, honey produces toxins. Milk that has been brought just to boiling and taken just before bedtime induces sleep and is highly recommended for *vata dosha*.

If you're reducing meat consumption in a standard Western diet, substitute lentils or split washed mung beans (served with rice) to supply a complete protein. To reduce the gas that beans can produce, clean, wash and soak them at least an hour and rinse them thoroughly again before cooking. Prepare them with onions, *ghee* and your favorite spices. Always rinse rice thoroughly before cooking.

Clarified butter, or *ghee* is preferable to butter or margarine. Although *ghee* does contain cholesterol, the absence of animal solids makes it a better choice for clean arteries and veins. According to *Ayurveda*, *ghee* is a superb source of *ojas* (life force) and facilitates improved absorption of the nutrients of any food it's cooked or served with. *Ghee's* healing properties make it a standard ingredient of rejuvenating tonics and an important part of any strength-building regimen.

For optimal health, some foods are best reduced or eliminated entirely from the diet. Try eliminating red meat of any kind, shell fish (all bottom-feeding scavengers), and white refined sugar. Reduce commercially prepared granola, breads containing yeast, highly processed cheeses and acidic foods. Limit your intake of such nightshade family vegetables as tomato paste, potatoes and eggplant. These contain substances known to cause joint pain and inflammation in some sensitive individuals.

Digestion is most efficient when the right nostril is activated. One to three cycles of *Nadi Shodhana* can accomplish this before a meal. A good quality, natural, full-spectrum multiple vitamin/mineral supplement every day is essential. To maintain healthy intestinal flora, take a pro-biotic, like acidophilus, daily.

Some form of gentle aerobic exercise should be undertaken every day. The exertion should be great enough to cause you to perspire—sweating out toxins from the body.

The Million Dollar Prescription

One of the most important steps you can take to enhance your overall well-being is to drink six to eight cups of plain hot water each day. The water should be drunk at the same temperature as hot coffee or tea. Do not add lemon or herbs. When consumed regularly, the hot liquid regimen will feel comforting. Hot water is generally used to clean dishes because it efficiently removes food residue. Similarly, hot water cleanses the entire urinary system and acts as a tonic. Any heat that you ingest above 98.6 degrees Fahrenheit offers instant energy to the body. Even after physical exercise, when the senses clamor for a cold drink, the more sensible option is a cup of plain hot water.

ADDITIONAL
AYURVEDIC PRACTICES

Nasal Wash

With its refined mechanism of hairs and mucous membranes, a healthy nasal filtering system is an important part of the body's immune defense system. Unfortunately, this filtering mechanism can become overloaded. In today's world, the body is asked to deal with a wide range of airborne chemicals and particulates. In addition, the Western diet favors foods that increase the body's production of mucus, often clogging the nasal passages and sinuses. Practicing daily nasal hygiene can be an important part of keeping the upper respiratory system functioning at peak efficiency.

Use a *neti pot* (nasal wash) morning and night to cleanse the nasal passages. Doctors and alternative health care practitioners around the world recommend the regular practice of nasal cleansing with a saline solution for health and well-being. Daily use of a *neti pot* helps keep sinuses clean and makes it easier to breathe freely. Most find the practice helpful in preventing colds and dealing with the effects of pollution, dust, allergies and the airborne spray of winter road salt.

Neti pots are available through the American Meditation Institute and most health food stores.

Tongue Scraper

Use a dry toothbrush or tongue scraper in the morning and evening. This practice easily removes *ama* and waste products that ordinarily accumulate on the tongue during sleep and throughout the day. Tongue scrapers are also available in most health food stores.

Oil Massage

Because of the frantic pace of our culture, *vata dosha*—in all people—tends to become unbalanced, increasing levels of anxiety, restlessness and dissatisfaction. One very pleasant remedy is the rejuvenating daily practice of *abhyanga*, massaging the body with warm sesame oil. This simple self-massage increases well-being by immediately rebalancing and stimulating the nervous and endocrine systems.

Traditional *Ayurveda* recommends *oil massage* as an early morning practice, but we suggest that you also consider it as a valuable addition to your preparations for evening meditation and sleep.

Pour a few tablespoons of refined sesame oil into a small cup or plastic squeeze bottle. Place the container in a pan of hot water until the oil is slightly warmer than body temperature. The amount of sesame oil to be used for the *oil massage* is small, but take precautions against spills and stains. This practice is best performed in the bathroom. When you finish the oil massage, rest for a few minutes while practicing *japa* and then take a warm bath or shower. (Leaving oil on the body overnight can also be nurturing, but if you experiment, be sure to take precautions against staining sheets and pillowcases.)

To begin this practice, place a small amount of warm sesame oil (or specially formulated oil for individual *doshas*) in the palm of the hand. Rub the hands together and begin your massage at the top of the head. Gently massage the scalp with small, circular motions. With your pinkie, place a dab of oil inside the ears and lightly massage the ears, temples, neck and throat.

Move downward to the shoulders, elbows, wrists and hands, massaging the joints in a circular motion and flat surfaces (such as upper arms and forearms) with longer up-and-down strokes.

Keeping a small amount of oil on the palms and using larger circular movements, massage the heart center, solar plexus, bladder region and sacrum.

Work downward with circular motions over the hips, knees and ankles. Use longer up-and-down strokes along the thighs and lower legs.

Finally, keeping a small supply of warm oil on the hands,

gently massage both feet. The soles of the feet contain a multitude of nerve endings, which, when stimulated, send beneficial messages to the entire body. Start the foot massage with the tips of the toes, moving in small, circular motions. Continue systematically to massage the balls of the feet, arches, heel and achilles tendon. Finish with a bit of oil on the palms and gently massage the entire sole of the foot.

DIETS
TO BALANCE YOUR DOSHAS

On the following pages, *Ayurvedic* diets appear for all *doshas* to guide you in your food selection.

You may note that the same food may appear on both the FAVOR list and the REDUCE/AVOID list for the *vata, pitta* and *kapha* diets presented on the following pages. These apparent conflicts can be explained by considering three factors: (1) the unique balance of *vata-pitta-kapha* of each person, (2) the unique balance of *vata-pitta-kapha* existing in each food, and (3) the fact that the lists are skewed because of the slightly differing effects experienced by the authors and other *Ayurvedic* authorities.

Whenever the same food appears on *both* the FAVOR list and the REDUCE/AVOID list, experiment and pay extra attention to the effects it has on your particular constitution.

Consider the sweet potato, which is almost equally *pitta* and *kapha*. Is it a *pitta* food or a *kapha* food? A *pitta-kapha* constitution may experience the sweet potato as a *pitta*-increasing inflammatory agent or as a calming *kapha* food. For the *pitta-kapha* person, the answer will come only with experimentation.

VATA DIETS

Vata Diet (FAVOR)
Vata types should favor these foods.
They tend to decrease vata.

Vegetables: artichoke, asparagus, avocado, beets, carrots, chilies, cilantro, garlic (cooked), green beans, mustard greens, okra, onions (cooked), parsley, radishes, seaweed, squash, sweet potatoes, turnips, watercress

Fruits*: apples (cooked), apricots, bananas, cherries, dates (fresh or rehydrated), figs (fresh or rehydrated), grapefruit, grapes, lemons, limes, mangoes, oranges, papaya, peaches, persimmons, pineapples, prunes (rehydrated), raspberries, strawberries
In moderation. Most vata types need to limit their fruit intake.

Grains: basmati rice, brown rice, couscous, oats, spelt, wheat

Beans: mung beans, tofu

Nuts and Seeds: All are acceptable in small amounts, but cashews are best; almonds, brazil nuts, cashews, coconut, filberts, pecans, pine nuts, pumpkin seeds, sesame seeds, sunflower seeds

Dairy: butter, buttermilk, cheese, cottage cheese, cream, ghee, kefir, milk, paneer, sour cream, yogurt

Animal Products: chicken, eggs, fish, turkey

Oils: almond, avocado, coconut, ghee, mustard, olive, peanut, sesame

Sweeteners: fructose, honey, maple syrup, molasses, raw sugar

Spices: asafoetida, basil, black pepper, cayenne, cardamom, cinnamon, cloves, coriander, cumin, fennel, fenugreek, ginger, horseradish, mint, mustard, nutmeg, rock salt, sea salt, turmeric

VATA DIETS

Vata Diet (AVOID/REDUCE)
Vata types should reduce or avoid these foods.
They tend to increase vata.

Vegetables: broccoli, brussels sprouts, cabbage, cauliflower, celery, cucumber, eggplant, leafy greens, lettuce, mushrooms, onions (raw), peas, peppers, potatoes, sprouts, tomatoes, zucchini, raw vegetables in general

Fruits: apples (raw), dried fruit, pears

Grains: barley, buckwheat, corn, dry cereals, millet, quinoa, rye

Beans: aduki, chick peas, kidney, lentils, lima, peanuts, pinto, soy (except tofu), split peas

Nuts and Seeds: none (see favor list)

Dairy: all dairy is acceptable

Animal Products: red meat (beef, lamb), pork

Oils: corn, margarine, safflower, soy

Sweeteners: white refined sugar

Spices: none

PITTA DIETS

Pitta Diet (FAVOR)
Pitta types should favor these foods.
They tend to decrease pitta.

Vegetables: asparagus, broccoli, brussels sprouts, cabbage, cauliflower, celery, cucumber, green beans, leafy greens, lettuce, mushrooms, okra, parsley, peas, potatoes, sprouts, squash, sunflower sprouts, sweet potatoes, zucchini

Fruits: apples, cherries, coconuts, figs, grapes, mangoes, melons, oranges, pears, pineapples, plums, prunes, raisins (all should be sweet and ripe)

Grains: basmati rice, brown rice (long grain), barley, blue corn, couscous, oats, quinoa, spelt, wheat, white rice

Beans: aduki, chick peas, kidney, mung beans, peanuts, split peas, tofu and other soybean products

Nuts and Seeds: coconut, pumpkin seeds, sunflower seeds

Dairy: butter, cottage cheese, cream, ghee, milk, paneer

Animal Products: chicken, egg whites, turkey (in small amounts)

Oils: coconut, olive, soy, sunflower

Sweeteners: all are acceptable except honey and molasses

Spices: cardamom, cilantro, coriander seeds, dill, fennel, mint, saffron, turmeric

PITTA DIETS

Pitta Diet (AVOID /REDUCE)
Pitta types should reduce or avoid these foods.
They tend to increase pitta.

Vegetables: avocados, beets, carrots, chard, chilies, corn, eggplant, garlic, hot peppers, onions (raw), radishes, seaweed, spinach, sweet potatoes, tomatoes, turnips, watercress

Fruits: apricots, bananas, berries, cherries, cranberries, grapefruit, lemons, limes, papaya, peaches, persimmon, strawberries (avoid fruits that come to market sour or unripe; green grapes, oranges, pineapple and plums should be sweet)

Grains: brown rice (short grain), buckwheat, corn, millet, rye

Beans: lentils

Nuts and Seeds: most (see favor list)

Dairy: buttermilk, cheese, ice cream, kefir, sour cream, yogurt

Animal Products: egg yolks, red meat, seafood in general

Oils: almond, corn, safflower, sesame

Sweeteners: all are acceptable except honey and molasses

Spices: asafoetida, barbecue sauce, basil, black pepper, catsup, cayenne, cinnamon, cloves, fenugreek, garlic, ginger, horseradish, mustard, nutmeg, pickles, salt, sour salad dressings, all spicy condiments, vinegar

KAPHA DIETS

Kapha Diet (FAVOR)
Kapha types should favor these foods.
They tend to decrease kapha.

Vegetables: asparagus, beets, bell peppers, broccoli, brussels sprouts, cabbage, carrots, cauliflower, celery, chilies, cilantro, garlic, green beans, leafy greens, mushrooms, okra, onions (cooked), parsley, peas, peppers, radishes, spinach sprouts

Fruits: apples, apricots, cranberries, pears, pomegranates (dried fruits are preferable)

Grains: barley, basmati rice, corn, millet, rye, spelt

Beans: mung beans are best (other beans are more difficult to digest)

Nuts and Seeds: almonds, pumpkin seeds

Dairy: skim milk (only if heated and rarely in *kapha* seasons or days)

Animal Products: chicken, turkey (white meat)

Oils: almond, corn, ghee, safflower, sunflower

Sweeteners: raw, unheated honey

Spices: all (hot spices like black pepper, ginger and cumin generally increase digestive fire)

KAPHA DIETS

Kapha Diet (AVOID /REDUCE)
Kapha types should reduce or avoid these foods.
They tend to increase kapha.

Vegetables: avocados, cucumbers, lettuce, seaweed, squash, sweet potatoes, zucchini

Fruits: bananas, cherries, coconuts, dates, figs, grapefruit, grapes, lemons, limes, mangoes, melons, oranges, papaya, peaches, pineapple, plums, raspberries, strawberries

Grains: brown rice, buckwheat, couscous, oats, wheat

Beans: mung beans are best (reduce or eliminate other beans)

Nuts and Seeds: most (see favor list)

Dairy: most (see favor list)

Animal Products: red meat and seafood in general

Oils: most (see favor list)

Sweeteners: most (see favor list)

Spices: salt

Part X

EASY-GENTLE YOGA

CHAPTER 37

Easy-Gentle Yoga

When you make the two into one, when you make the inner like the outer, and the upper like the lower, when you make the male and the female into one, so that the male will not be male and the female will not be female . . . then you will enter the kingdom.

JESUS THE CHRIST (THE GOSPEL OF THOMAS)

One can find many mysterious passages in the scriptures, but Jesus the Christ is never more cryptic than when He advises in the Gospel of Thomas that we must "make the male and female into one" in order to enter the kingdom of Heaven. What is He talking about and what is the connection between these words and the practice of *Easy-Gentle Yoga*? For the earnest seeker, the answer to this riddle lies in understanding the origins of the physical exercises known as *hatha* and their relationship to the broader science of yoga.

There are various yoga paths, each appropriate to people of a particular temperament and capabilities. The major paths include *bhakti yoga* (devotion), *jnana yoga* (intellectual knowledge), *karma yoga* (selfless service), and *raja yoga* (the "royal path" because it includes teachings from all yogic paths). *Hatha yoga* is a spiritual path for those who find the physical body to be their most natural passageway to the Divine, but as part of a balanced *sadhana*, it is a valuable tool for all. Its concentrated physical discipline can prepare one to realize, through direct experience, that the *Atman* (the soul of the individual) is, as it always has been, none other than the One Supreme Reality.

If you were to ask the average person to define the word yoga, your request would probably conjure up images of exceptionally limber people bending their bodies into unusual shapes. However, the physical yoga with which most people are familiar developed from one aspect of a greater oral tradition that dates back some five thousand years—the eight-fold path codified by Patanjali (see *Eight Steps of Yoga Science*, Chapter 1).

Yoga was already an ancient and comprehensive science when, around 1000 A.D., a specialized branch emerged. The new *hatha* yoga, emphasizing only the *yamas, niyamas, asana* and *pranayama*, was adopted primarily as a health regimen for the body and mind. Although *hatha* did originally teach breath awareness as a method of reaching *samadhi*, it gave little attention to meditation and mastery of the senses—those aspects of *raja* yoga it had traditionally supported. This new branch (which initially consisted of only a few postures) maintained a small but enduring presence until the turn of the twentieth century when it blossomed, in the West, into the largely American synthesis of stretching, strengthening, balancing and relaxation we are familiar with today.

The etymology of the Sanskrit word *hatha* offers some important insights into the traditional relationship between *hatha* and yoga science. The word *ha* means sun. It represents the active, masculine principle lying within the right nostril breath (*pingala*). The word *tha* means moon. It represents the intuitive and passive feminine principle that manifests through the left nostril breath (*ida*).

When *asanas* (physical postures) and *pranayama* (breath exercises) facilitate an equal volume of air passing through the right and left nostrils, the *wedding of the sun and moon* takes place—balancing the male and female energies. This balance induces the central *sushumna* channel in the subtle body (*pranamaya kosha*) to swell—allowing the creative energy of *shakti* (also called *kundalini*) to rise from the lower *chakras* to the higher *chakras* in preparation for meditation and the awakening of Divine consciousness.

Similarly, in the Gospel of Thomas, Jesus the Christ teaches that Self-realization, or *Christ-consciousness*, can occur only "When you make the two into one, when you make the inner like the outer, and the upper like the lower, when you make the male and the female into one, so that the male will not be male and the female will not be female . . . then you will enter the kingdom."

Many passages from the Bible appear to have hidden meanings. In this case, however, yoga science makes the words crystal clear. Jesus the Christ is first explaining that we attain liberation by putting aside our *raga/dveshas*—our attractions and aversions to the relative truths we cherish. True freedom occurs naturally when we are no longer enslaved to alluring pairs of opposites like good and bad, pleasant and unpleasant. Additionally, it appears that He may be reminding us that *hatha* is the means to establishing the *wedding of the sun and moon*. By purifying and balancing the male and female aspects of our body, breath and mind through *hatha*, a seeker is prepared for concentration, meditation and, ultimately, *samadhi* (union with the Divine).

Unfortunately, without a basic underlying understanding, *hatha*, like any other exercise program, runs the risk of reinforcing desires for physical accomplishment and short-term emotional highs. Without practicing the complete philosophy of yoga science, *hatha* may become just another form of ego gratification or a feel-good experience. We can become fixated on testing our physical skills or competing against others.

This narrow perspective can produce an effect no more profound than would swimming, tennis, golf or running. *Hatha* may free us from dis-ease in the short term, but unless it's understood as an integrated practice of yoga science, it cannot become the cure for our stressful condition.

In *hatha* yoga the body and the subtle energy within the body become the focus of our concentrated attention, in the same way we use the *mantra* in seated meditation. When the body assumes a specific position (*asana*) we find that certain thoughts, emotions, memories and attachments arise in our conscious mind. Each is welcomed, witnessed and honored and then surrendered back to the Origin from which it has come, and we then redirect our attention back to the body and its energy.

Valuable information can be gleaned by making physical yoga a meditation practice. During your *contemplation* (a quiet time during the day), review the thoughts, desires and emotions that have come forward during your *hatha* practice, just as you review the attachments revealed in your seated meditation practice. By analyzing these issues and feelings in light of the four primitive urges for food, sex, sleep and self-preservation, you will gain great insight into how your vital energy can best be used. (see *Contemplation*, Chapter 39).

By consciously integrating your *hatha* practice into your *sadhana*, you will accelerate the transformation of previously debilitating forces into positive reserves of energy, will power and creativity. In this way, *hatha* becomes a means of union—a yoga—serving both your spiritual growth and your current daily needs.

Hatha, like the larger science of yoga from which it grew, requires continuous *abhyasa* (practice) and *vairagya* (non-attachment and surrender). The importance of consistent practice is an obvious part of any physical training, but the value of sacrifice in *hatha* may not be as readily apparent. In *hatha* we surrender the habitual way we look at life and ourselves. As we focus on what appears in the moment, rather than what our preconceptions tell us, we recognize that our bodily stiffness is actually the physical evidence of our own mental conditioning. In *hatha*, our willingness to let go of attachments facilitates a total absorption and joy in the appreciation of what presents itself in the moment. Together, this acceptance and surrender offer us the freedom to experience the bliss of total engagement and the blessings of our innate fullness. In order to gain anything, we must first sacrifice something. Giving up our addictions to habitual desires and the gratification of the ego and senses frees us to reap the full benefits of *sadhana*.

The *law of karma* implies that dis-ease arises in our lives as a consequence of previous action. For every action there is an equal reaction. All the practices of yoga science are designed to free us from the bondage of this cycle through attention to conscious and discriminating choices. *Hatha* yoga, practiced with an understanding of the great science of which it is a part, offers us both a tool for *svadhyaya* (Self-study) and a means to the attainment of our highest goal: the freedom and inner balance that accompany our conscious union with the Divine within.

Begin with the Right Attitude

When beginning any exercise program, ask yourself, "Who has made the decision to exercise? Who am I?"

Under ordinary circumstances, you might describe yourself by your physical appearance, occupation or emotional state. You have certain likes and dislikes, impulses and desires, but these are not the real you. You are the Eternal Witness. These descriptions of your perceived condition are all objects appearing in your awareness. They are part of an ever-changing landscape of transitory images, ideas, desires and feelings. None of them are you—the real, observing Self.

Once focused on the question, "Who am I?" you immediately become aware that you have a body, but that you are not the body. You have a mind, but you are not mind. The Lord of Life, being omnipresent, resides within you. With this understanding, your body becomes what it really always was: a shrine that houses Eternity.

Remember, your daily exercise or *asana* practice is an essential element of your *sadhana*. Begin with your centering process and, if it is your habit, with prayers. Don't impatiently rush through your daily exercises without preparation. Without first acknowledging the Eternal Witness, you cannot experience fully the profound and lasting benefits of *Easy-Gentle Yoga*.

When you are centered in your Essential Nature (*Sat-Chit-Ananda*) remember *ahimsa* (non-injury, non-harming). In your practice of *Easy-Gentle Yoga* you should never cause yourself injury. If you are completely focused on the messages emanating from the body, you will be aware when you are approaching the threshold of pain. At that point, welcome and honor this limit, surrender your emotional involvement or judgment, and gently release from the posture.

EASY-GENTLE YOGA

We are offering a simplified and condensed two-part program that provides the benefits of a much more complex and time-consuming *hatha* practice. It is practical, effective and suited to self-directed *sadhana* in an active American life.

As with any exercise program, consult your medical physician before beginning these practices.

Easy-Gentle Yoga: Part I
(For the lymphatic system, joints and glands)

These exercises stimulate and massage the lymphatic system, joints and glands, and should be used in preparation for meditation twice a day—prior to *Part II*, described later in this chapter.

Part I begins at the top of the head and continues systematically down to the toes. In this program, the cleansing action of the lymphatic system is stimulated, and the joints and glands are toned and supplied with increased blood supply to ensure healthy functioning.

The lymphatic system is a complex network that appears throughout the body—just beneath the skin, but over the muscle sheath. Its responsibilities include transporting digested fat from the intestine to the bloodstream, removing and destroying toxic substances and preventing the spread of disease through the body. Stimulating the joints, glands and the lymphatic system also enhances blood circulation—thereby facilitating the cleansing and nourishing activities of the body.

These exercises are highly recommended for individuals suffering from arthritis or general stiffness. They provide a safe and simple way to get started on the path to better health (or to maintain an already healthy body) and keep the mind tranquil.

When you practice *Easy-Gentle Yoga*, be regular and move slowly, with concentration. Keep the breath full, even and diaphragmatic—without any jerks, pauses or sounds.

At the conclusion of each individual exercise, close the eyes and focus your attention on the body and the energy of the body. Ask yourself, "What do I feel and where do I feel it?" Allow yourself to be present with whatever might appear and all that it might concern—without any expectations or judgments. When you are ready, proceed to the next position.

Easy-Gentle Yoga, Part I
(begins on page 370)

Repeat each exercise three times and respect your comfortable capacity. That capacity will increase with consistent practice. If you ever feel a strain, stop and relax, then proceed more gently. As always, remember *ahimsa*. Be gentle and kind with yourself.

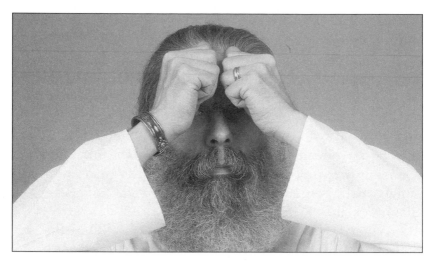

1. Forehead, Ears, Neck

With hands in a loose fist, position the thumbs against the forehead. Using the fleshy part of the hand below the thumb as a squeegee, gently drag the fist across the forehead, up, over and around the back side of the ears, and down the side of the neck.

Repeat each exercise three times

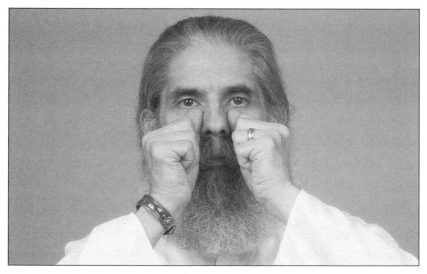

2. Cheeks, Ears, Neck

With the same loose fist, position the thumbs under the corners of the eyes. Using the fleshy part of the hand below the thumb as a squeegee, gently ski down the nose with your fists, go under, and then up the outer side of the cheekbone; continue up, over and around the back side of the ears, and down the side of the neck.

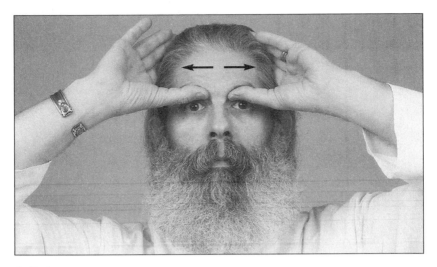

3. Eyebrow

Using the fleshy part of the thumbs, and pressing upward, gently work the thumbs across the upper rim of the eye socket outward toward the temples. Never push the thumbs in toward the eyes.

Repeat each exercise three times

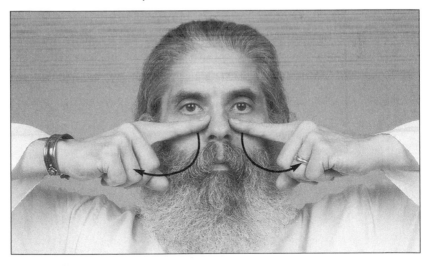

4. Windshield Wiper

Position the index fingers at the corners of the eyes. Then, follow a gentle, semi-circular sweeping motion around and under the cheekbones, like a windshield wiper.

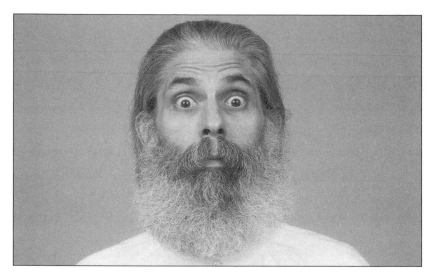

5. Eyebrow and Forehead
Keeping the head and shoulders stationary, raise the eyebrows—furrowing the forehead. Relax completely.

Repeat each exercise three times

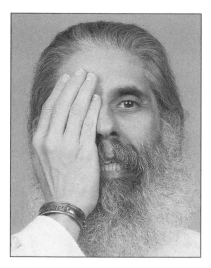 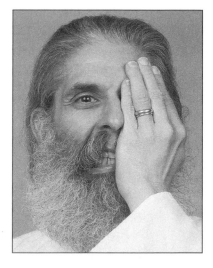

6. Half-Face Contraction (two parts)
Cover the right side of the face with the right hand. Contract the muscles of the exposed side of the face (squinting the eyes and contracting the neck muscles) as if you were a growling dog. The covered half of the face remains relaxed. Then, repeat the exercise covering the left half of the face. Between contractions, relax completely.

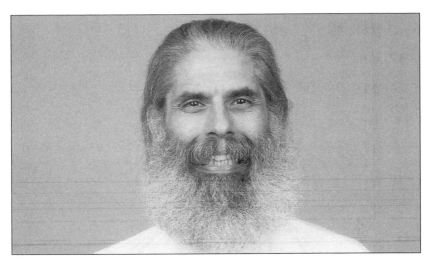

7. Full-Face Contraction

Contract and tense all the muscles of the face as if your eyes and mouth were being drawn toward your nose. Be sure to squint the eyes and contract the muscles of the neck. Relax completely.

Repeat each exercise three times

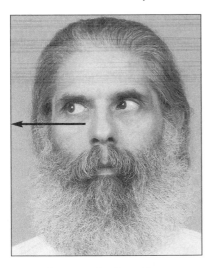 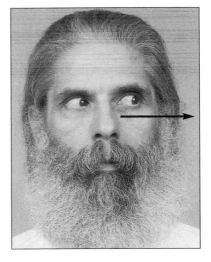

8. Eye Movement (horizontal)

Keep the head and shoulders stationary and facial muscles relaxed during all eye exercises. Gently move the eyes to the far right and then back to the center. Next, gently move the eyes to the left and again back to the center. Never strain your eye muscles.

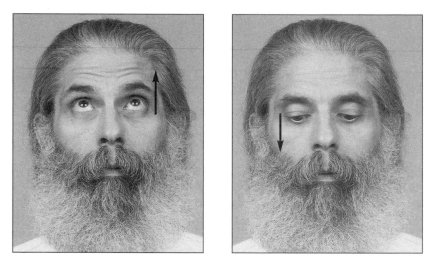

9. Eye Movement (vertical)

Alternate the vertical movement of your eyes. Start by gently moving the eyes up to twelve o'clock and then back to the center. Then gently move the eyes down to six o'clock and again back to the center. Never strain your eye muscles.

Repeat each exercise three times

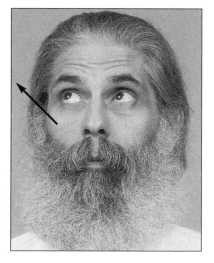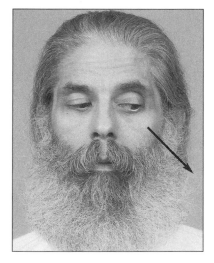

10. Eye Movement (diagonal-right to left)

Gently move the eyes up to the right and then down to the left in a diagonal manner. Never strain your eye muscles.

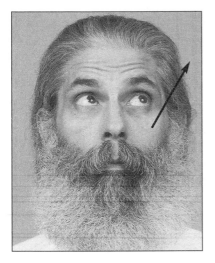
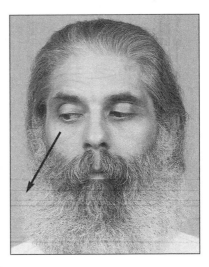

11. Eye Movement (diagonal-left to right)

Gently move the eyes up to the left and then down to the right in a diagonal manner. Never strain your eye muscles.

Repeat each exercise three times

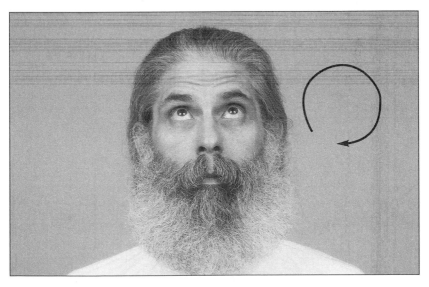

12. Eye Movement (clock rotation)

First, bring the eyes up to twelve o'clock and then rotate the eyes clockwise three times—being certain to visualize every hour. Close and rest the eyes for a few seconds. Then, repeat the exercise three times counter-clockwise. Never strain your eye muscles.

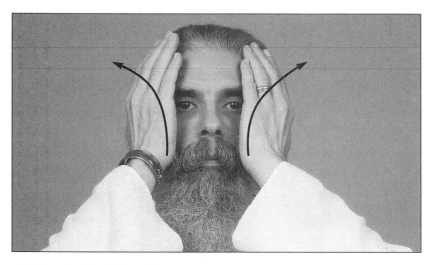

13. Face, Head and Chest Massage

Using your hands in a gentle sweeping motion, begin at the chin, move up over the face, around and down the back of the ears, down the side of the neck and over the front of the chest. *(Recent studies suggest that gentle massage of the breasts may reduce the incidence of some cancer.)*

Repeat each exercise three times

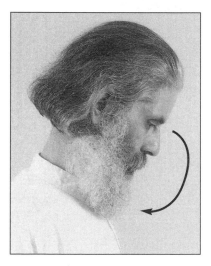

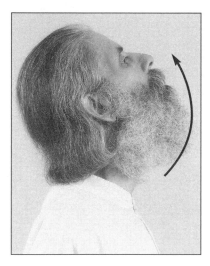

14. Head and Neck Movement

With shoulders stationary, exhale as you bend the head and neck forward—tucking the chin to the chest. Then inhale as you lift the head—tilting backward slightly. Be very mindful and gentle and observe the relaxing of the muscles.

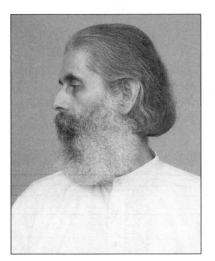
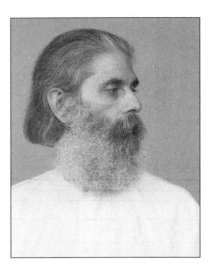

15. Chin over Shoulder

With shoulders stationary, exhale as you turn the head far to the right until the chin is over the shoulder. Then inhale as you turn the head back to center. Repeat the same motion to the left, and then back to center. Then, observe the relaxation of the muscles.

Repeat each exercise three times

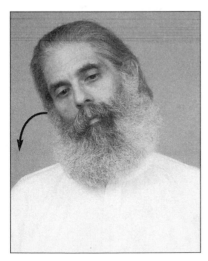
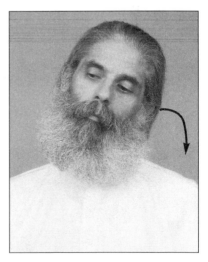

16. Ear to Shoulder

With shoulders stationary, exhale as you lower the right ear toward the right shoulder. Then inhale as bring the head back to the upright position. Repeat the same motion on the left side. Observe the relaxation of the muscles.

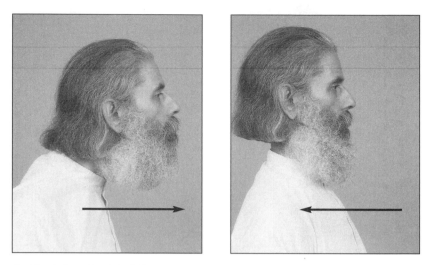

17. Turtle into Double Chin

With shoulders stationary, mouth closed and teeth together, exhale as you *slowly* thrust the head and neck as far forward as possible. Then inhale as you slowly pull the head back into a double chin (chin tucked into the neck).

Repeat each exercise three times

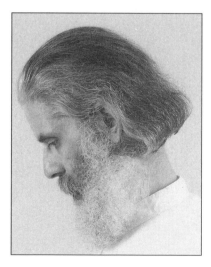
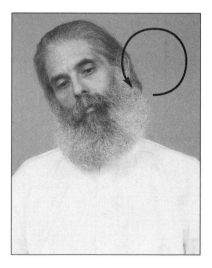

18. Neck Rolls

Lower the chin to the chest and *slowly* rotate the head in a clockwise direction—inhaling going up and exhaling coming down. Then, reverse the exercise by rotating the head in a counter-clockwise direction. Allow the head to be relaxed and to rotate freely and loosely.

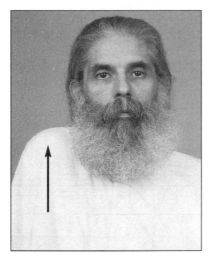 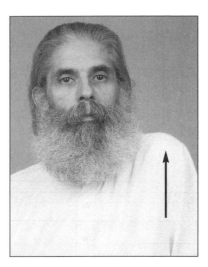

19. Shoulder Lifts

With arms hanging loosely at your sides and without moving the head or neck, lift the right shoulder to the right ear. Squeeze upward in that position for three seconds and quickly release—dropping the arm to a relaxed position at your side. Repeat the exercise with the left shoulder. Then, lift both shoulders as close to the ears as possible, hold for three seconds, and release *slowly* this time—returning the relaxed arms to your sides.

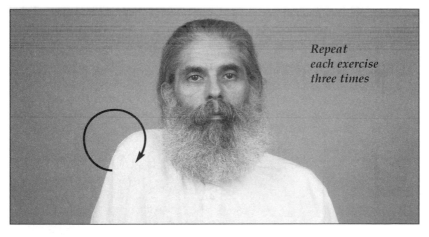

Repeat each exercise three times

20. Shoulder Rotations

With arms hanging loosely at your sides, begin to rotate the right shoulder forward in a large circle—*slowly* moving the shoulder up, forward and then backward in a clockwise direction. Then, reverse direction by *slowly* rotating the shoulder up, backward and then down. Repeat the same sequence with the left shoulder. Finally, repeat the forward and backward rotations with both shoulders simultaneously.

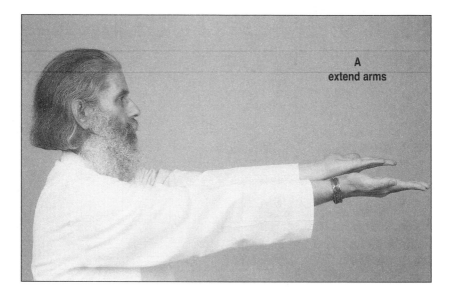

Repeat each exercise three times

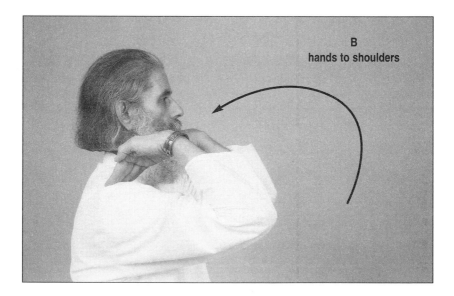

21. Arm Extensions
Reach arms straight out (palms up) and then bring fingertips to the shoulders.

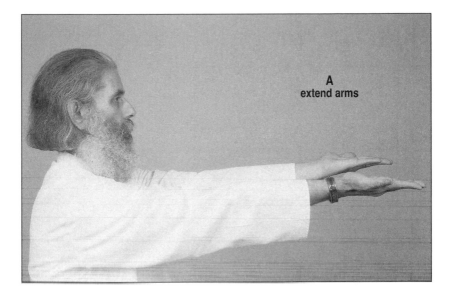

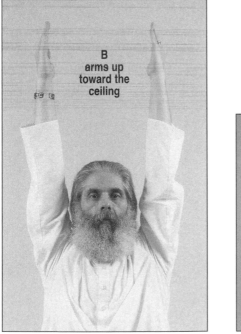

*Repeat
each exercise
three times*

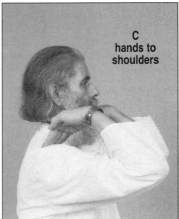

22. Arm Extensions

Reach arms straight out (palms up), extend arms up toward the ceiling (palms facing up) and then drop the hands to the shoulders. Repeat three times.

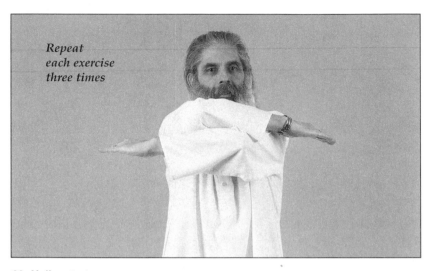

Repeat each exercise three times

23. Helicopter

Raise and extend arms out to the sides, horizontal to the floor. Exhale as you swing arms forward (crossing the left over the right). Then inhale as you reverse the process, again extending arms to the sides. Each time you swing the arms forward, alternate which hand crosses over the other.

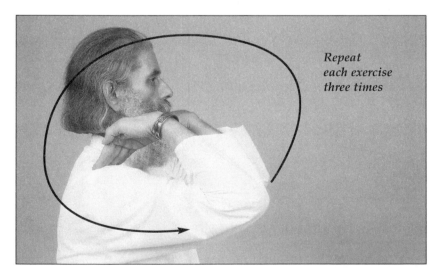

Repeat each exercise three times

24. Shoulder Circles

With arms bent and hand on shoulders, *slowly* draw a large zero with your elbows—moving the elbows up, around and then backward in a clockwise direction. Then, reverse direction by rotating in a counter-clockwise manner—*slowly* moving the elbows up, around and then down.

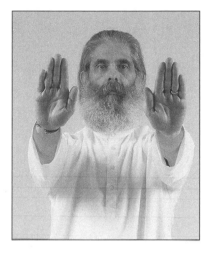

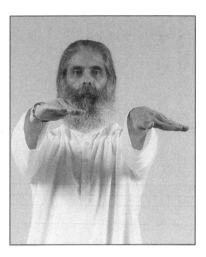

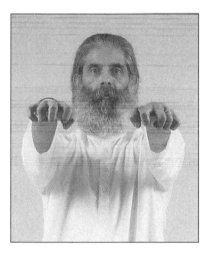

Bear-Claw Position

*Repeat
each hand position
three times*

This exercise is recommended for anyone who engages in repetitive tasks, such as computer data entry.

25. Hands, Wrists and Arms

Stretch the arms out in front of the body with fingers toward the ceiling. Then, follow this sequence with both hands simultaneously:

1. Down to six o'clock and up to twelve o'clock.

2. To the left and back to center.

3. To the right and back to center.

4. Rotate the hands toward each other at the wrists (the right hand in a counter-clockwise direction and the left hand in a clockwise direction).

5. Rotate the hands away from each other at the wrists (the left hand counter-clockwise and the right hand clockwise).

6. Rotate both hands simultaneously to your left in a counter-clockwise direction.

7. Rotate both hands simultaneously to your right in a clockwise direction. When complete, bring the arms down to your side and rest.

8. Repeat the entire *"Hands, Wrists and Arms"* sequence (positions 1-7) with the hands in a bear-claw position.

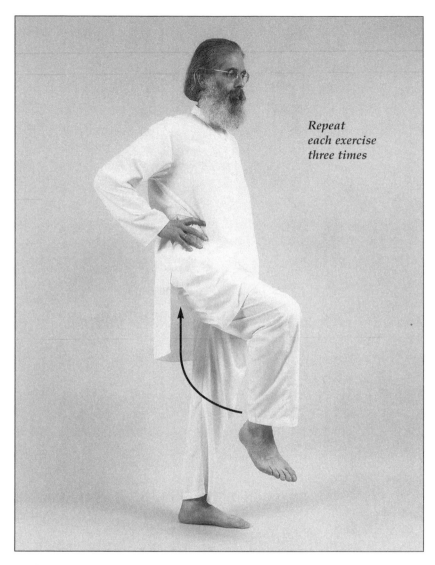

*Repeat
each exercise
three times*

26. Leg Kick

Stand with head, neck and trunk straight and place hands on hips. Lift the right foot until the thigh is parallel to the floor—balancing yourself on the opposite foot. Then, with a whip-like action, gently kick yourself in the buttocks three times. Repeat the exercise with the left leg lifted.

Do not attempt this exercise if you have knee or hip problems. Rest your hand on the back of a chair if you need an assist in balancing.

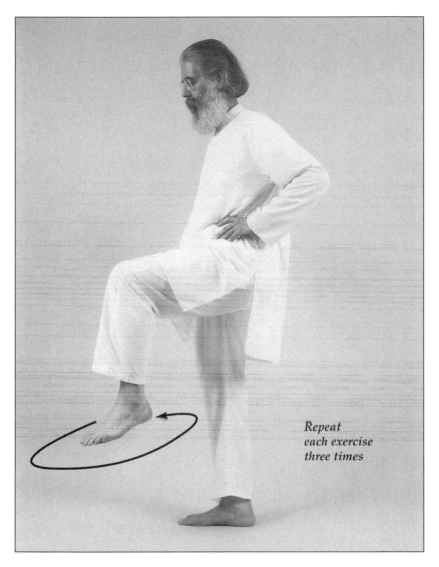

*Repeat
each exercise
three times*

27. Knee Swirl

Use the same stance as in the previous exercise. When the right leg is lifted and the thigh is parallel to the floor, gently swirl the lower leg in a circular motion—first clockwise and then counter-clockwise. Keep the ankle stationary—performing the circular motion from the knee (as if you were stirring a drink). Repeat the exercise with the left leg.

Do not attempt this exercise if you have knee or hip problems. Rest your hand on the back of a chair if you need an assist in balancing.

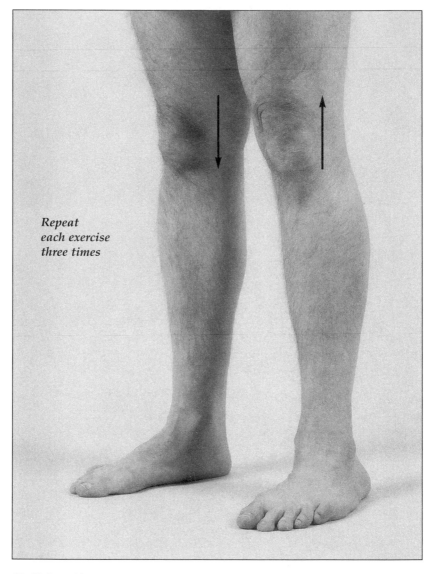

*Repeat
each exercise
three times*

28. Tighten Kneecaps
Stand with the feet spread shoulder width apart. Tighten and lift the muscles surrounding the left knee cap (raising the knee cap slightly), then relax the knee completely as you tighten and lift the muscles surrounding the right knee cap. Alternate back and forth at a moderate rate of speed, always remembering to tighten and loosen the knee cap completely.

Do not attempt this exercise if you have knee problems.

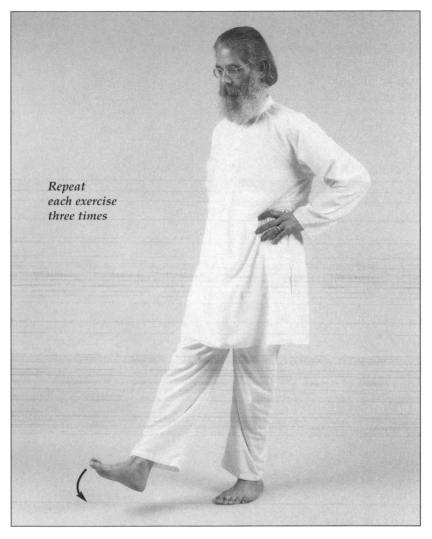

*Repeat
each exercise
three times*

29. Foot and Ankle

Stand with head, neck and trunk straight and place hands on hips. Lift the right foot a few inches off the floor—positioning the toe up and the heel down. When ready, begin this sequence with the right foot—repeating each position three times: 1. Down to six o'clock and up to twelve o'clock; 2. To the left and back to center; 3. To the right and back to center; 4. Rotate the foot in a circular motion counter-clockwise; 5. Then rotate the foot in a circular motion clockwise. Bring the right leg down, rest completely and repeat the exercise with the left leg.

Do not attempt this exercise if you have knee or hip problems. Rest your hand on the back of a chair if you need an assist in balancing.

30. Upper Body Rotation

Position the feet a little wider than shoulder width apart with the hands on hips. Bend at the hips until the body tells you it has reached its comfortable limit at the six o'clock position.

Now, gently rotate the torso in a continuous counter-clockwise pattern. Moving from the hips, inhale as you slowly raise up toward your right (nine o'clock). Then bend backward slightly as you approach the twelve o'clock position. Exhale as you begin your descent back toward the six o'clock position—slowly lowering the body to your left. **Repeat the same movement in the clockwise pattern.**

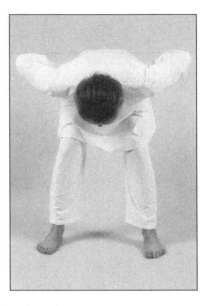

Repeat each exercise three times

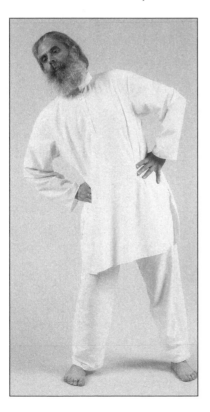

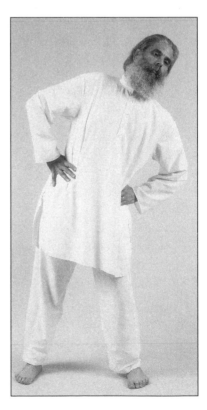

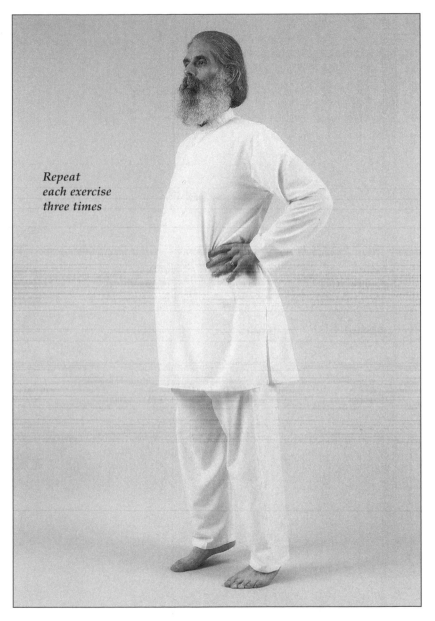

*Repeat
each exercise
three times*

31. Toe Balance

With feet fairly close together and hands on hips, rise onto the balls of the feet and remain balanced in that position for thirty seconds or to your comfortable capacity. Then, return to the normal standing posture. To help balance, stare at one point on the wall.

32. Spinal Twist

Again, assume the "Toe Balance" position. Then, raise your arms straight out in front of your chest (arms parallel to the floor and palms down). Exhale and slowly turn to the left as far as possible while balancing on the balls of your feet. As you twist, the head will turn (eyes following your left hand) until the chin is positioned over the left shoulder. The right elbow will bend until the right hand touches the chest.

Inhale as you twist back to the center, and then turn to the right in the same manner. Gently twist back and forth. To improve balance during the twist, stare at any horizontal landmark in the room, such as the bottom of picture frames, a chair rail or the top surfaces of furniture.

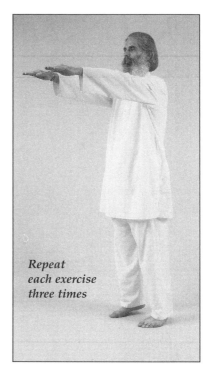

Repeat each exercise three times

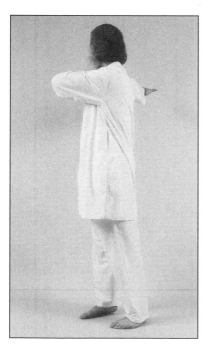

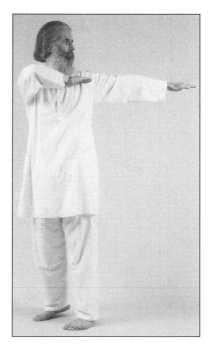

Easy-Gentle Yoga: Part II

Always stand with your feet perfectly parallel and a comfortable distance apart. Begin with the feet twenty-four to thirty-six inches apart. The wider your stance, the fuller will be the stretch. You will consciously be supporting the upper body with the lower body in these postures. Keep your hips, thighs and ankles firm, kneecaps lifted, and hamstrings and calves engaged. Be mindful of the entire body at all times and respect your limits. Yoga is not a competition. Constantly listen to the whispers of your body so you'll be able to hear when the torso has bent as far as is comfortable. Remember, throughout these exercises, your body is your *mantra*—the focus of all your attention.

When twisting and bending to the left, mindfully feel the muscles and joints of your left leg contract. Firm your ankle, calf, knee, thigh, hip and left buttock. As you begin to bend your upper body toward the left, your left side will contract and you will feel a healthy stretch all along your right leg. Soften the belly, breathe diaphragmatically into the navel region and feel the tension roll off the body with each exhalation.

When twisting and bending to the right, mindfully feel the muscles and joints of your right leg contract. Firm your ankle, calf, knee, thigh, hip and right buttock. As you begin to bend your upper body toward the right, your right side will contract and you will feel a healthy stretch all along your left leg. Breathe diaphragmatically into the navel region and feel the tension roll off the body with each exhalation.

After you have completed your bend, begin your ascent slowly and consciously—with the buttocks contracted for extra support. When you attain the vertical standing position, maintain a slight arch of the back, keep your head up slightly, lengthen the spine upward and slightly lower the shoulders.

Now, allow the heart center to be open as you gently and lovingly lift your chest toward the ceiling. As you experience the feeling of lift, imagine your body is made of Turkish taffy and you are stretching it—increasing the spaces between all the cells in the body.

Throughout each bend and lift, keep the legs firm, feet parallel, and maintain a complete spinal twist on both the descent and ascent. When you lower the upper body in the spinal twist, blood is gently wrung out of the internal organs like water from a sponge. As you commence your ascent, a nourishing transfusion of freshly oxygenated blood rushes into the organs bringing renewed vitality and energy.

As you start these exercises, refer to the illustrations provided. Be conservative and patient—content to make progress a week at a time rather than each day. Think of each movement as part of a journey. Moving into the position is the journey and holding that posture for several breaths is the short-term destination. Make the journey, observe the surroundings and enjoy both the journey and the destinations.

When you have memorized the positions of *Easy-Gentle Yoga Part II*, and if you are very sure of your balance, try doing them with your eyes closed. You will have greater concentration if your sense of sight is disengaged.

As always, remember *ahimsa* as you make *Easy-Gentle Yoga* an integral part of your *sadhana*. If you are aware of any physical problems or injuries, seek a physician's approval *before* you begin these exercises.

All of yoga science stresses balance and flexibility. To ensure these, and to avoid the formation of undesirable habits of the body, follow this alternating plan:

On odd numbered days of the month, twist to the left side first, then the right and conclude with the forward facing position.

On even numbered days of the month, twist to the right side first, then the left and conclude with the forward facing position.

Sequence for Easy-Gentle Yoga Part II

The following sequence applies to each of the seven starting positions beginning on page 394. This example demonstrates starting position #1.

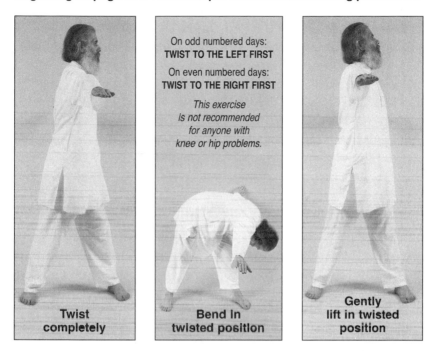

On odd numbered days:
TWIST TO THE LEFT FIRST

On even numbered days:
TWIST TO THE RIGHT FIRST

*This exercise
Is not recommended
for anyone with
knee or hip problems.*

Twist completely

Bend in twisted position

Gently lift in twisted position

After you assume the starting position (for each of the seven postures): twist completely ninety degrees; bend in the twisted position and then lift to the vertical position. Then twist to the other side, bend in the twisted position and then lift to the vertical. Return to center position and bend forward, rise to the vertical, and gently lift toward the ceiling and relax.

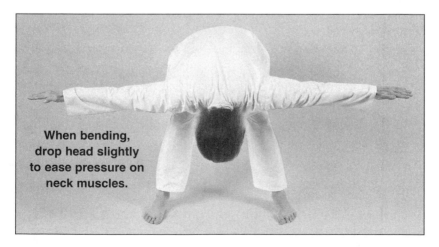

When bending, drop head slightly to ease pressure on neck muscles.

The example below is for ODD numbered days of the month
Reverse the sequence for EVEN numbered days of the month.

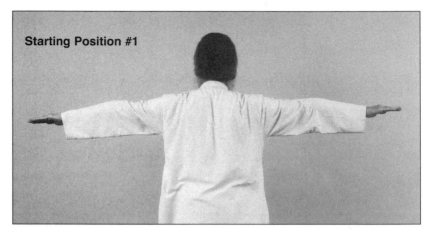

Starting Position #1

Position 1. Place both arms straight out to the sides—parallel to the floor, with all the fingers and thumb touching and palms facing down (see illustration). Maintain this arm placement throughout this first position.

Now, mindfully twist the entire torso as far to the left as is comfortable. When you reach the limit of the spinal twist to the left, slowly and mindfully bend forward, maintaining that twist, until the body tells you that it has reached its limit. Once in the forward bent position, lower the head to release tension in the neck muscles. Remain in the bended, twisted position (to the left) for two to six breaths, or as long as is comfortable.

When you are ready to rise, slowly lift the torso, maintaining the spinal twist, until you reach the vertical position and gently stretch or lift the entire body toward the ceiling.

Then, relax and slowly twist the entire torso to the right as far as is comfortable. When you reach the limit of the spinal twist to the right, slowly and mindfully bend forward, maintaining that twist, until the body tells you that it has reached its limit. Once in the forward bent position, lower the head to release tension in the neck muscles. Remain in the bended, twisted position (to the right) for two to six breaths, or as long as is comfortable.

When you are ready to rise, slowly lift the torso, maintaining the spinal twist, until you reach the vertical position and gently stretch or lift the entire body toward the ceiling.

Then, relax and slowly face forward. Slowly and mindfully bend forward from the hips until the body tells you that it has reached its limit. In the forward bend, lower the head to release tension in the neck muscles. Remain in the forward bend for two to six breaths, or as long as is comfortable. Rise slowly until you reach the vertical position and gently stretch or lift the entire body toward the ceiling.

Relax completely and observe the entire body. Ask yourself, "What do I feel and where do I feel it?" without any expectations or judgments. When you are ready, begin the second position.

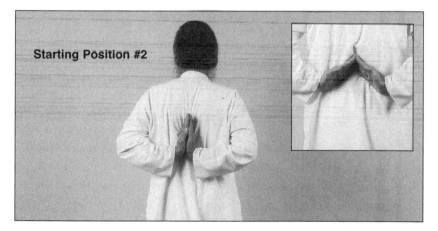

Starting Position #2

Position 2. Place the hands in prayer position behind the back—fingers pointing toward the ceiling (see illustration). Try to keep the palms together and lift the joined hands comfortably to the center of the back. If you are unable to join the palms completely, just make contact with your fingertips, at the waist. *Ahimsa* requires that you be free of pain while doing these postures, so experiment until you find a position that is comfortable. In this posture, follow the same instructions described in position one: twist left, bend forward left, rise and lift twisted left. Twist right, bend forward right, rise and lift twisted right. Face forward and bend forward from the hips, rise and lift.

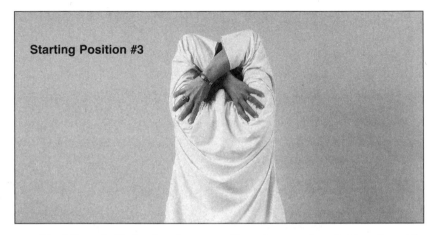

Position 3. Raise both arms directly overhead. Reach with the left hand behind the neck and grab the right shoulder (see illustration). Then reach with the right hand behind the neck (bending the elbow) and grab the left shoulder. *(On even days of the month, the right hand will grab the left shoulder first, followed by the left hand grabbing the right shoulder.)* In this posture, follow the same instructions described in position one: twist left, bend forward left, rise and lift twisted left. Twist right, bend forward right, rise and lift twisted right. Face forward and bend forward from the hips, rise and lift.

Position 4. Clasp the hands together behind the back, interlacing the fingers (see illustration). Press the palms together, lock the elbows and raise the arms a comfortable distance away from the tailbone. Depending on your level of flexibility you may be able to raise your clasped hands and arms one to six inches or more away from the tailbone. Don't be discouraged, however, if you need to rest your clasped hands on the sacrum

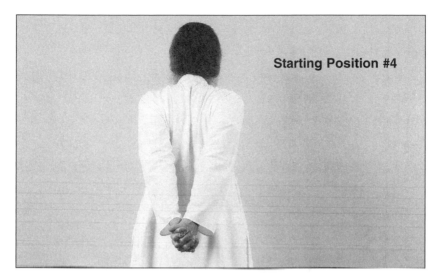

Starting Position #4

or if you cannot press the palms of the hands completely together. Remember *ahimsa* and just honor the current limitations of the body—which is *not* you.

In this posture, follow the same instructions described in position one: twist left, bend forward left, rise and lift twisted left. Twist right, bend forward right, rise and lift twisted right. Face forward and bend forward from the hips, rise and lift.

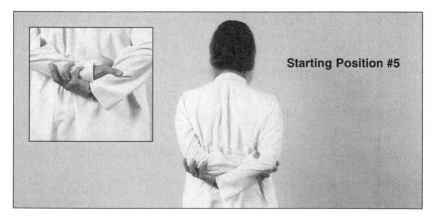

Starting Position #5

Position 5. Bring your left hand behind your back and clasp your right elbow (see illustration). Then bring your right hand behind your back and clasp your left elbow.

(On even days of the month, the right hand will grab the left shoulder first, followed by the left hand grabbing the right shoulder.) If you cannot grasp the elbow, clasp the forearm. In this posture, follow the same instructions described in position one: twist left, bend forward left, rise and lift twisted left. Twist right, bend forward right, rise and lift twisted right. Face forward and bend forward from the hips, rise and lift.

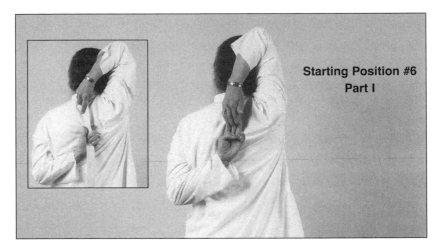

Starting Position #6
Part I

Position 6. Position number six has two parts and may require the use of props. Please read the entire instruction before beginning.

For Part I: Place your left hand in the center of the back between the shoulder blades with the palm facing out. With your right arm, reach up from the shoulder, bend the elbow and try to join the two hands—interlocking the fingers of both hands, gently pulling the right elbow behind the head (see illustration). If the fingers of your two hands will not meet, a belt, scarf, rope or yoga strap can be used, as illustrated. In this posture, follow the same instructions described in position one: twist left, bend forward left, rise and lift twisted left. Twist right, bend forward right, rise and lift twisted right. Come to the center, forward facing position and bend forward, rise and lift.

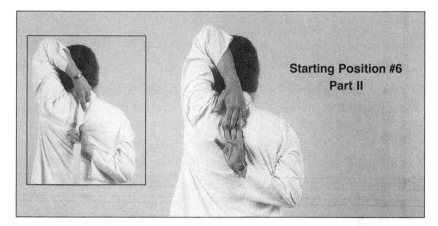

Starting Position #6
Part II

For Position 6, Part II: Place your right hand in the center of the back between the shoulder blades—palm facing out. Extend your left arm up from the shoulder, bend the elbow and try to join the two hands—interlocking the fingers of both hands, gently pulling the left elbow behind the head. In *Starting Position #6 Part II*, follow these instructions: twist right, bend forward right, rise and lift twisted right. Twist left, bend forward left, rise and lift twisted left. Face forward and bend forward from the hips, rise and lift. *(On even numbered days of the month, reverse the grabbing sequence. Place the right hand in the center of the back, clasp with the left hand and twist and bend first toward the right.)*

Position 7. The final position varies slightly from the others. Place the hands on your hips with the elbows back, thumbs on your back and fingers forward (see illustration). In this posture, twist completely to the left, then bend slightly forward, about thirty degrees, and arch the upper torso, keeping the head slightly lifted without pinching the muscles at the back of the neck. Next, while remaining twisted to the left, rise to the vertical position and lift gently toward the ceiling as in the other positions. Relax and twist completely to the right, bending slightly forward, about thirty degrees, and arching the upper torso. While remaining twisted to the right, rise to the vertical position and lift gently to the ceiling. Relax and face forward, then bend slightly forward, about thirty degrees and arch the upper torso, keeping the head slightly lifted without pinching the muscles at the back of the neck.

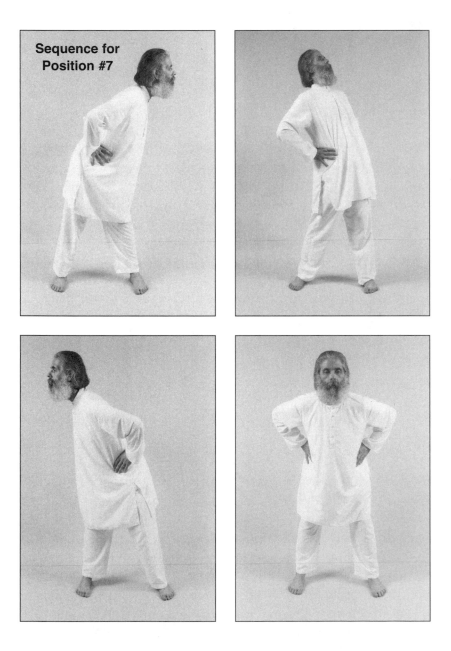

Sequence for Position #7

Additional Practices

In addition to the *Easy-Gentle Yoga Parts I and II*, try to incorporate the following practices into your daily routine. In our experience, they are very beneficial.

Swimming Exercise

If you suffer from stiffness or pain in the lower back, this exercise is a must for your daily *sadhana*. The swimming exercise should be practiced first thing in the morning—before you get out of bed—and on the floor after your *Easy-Gentle Yoga* exercises and before your evening meditation and sleep.

Upon waking in the morning, move the body slightly toward the foot of the bed to avoid hitting your hands against the headboard during this practice. Lying on your back, simultaneously raise your bent left knee to your chest and lift your right arm over your head so that the hand rests on the pillow (it's okay to bend the elbow) as you turn your head to the right as if looking into your right armpit. Then, as you lower the left leg and right arm, simultaneously raise your bent right knee to your chest, lift your left arm over your head so that the hand rests on the pillow, and turn your head until it faces your left armpit. Now, in a methodical, concentrated and fluid motion, continue to alternate the movements described (as if swimming) for a total count of twenty repetitions (ten on each side).

The swimming motion will help move fluids that have settled in the tissues along the spinal column during the night, thereby improving morning flexibility of the back. The neurological stimulation of performing the swimming exercise is also said to sharpen and synchronize communication between the left and right brain to help you begin the day with greater clarity and concentration.

Walking

Brisk, twenty minute *mantra walks*, early in the morning

and in late afternoon or early evening, are the most healthful and non-injurious exercises you can practice on a regular basis. Physicians agree that for many adults, frequent running can be the cause of damage to hips, knees, ankles, feet and kidneys. As the human body ages, the drying air and space elements of the *vata dosha* are increased and the lubricating water and earth elements of the *kapha dosha* are diminished. So please consider this gentler alternative. A brisk *mantra walk* clears the mind, oxygenates the blood, builds stamina and lung capacity and has powerful mood-lifting effects.

Kegel Exercise

The *Kegel exercise*, traditionally prescribed for women as a means to strengthen pelvic floor muscles and to overcome incontinence, is also an excellent practice for men. It's among the very few exercises that massage the prostate gland. Perform the *Kegel exercise* by alternately tightening and relaxing the urinary sphincter (the muscle used to stop and start the flow of urine). Practice this exercise daily for twenty-five to fifty repetitions. Contract the muscles strongly and completely for a count of four and then relax completely for a count of four.

Part XI
PULLING THINGS TOGETHER

CHAPTER 38

Two Wings of Yoga

Attachment is a state of ignorance based on a memory of pleasure.
PATANJALI - CODIFIER OF YOGA SCIENCE

In order to save oneself from being boiled in a boiling kettle, it is proper to jump out of it; to remain attached to the kettle is foolish.
SWAMI RAMA TIRTHA

In the ancient texts, yoga is often metaphorically described as a bird. In order for the bird to take flight and successfully fulfill its potential, its two wings must function proficiently and in unison. The two wings of yoga are the complementary practices of *abhyasa* and *vairagya*.

Constant Practice: *Abhyasa*

The sages remind us that pain, misery and bondage are caused by ignorance. They are the consequences of ignoring the Divine Reality when taking an action. Yet the elders of every tradition also teach the good news: such ignorance will ultimately yield to our sustained earnestness and devotion to practice. Moment-by-moment and thought-by-thought, we are asked to welcome and attend to each relationship as it appears. By being awake to the present moment, as the Compassionate

Buddha teaches, we learn to coordinate the four major functions of the mind—creating a global skill that helps us consistently serve the *shreya* and surrender the *preya* in mind, action and speech.

Dedication to purification of the mind is the first step toward freedom. Unless we earnestly seek to purify the mind, our deepest *samskaras* will continue to motivate actions that bring about painful consequences. Constant practice, in every waking moment, is called *abhyasa*. It is through *abhyasa* that the limiting power of the unconscious is transformed into the energy, will power and creativity necessary for liberation.

Two objects cannot occupy the same space at the same time. Obviously, in order to be constantly practicing, something must be given up. *Abhyasa* always involves some *renunciation*, the surrender of some fleetingly attractive *preya*. This ongoing process effectively places the reins of the mind in the hands of the *buddhi*, ensuring that mind, action and speech function as instruments of Divine wisdom.

Detachment: *Vairagya*

Right now, today, there is something you can do to experience peace and happiness. That's right. Within twenty-four hours you can be living your life with a greater contentment and joy than you have ever imagined—no matter what trials you may be currently facing.

Human birth provides each of us immense resources that, by our conscious choice, can instantaneously transform our lives. But there is a catch! We do have the capacity to choose Happiness, but first we must know how to make the correct choice, and choosing correctly is not always a simple matter. The charm of immediate sense or ego gratification is very often more tempting than the Divinely deferred blessing of the *shreya*.

Even though we may think otherwise, our pain results from our own everyday human behavior—behavior that reflects a chronic capitulation to the ego and senses rather than an homage to our Divine nature. Most of our daily human activities (like eating, sleeping, working, playing and sex) are generally undertaken without an understanding of the true purpose of life. That purpose, the sages remind us, is *moksha*—the enlightened consciousness that brings the end of all sorrow.

In order to gain the kind of freedom the sages speak of, we must understand and practice the philosophy of *vairagya*: detachment or non-attachment. In this culture, when we hear the word detachment we think of people who are callous, aloof, indifferent or uninvolved, but yoga science teaches us that *vairagya* actually means just the opposite.

In practical terms, *vairagya*—the second wing of yoga—means love in action. We're not required to renounce the things of the world nor the fulfillment of our genuine needs, but we are asked to perform our duties lovingly, skillfully and selflessly—remaining unattached to the fruits of our action.

What we're really detaching from is the demands of our own ego, whose tyranny has made us believe that happiness comes only when events and people serve our *raga/dveshas* and self-willed desires. *Vairagya* grants us the freedom to set aside our own limitations and those of others—before we commit to taking a specific action that will yield a specific consequence. St. Francis of Assisi reminds us "it is in giving that we receive." In order to become the beneficiary of something worthwhile, like unbounded Happiness, we must be willing to give up our attachment to the likes and dislikes we treasure.

When we are faced with a choice of what to think, say or do, the philosophy of non-attachment helps create a space between our first habitual reaction—based on the limitations of our deep *samskaras*—and our ultimate response. When practicing *vairagya*, the stored power of the *mantra* comes forward with love, fearlessness and strength. Then, even in the face of *preya*'s charms, detachment provides us the freedom to re-center ourselves in our Essential Nature (*Sat-Chit-Ananda*). In that fullness, we discover the resources and encouragement that allow the discriminating *buddhi* to guide mind, action and speech for our highest and greatest good.

The Power of Donuts

Eknath Easwaran tells the story of a man who was troubled by his recent weight gain. Trying to explain how he got so heavy, the overweight man confessed to a friend that every morning he passed an enticing bakery as he walked to work. The aroma was so tempting that he couldn't resist buying a little bag of donuts. In desperation he asked the friend for some advice.

After pondering a bit, the friend suggested that the man leave his wallet at home on the days he walked to work. At this, the overweight man recoiled in shock. "You mean you want me to *steal* the donuts?"

The practices of *renunciation* and *vairagya* (non-attachment) are often misunderstood. Freely giving up anything attractive is usually associated with the unhealthy repression of normal desires. But the philosophy of non-attachment does not involve repression, nor does it require or endorse asceticism. On the contrary, *vairagya* helps us to enjoy the delights of the world, with discrimination, and without the bondage of attachment and its painful consequences.

In the *Bhagavad Gita*, Shri Krishna (representing the Lord of Love as our spiritual guide) teaches the philosophy of non-attachment to Arjuna (representing every human being facing the daily challenges of life). Through his clear and practical message, Krishna explains to Arjuna that only by understanding yoga science and practicing *vairagya* sincerely, systematically, and with sustained enthusiasm will his physical, mental and emotional problems find resolution; only then will he be at peace:

> *When you keep thinking about sense-objects, attachment comes. Attachment breeds desire, the lust of possession which, when thwarted, burns to anger.*

Anger clouds the judgment and robs you of the power to learn from past mistakes. Lost is the discriminative faculty (buddhi), and your life is utter waste. But when you move amidst the world of sense, from both attachment and aversion freed (vairagya), there comes the peace in which all sorrows end, and you live in the wisdom of the Self.

The *Gita* teaches that whenever we indiscriminately direct our attention toward a sense object, a desire for the object grows in the unconscious mind (*chitta*). This desire then gives rise to powerful cravings—born of the misconception that the object or relationship sought has the capacity to bring us happiness or eliminate pain.

If this desire is not fulfilled, we can be swept away by a turbulent sea of anger. Anger creates a cloud of delusion that obstructs our access to pertinent memories, imagination and the logic of cause and effect. Lacking both hindsight and foresight, we suffer from psychological blindness that obscures the intuitive facility of the *buddhi*. When anger blocks access to the superconscious mind, our thoughts, words and deeds serve the *preya* of habitual fear, anger or self-willed desire, and the *karmas* (consequences) of these actions enslave us to a whirlpool of dis-ease and pain.

Lesson of the Samurai Warrior

A bold and handsome young Samurai warrior stood respectfully before the aged Zen master and asked, "Master, please teach me about heaven and hell." The master snapped his head up in disgust and said, "Teach YOU about heaven and hell? Why, I doubt that you could even learn to keep your own sword from rusting! You ignorant fool! How dare you suppose that you could understand anything I might have to say?"

The old man went on and on, becoming even more insulting, while the young swordsman's surprise turned first to confusion and then to hot anger, rising by the minute. Master or no master, who can insult a Samurai and live? At last, with teeth clenched and blood nearly boiling in fury, the warrior blindly drew his sword and prepared to end the old man's sharp tongue and life. At that instant, the master looked straight into his eyes and said gently, "Now, that's hell."

At the peak of his rage, the Samurai realized the importance of this teaching; the Master had hounded him into a living hell of uncontrolled anger and ego. The young man, profoundly humbled, sheathed his sword and bowed low to this great spiritual teacher. Looking up into the wise man's beaming face, he felt more love and compassion than he had ever felt in his life—at which point the master raised his index finger as would a schoolteacher and said, "And that, my son, is heaven."

Yoga science reminds us that our rigid attachments cause pleasure and pain—both of which limit our range of action. When we become habituated to likes and dislikes (*raga/dveshas*), we cut ourselves off from the fullness of our Divine source and consequently fail to employ our intuitive creativity and to enjoy our innate Happiness.

The wise and loving person, however, guided by the philosophy of non-attachment, is ever aware of the true Self, and is able to enjoy the unchanging bliss and fullness of That which is perfect freedom. *Vairagya* teaches us how to love and be loved, whether things are going our way or not. If we can constantly be aware of the Absolute Reality within and learn to practice *vairagya* at all times—in the midst of every relationship—the promise is that we will be liberated from all forms of sorrow, here and now, in this lifetime, and that everything we need will come to us.

Through *abhyasa* and *vairagya*, we go beyond a mere intellectual understanding of yoga science. Each of our thoughts, words and actions becomes a powerful expression of that sage prescription for Happiness—*namaha Shivaya*: nothing belongs to me, everything belongs to Thee. Everything is here for me to use and enjoy, but not to possess nor to be possessed by.

Tiramisu

The practice of *vairagya* does not require that we deny ourselves the pleasures of life. As a child, my principal Ayurvedic *dosha* was (and still is) *kapha*. Like attracts like, and consequently, I was very fond of *kapha*-producing foods, including ice cream, cheese and wheat products—especially bagels. Over the years I consumed a lot of them—placing an undue burden on my body. As a result, I gained weight, suffered allergies and often lacked sustained energy.

Now, as part of my *sadhana*, I rarely bring those foods into the house, although I'm still very fond of them. Instead, I surrender my attachment to them so that by balancing my *doshas*, I can move closer to attaining my deepest driving desire for unbounded Life, Liberty and Happiness.

Yet when I visit an Italian restaurant, I look forward to ordering one of my favorite *kapha* desserts—tiramisu. On those special occasions I thoroughly enjoy the mouth-watering treat—without one bit of guilt!

The detachment of *vairagya* does not mean denial. At the present time we know the satisfaction that comes from fulfilling a desire, but we have not yet experienced the joy that comes from sacrificing a desire. Because I've been willing to experiment, I no longer feel I must fulfill every desire. I can enjoy things of the world, with discrimination, and still be free. Through the practice of *vairagya*, I am freed from many once-powerful desires that never served me well.

Vairagya means freedom—the freedom to choose consciously and wisely.

Two Monks

Two monks on a journey were silently enjoying the splendor of nature as they walked. The holy men came to the bank of a river where they met a beautiful woman who appeared to be in considerable distress. She told them that despite her many attempts, she was unable to cross the swiftly flowing river by herself. Recognizing her dilemma, the stronger of the two picked up the woman in his arms and carried her across the river—setting her down politely on the opposite shore. He humbly accepted her thanks and she continued her journey in one direction while the two monks continued theirs in another.

As the two walked on for hours in silence, the monk who had observed his brother carry the beautiful woman across the river grew agitated and then angry. Finally, losing his discrimination and equanimity, he began to berate his fellow renunciate. "You know that we are celibates. We have taken sacred vows—never to entertain impure thoughts of women. And yet you knowingly held a beautiful woman close in your arms—holding her as if your two bodies were one as you slowly crossed the river. It's a shocking violation of our vows of chastity!"

During this firestorm of criticism, the first monk examined his own actions as well as the disparaging remarks of his companion. "You're right." He responded. "We are renunci-ates, having taken vows of chastity, and yes, I did pick up the woman in my arms and I did carry her across the river. She could not cross the river by herself. By her own admission she needed assistance, and I realized that I had the capacity to help. With pure intentions, I picked her up, carried her across the river and set her down on the shore. However, you, my dear brother, are still carrying her."

To fully assimilate and understand the practice of *vairagya*, always be aware of your own intentions. The monk in this story had no intention of breaching his vows. His sole purpose was to assist another human being. The fact that the benefici-ary of his action was a beautiful woman was incidental. Regardless of any external circumstances or appearance, the choice of action for a yoga scientist is always to serve the Divine counsel of the *buddhi*.

St. Francis and Perfect Joy

One day St. Francis asked his close disciple, Brother Leo, to write down his understanding of perfect joy. "I cannot," Leo replied with great honesty. "Can you teach me about perfect joy, Father?"

"Well," Francis replied, "if all the masters of every spiritual tradition in the world were to come together to help us in our work, we would not have attained the secret of perfect joy. And even if we were granted magical powers to heal the sick and perform all sorts of miracles, we would not have found perfect joy."

Eager for a genuine understanding, Brother Leo urgently pleaded to St. Francis, "Then what is the secret of perfect joy?"

Finally the master replied. "Brother Leo," Francis said, "imagine that in the middle of a cold, winter night you are returning from the mountains back home to Assisi. The weather is so nasty that icicles form at the edges of your habit—striking your legs at every step. And when you arrive at the monastery, seeking food and warmth for the night, an irrational gatekeeper confronts you with mean-spirited accusations and physically throws you back out into the winter storm. Then, Brother Leo, in the face of such pain and insult, if you can surrender your outrage and lovingly say, 'Bless you in the name of Jesus,' then *you* will have found the secret of perfect joy."

Clearly none of us has control over what comes to us, but we always have the ability to choose our reaction. Yoga science teaches us that every relationship comes to us through the grace of Divine Providence as an opportunity for our spiritual unfoldment. The *ahamkara* (ego) might habitually try to assert its dominion by encouraging us to seize the pleasant or avoid the unpleasant, but the sages remind us that these pairs of opposites are not what they seem.

That which appears as pleasant eventually will become unpleasant. Any pleasant sense gratification indulged without discrimination will inevitably yield to a painful experience. That which appears as unpleasant can, on the other hand, yield unimagined blessings. *Vairagya* extends the time between stimulus and response so that we can make discriminating choices that allow us to know perfect joy and contentment.

CHAPTER 39

Contemplation, Repentance and Prayer

*Contemplation for an hour
is better than formal worship for sixty years.*

MUHAMMAD

The *law of karma* states that for every action there is an equal reaction. It follows then, that our every act—from the most subtle movement of the mind to the most complicated action of the body—contains creative power. Every act moves us either closer to our goal of life, or farther away.

In yoga science, a *sadhaka* (spiritual aspirant) is often likened to an archer. His actions, described metaphorically as arrows, are of three distinct categories. Some arrows have already been shot in the past; one is in the bow now, in the present, and the remaining arrows are stored in the quiver for future use.

In every moment we have control over two of the three types of *karma*, or arrows. The first arrows represent the actions we have already taken. Even though we no longer have control over these arrows, we will still reap their consequences. The second arrow is the one presently positioned in our bow, ready to be shot. We do have control over this arrow. The arrows stored in our quiver represent the actions not yet taken. We have control over these arrows as well.

Contemplation

As an integral part of *sadhana*, the daily practice of contemplation helps us grasp the consequences of the arrows we have already shot and evaluate the potential trajectories of the arrow now in our bow. It also allows us to consider the possibilities represented by all those remaining in our quiver. In *contemplation*, we review the thoughts, words and actions of the day by asking ourselves which have been helpful and which have created obstacles to fully realizing unbounded Life, Liberty and Happiness. Through *contemplation* we recognize which of our actions have been in service to the *shreya* and which have been in service to the *preya*.

In Western traditions, some confusion exists concerning the meanings of the words *contemplation* and meditation. When an individual has a weighty issue hanging over his head, he might use the phrase, "I'll meditate on that." But, according to Eastern traditions, he is actually engaging in the practice of *contemplation*. Meditation always refers to the practice of consciously placing all of one's attention on a single object, to the exclusion of all other objects, for the purpose of calming and training the mind, and experiencing the eternal truth beyond the mind.

For your *contemplation* practice, choose a time and place not encumbered by the demands of your everyday responsibilities. Sit in a clean, quiet, comfortable environment and systematically review your thoughts, words and actions of the past twenty-four hours.

Contemplation helps you take stock of where you are—in relation to where you want to be. Imagine for a moment that you live in Albany, New York and the thought comes to you that you'd like to drive to Boston, Massachusetts. As you give attention to the thought, a desire begins to grow in your awareness, and you decide to drive to Boston.

You get into the car and drive for several hours. Not reaching your destination by nightfall and feeling tired, you decide to spend the night in a motel. When you awake in the morning ready to complete your trip, you discover, to your amazement, that you're in Cleveland, Ohio!

All the time you were intending to drive to Boston, you were actually headed in the wrong direction. *Contemplation* is the practice of reviewing all your actions to evaluate whether they've gotten you closer to, or further away from your goal. If you practice *contemplation* and discover that some of your actions have been in service to the *preya*—and you will—it doesn't mean that you have failed. It means you have something valuable to learn from those experiences.

During *contemplation*, always remember *ahimsa* (non-injury, non-harming). Do not continue to entertain any thought that is unkind to you. An error you've made in the past is a reflection of the limitations of your consciousness that existed in a particular moment. Now your consciousness has changed. Forgive the mistake, recognize its significance and be grateful for the lesson. Every experience is a valuable experience on this path. Thanks to your *contemplation* practice, you will be able to exhibit the will power necessary to serve the *shreya* and surrender the *preya* the next time you are faced with a similar decision.

The key in all of yoga science is your intention. "Blessed are the pure in heart, for they shall see God," Jesus the Christ teaches. Regardless of the short-term outcome, your mind will continue to be purified and you will continue to make progress along the path of fire and light, if you are earnest. If you're willing to take responsibility for your consciousness, there is always a benefit.

The Meaning of Sin

In the West, the concept of sin conjures up many frightening and sorrowful images. It's interesting to note that the word sin was used as an archery term in ancient Greece. At public competitions, when an arrow went astray, the judge would call out "sin," to indicate that the archer had missed the target.

That original concept of sin—missing the target—is important to the practice of yoga science. In *contemplation*, we are asked to routinely examine the habits of the mind. We learn which of our thoughts, words and actions have hit their intended target of *shreya*, and which of our arrows have missed the mark by serving the *preya*. Daily *contemplation* brings us the clarity and wisdom to redirect the flight of the next arrow so that every action can hit the intended target.

Neil Armstrong and the Lunar Module

In 1969 when Neil Armstrong was hurtling toward the surface of the moon in the tiny lunar module, on-board computers were continuously reading bits of flight information and transmitting the data back to the Johnson Space Center in Houston, Texas. Almost instantaneously, the powerful computers at the command center analyzed the data and radioed instructions back to astronaut Armstrong. "Fire your first retro rocket .2 seconds. Fire your second retro rocket .75 seconds, and fire your third retro rocket one complete second—and not 1/1000th of a second more or less." Why all the precision? So Armstrong and the lunar module could make a soft landing on the moon.

The sage, Ramakrishna, advised: if you want to travel east, don't go west. Through the practice of *contemplation*, each of us is able to gather pertinent information about ourselves to determine if we are headed in the right direction.

Contemplation is like a pre-battle intelligence briefing. The process makes you aware of how you expend your vital energy. Once you recognize the *preyas* you've been serving and the primitive fountains (food, sex, sleep or self-preservation) from which they've sprung, you'll be better prepared to serve the *shreya* and surrender the *preya* the next time you face similar attachments on the battlefield of life.

Analyzed in the light of *buddhi*, the knowledge gathered in *contemplation* leads you to make inspired decisions and experience a comfortable and enjoyable soft landing in every circumstance.

Repentance

Let's face it, your daily *contemplation* will sometimes uncover and examine situations in which you simply could not muster the requisite will power to choose the long-term benefit of *shreya*. The practice of *repentance* asks you to face these attachments courageously and to pledge to your Self, the Eternal Witness, that you will not repeat the thought, word or action the *buddhi* has defined as *preya*.

As you silently rededicate your efforts, reaffirm the pledge of *sankalpa*: "I want to do it. I can do it. I have to do it. I am going to do it. No matter what!" A firm resolve is essential to developing *vairagya*—the detachment that allows you to surrender fears, anger and selfish desires and to transform their inherent powers.

The practices of *contemplation* and *repentance* are found in every religious tradition. In Catholicism, the season of Lent asks the faithful to surrender some personal attachment and to contemplate the kinds of sacrifices Jesus made in preparation for becoming fully Christ-conscious. The Jewish tradition celebrates the annual holy days of Rosh Hashanah and Yom Kippur—asking its faithful to contemplate and repent for all their various sins of omission and commission. Similarly, the Muslim tradition celebrates the sacredness of Ramadan—a time for inner reflection, devotion to God and self-control. Unlike these annual holy days, yoga science calls for daily self-examination.

Interestingly, all three traditions incorporate some form of fasting (a form of *renunciation* and sacrifice) as a means of ascendancy to our true spiritual nature. For all traditions, holidays that institutionalize the practices of *contemplation* and *repentance* become opportunities to experience the intuitive wisdom that "it is in giving that we receive."

Remember *Ahimsa*

In addition to specific issues and themes that come to light in your spiritual practice, you will also be dealing with personal judgments, frustrations and even pride-filled satisfaction. As your *sadhana* deepens and you feel better physically, mentally and emotionally, you risk becoming puffed up with the *preya* of pride. Or, if like most human beings you are dealing with a deep *samskara* of impatience, you may become dissatisfied because changes are not coming quickly enough.

In the face of these ego-centered assessments, remember that every thought is only a suggestion. No one is commanding you to give every single thought your attention. Whenever consternation appears in your awareness, it means you're dealing with your thoughts from the limited perspective of the personality. Such inner conflict indicates that you are being swayed unduly by the *ahamkara*—that function of the mind that separates you from your Divine Self.

At such times, don't be upset about your habitual thought process. Don't become angry or belittle yourself by saying, "Oh, I'm an impatient person. I'm a lousy meditator. Yoga science is not working for me." Just remember *ahimsa*— non-injury, non-harming. During these moments especially, charity must begin at home.

Be kind and learn to love yourself by acknowledging that for a brief moment you simply forgot the truth of your eternal, bliss-filled nature. Then, re-center yourself and seek the Divine wisdom of the *buddhi* to determine if that thought you were entertaining is really worthy of your continued attention.

If the *buddhi* tells you that the thought is a *preya*, willingly, lovingly and humbly follow the example of the Compassionate Buddha by offering the thought back to the Origin from which it has come. "No thank you, Father (or Mother or Jesus or Inner Dweller; no thank you, Lord; no thank you, Buddha; no thank you, Allah). I have no use for this debilitating thought right now. Therefore, I am lovingly returning it to You—the Source of all."

Prayer

No matter what your religion, or lack thereof, prayer can become a valuable part of your daily practice. In yoga science, *contemplation, repentance* and *prayer* are often grouped together because, in concert, they enhance every aspect of spiritual life. Even if you are an agnostic or avowed atheist, *prayer* can become a powerful force for personal transformation.

In the dualistic paradigm, God is conceived of as a super-force, separate and apart from the human being. In yoga science, however, the two are One; there is no "other." Although traditions and individuals may differ in their definition of God, everyone acknowledges his or her own existence and capacity to witness. For each of us, based on our experience and memory, there has never been a time when the concept "I am" was not true.

According to yoga science, this *I-amness*, our capacity to be present to witness, is the doorway to experiencing union with One Divine Reality. According to yoga science, the *I-amness* of which all traditions speak is an aspect of the One Absolute Reality, and it is to that Eternal Witness within each of us that the lower self, or personality, offers its prayer.

Ego-Centered Prayer

The most familiar form of prayer is ego-centered prayer. This kind of petitioning is learned in early childhood. Generally, it begins in this manner: "Mommy, may I have a cookie? Mommy, may I please have a cookie? Please, Mommy, may I have a cookie? Please. Please, Mommy!" "Okay, honey, Mother replies. "Here's a cookie." You're such a good boy. Mommy loves you." "Thank you, Mommy."

In real terms, this kind of learned behavior quickly teaches the child to become a beggar. Motivated by the delusion that each of us is a separate individual, we begin petitioning a variety of authority figures at a very early age in hope of securing the objects and relationships we believe will bring us happiness or eliminate our pain.

As we mature into adulthood, certain desires take on great importance in our lives. Perhaps we have an opportunity to get a new, better-paying position at work. In furtherance of that desire, we update our resume, complete the application and interview for the position. Then, after we have done all in our power, we might call on the Supreme authority figure for Divine intervention. In other words, we pray—in the same manner the child learned to beg for cookies. "Dear God, please let me get this job. Please let me get this job. *Please*, God. *Please!*"

If we are sufficiently creative and resourceful, we might even bargain with the Supreme authority figure as if we were playing *Monopoly*. "Dear God, if you give me this job . . . I will start doing this and I will stop doing that." In modern business vernacular, we try to cut a deal.

Unfortunately, this subservient, ego-centered, petitioning attitude increasingly alienates us from the One Divine Reality as it reinforces the divisive power of the ego (*ahamkara*). Regardless of the immediate outcome, the *samskaras* created as a consequence of this repetitive begging enslave us to further rounds of pain and bondage.

God-Centered Prayer

God-centered prayer recognizes that on the highest level of consciousness only One Absolute Reality exists. Unlike the dualistic paradigm that represents man's relationship with God as "I and Thou," yoga philosophy maintains that I and my Father are truly One; that the Divine Reality resides within each of us as the Eternal Witness (*Sat-Chit-Ananda*). Accordingly, the only thing an earnest seeker can legitimately pray for is strength.

Why strength? Because as a yoga scientist you learn through experience that when thought, word and action are in harmony with *buddhi*, you are always led for your highest and greatest good.

Therefore, in *God-centered prayer*, speak to that aspect of the

Divine Reality closer to you than your own breath. "Dear Lord, Dear Jesus, Dear Inner Dweller, Dear Divine Mother, O Great Spirit, Dear Higher Power (whatever phrase feels most comfortable to you based on your personal religious or non-religious upbringing) . . . please grant me the strength to do Thy will—to serve the *shreya* and surrender the *preya*."

The agnostic will fashion a prayer in an entirely different manner than will the Christian or a person from the Jewish tradition, but the form is not as important as your intention.

Remember, words are just pointers. Yoga science does not ask anyone to abandon his or her faith or belief and adopt another, nor should you ask your friend or loved one to use the prayer that you use. To be meaningful and effective, prayer must be a very personal experience and spoken in the language of love—the same language the mother or the father uses with the newborn baby. Avoid using memorized passages that do not have an intimate, heart-opening meaning for you.

Don't feel pressured to construct a long, formal, poetic or grammatically correct prayer. Merely speak lovingly to that Inner Dweller residing in the *cave of the heart* in a simple, direct, open and honest manner.

Make an Offering

Remember, the sages teach that "it is in giving that we receive." Instead of begging for something, as in ego-centered prayer, *God-centered prayer* is an opportunity to give away something you're holding on to—something that is separating you from the Divine Reality. No one knows better than you what your attachments are. Therefore, in your prayer, openly share with the Absolute Reality how difficult it may be for you to give up the worry, anger or unfulfilled selfish desire presently calling your attention and blocking your path.

In the process of making an offering, welcome, witness and honor your attachments dispassionately. Remember, they were created by your previous attention. They're part of the bundle of habit patterns known as your personality. Then, with all the strength and will power you can marshal, make an offering of the contracting *preya* back to the Origin from which it has come. Make the offering lovingly, willingly and joyously as part of your *sadhana* and ask the Inner Dweller to accept this gift of a dedicated seeker, to transform its power and to lead you for your highest and greatest good.

The more you can consciously and willingly surrender your attachments in *God-centered prayer*, the weaker the *samskaras* become, and the less control they will have over your future actions.

Sample God-Centered Prayer

To encourage your own creativity, we have prepared a sample *God-centered prayer*. Please don't consider this something you should memorize. If certain passages speak to your own situation and heart, feel free to incorporate them into your own prayer. If other phrases feel uncomfortable to you, perhaps they might at least help clarify what you're really feeling. Remember, earnestness is the key. As spiritual food for thought, the following is suggested:

> "O Lord of Life, O, my Inner Dweller, Thou Who gives me Light, that I might see, Who gives me power to hear, to smell, to taste, to touch, to think, to analyze, Who gives me power to walk, energy to walk, to do things in the external world; O that Center of Power within me, let me draw strength directly from You. You are my only source of strength.

> O Inner Dweller, Light of Light and Holy of Holies, with a grateful heart for the bounty and blessings of creation that You unceasingly provide, I humbly pray that your Presence come forward into my awareness and that you lead me in my meditation and my practice.

Teach me to receive with equanimity the pleasant and the unpleasant, remembering that You are the Origin of all; that everything is here for me to use and to enjoy but not to possess, nor to be possessed by.

O Inner Dweller, help me to purify this body, mind and senses that I might become an instrument of love, forgiveness and compassion, to do Thy will—even in the face of my own likes and dislikes.

O Inner Dweller, though I am attached to the charms, attractions and temptations of this material world, I desire to surrender all my attachments back to You: I surrender my very breath, body, mind and senses. I surrender every concept of I, and me and mine. I surrender all fear and worry, anger and selfish desire. I surrender the ignorance of separateness and the illusion of personal doer-ship. On the altar of surrender I offer You my expectations, anticipations and intentions, my judgments and criticisms, conclusions and opinions—every thought, every word, every deed. I make this offering lovingly, humbly and earnestly, and pray that You will consume this offering in the fire of your compassionate Light. Lead me from the unreal to the Real. Lead me from the darkness to the Light. Lead me from mortality to immortality.

O Inner Dweller, I pray for your strength. I humbly pray for your grace. I pray for your grace through the scriptures. I pray for your grace through those teachers who bring me knowledge. I pray for your grace through the Absolute Reality within. May the voice and light of the Divine Reality Within grow in my awareness. Grant me an ear to hear and eye to see, at all times, in every relationship and every circumstance, that I might declare with full faith, in this lifetime: I and my Father are One."

CHAPTER 40

Seeing Discipline as a Joy

Enter in at the strait gate: for wide is the gate and broad is the way that leadeth to destruction, and narrow is the way which leadeth unto life, and few there be that find it.

JESUS THE CHRIST

New students invariably cringe at the first mention of the dreaded "D" word—Discipline. That's because most people equate discipline with losing the freedom to enjoy something pleasant. Nothing could be further from the truth. Lack of self-discipline is not real freedom, but rather an expression of the fear of accepting responsibility. Real freedom and unbounded Happiness are realized only when we go beyond the enslaving and debilitating consequences of habitually acting from our fear, anger or self-willed desire.

Despite our physical, mental or emotional dis-ease, yoga science never describes the human being as imperfect. Rather, individuals are considered incomplete—unfinished works in progress. The word yoga means unity or union. To make ourselves complete and to fulfill our true purpose of uniting with the Divine (God-realization), each of us has been granted this human life.

If we can establish a philosophy of life that helps us exercise discrimination in thought, word and deed, we eliminate obstacles to our path and come to know genuine Happiness.

"You are the architect of your life," Swami Rama of the Himalayas teaches, "and you determine your destiny." But in order to know a healthy, creative, loving and rewarding destiny, yoga science requires a commitment to the ongoing examination, understanding and stewardship of your greatest resource: the power of the mind.

Those who habitually avoid discipline in favor of serving the *preya*, mistakenly believe they will experience happiness as a result. But they never do. In real life, just the opposite occurs. The situation is like the Chinese finger torture: the harder you pull your fingers apart, seeking freedom, the more enslaved you become.

When a seeker begins to practice self-discipline, the four major faculties of the mind are coordinated—all in service to the higher knowledge of the Inner Dweller. Self-discipline facilitates the transformation of the inherent power of habit patterns into strategic reserves of energy, will power and creativity. Instead of remaining enslaved to the charms of the world, the *sadhaka* employs the *buddhi* to reduce inner conflict. When your inner conflict is resolved, outer conflict disappears.

The sages of all traditions remind us that fulfillment of desire does not bring true Happiness. In fact, the fulfillment of one desire simply gives rise to another desire, and to the fear that we might lose what we have. Rather, it is our introspection and coordination of the functions of the mind in service to the Divine wisdom within that bring lasting peace and Happiness.

The Challenge of Siblings

Several years ago an acquaintance sent me an e-mail written by Brian Drew Chalker. The message suggested that when people come into our lives it is for "a reason, a season, or a lifetime." When we figure out which category describes a particular relationship, Chalker wrote, we will better know what we are to do to make that relationship harmonious and rewarding.

When a relationship lasts an entire lifetime it means that major lessons are to be learned, and some of our most important lifetime relationships are with siblings. Because of their intensity and duration, these relationships are well-suited to presenting the karmic issues we are destined to face in this life. They can be especially challenging because brothers and sisters are likely to possess intimate knowledge of how and when to push our emotional buttons. These lifetime relationships often remain problematic and painful until we can detach ourselves from our habitual reactions. When that lesson is learned, with the aid of self-discipline, we become free to act skillfully in mutually rewarding and beneficial ways.

My sister and I were the only two children in our family. Carol was three years older, and from early childhood I wanted to share every new observation and insight with her, my confidant and sounding board in a world populated with adults. As we grew, she naturally began to look beyond our sibling relationship for stimulation, fulfillment and acceptance. But the desire to share my latest discoveries with her only increased as Carol began to spend more time away from the family.

As a teenager, this desire to share experiences and perceptions centered on the usual litany of adolescent concerns like music, movies, crushes and athletic and academic achievement. As years went by, I studied, practiced and benefited from meditation and its allied disciplines, and, as usual, I was eager to share my experiences with my sister. But as a consequence of serving this desire without discrimination, a problem developed.

On some occasions when I enthusiastically attempted to discuss the benefits of yoga science, Carol responded as though my comments were a criticism of her and her chosen lifestyle. Her misperception, and my inability to heal it, drove a wedge between us and dampened our relationship.

Because of the pain we were both experiencing, I began to contemplate and question the worthiness of serving a desire that had brought dis-ease to my sister. Even though I never intended to hurt her, the *buddhi* was telling me that my actions were *preya*, and as such, not in harmony with *ahimsa*.

Acknowledging the pain my words were causing, I under-took an experiment in self-discipline. As part of my *sadhana*, I willingly sacrificed the desire to speak about my yogic experiences with my sister. What followed was very interesting.

At first, I felt some resentment about giving up an innocent desire to share the benefits of meditation and yoga philosophy. But when I was able to skillfully surrender those self-centered *preyas*, I became less concerned with what I desired to say and more open to hearing what Carol was actually saying.

It's not easy to refrain from serving a lifelong desire, but my self-discipline turned out to be very fulfilling. When I remained centered as the Inner Witness—really listening to my sister rather than serving my own agenda—my heart became more receptive to her needs. By practicing self-discipline and serving the Divine wisdom of *buddhi* I discovered wellsprings of compassion and concern within both myself and my sister that have helped heal and expand the nature of our relationship.

This personal experience with self-discipline proved to be a perfect illustration of the practical and profound prayer of St. Francis.

Lord, make me an instrument of thy peace.
Where there is hatred, let me sow love.
Where there is injury, pardon.
Where there is doubt, faith.
Where there is despair, hope.
Where there is darkness, light.
Where there is sadness, joy.
O divine master, grant that I may not so much seek
To be consoled as to console,
To be understood as to understand,
To be loved as to love.
For it is in giving that we receive,
It is in pardoning that we are pardoned,
It is in dying [to the small separate sense of self]
That we are born to eternal life.

Self-discipline fosters the capacity to observe mindfully all that is happening in both the external and internal worlds so we can make the conscious, discriminating choices that lead us to freedom.

At the present time, the mind and its habits still have most human beings enslaved. The secret of successful living is to recognize that we are actually citizens of two worlds. Therefore, we are to live in the world, yet remain the Inner Witness, aware of the Divine Reality in all circumstances and relationships. How? When you look around your world and bemoan the fact that so many things are "bad," go deeper within until you identify the Witness of that thought. Whenever there is consternation in the mind, it means that the ego is in charge—condemning you to the delusion of separateness, judgment and want.

Now, knowing the bliss and fullness of your own true Self as the Eternal Witness, stop identifying with your thoughts and the objects of the external world, and let your mind, action and speech be guided dispassionately by the *buddhi*. Through this discipline, suffering ends.

Starting today, learn through your daily *sadhana* to become a discriminating instrument in service to the Divine intelligence that is both within you and *is* You . . . having this human experience. As you continue a consistent and dedicated spiritual practice, you will come to recognize that self-discipline is not an onerous denial of satisfaction, but rather the pathway to life's greatest joy.

CHAPTER 41

Entering the Crucible of Change

Take my yoke upon you and learn of me . . . and ye shall find rest unto your souls. For my yoke is easy, and my burden is light."

JESUS THE CHRIST

Pain is your best friend. It is infinitely more honest with you than pleasure. Despite what you might think, the painful experiences you have had benefit you far more than the pleasurable ones, even though most of us spend our lives trying to duck and hide from them. But when you can center yourself and be open to look pain dead in the eye, then you have transcended the limits of your ego and this humanity. It is then that you enter into the possibility of becoming a great being.

SWAMI CHETANANANDA

If you want to be given everything, give up everything.

LAO TZU

July 26, 1995

It was unusually hot and humid on that first day of thoroughbred racing in Saratoga Springs. For the nineteenth year in a row, we had completed the arduous three-day task of hanging our annual exhibition of paintings and preparing for the opening reception. Satisfied that all was ready, we left the gallery and tried to unwind during the fifty minute drive back to our home in Averill Park.

As we drove, we began to reminisce and take stock. As usual, the final days of preparation were physically and emotionally draining. We weren't kids anymore, and the pressure had been building for months. Painting, framing, transporting and hanging seventy-five works of art had made us, at the age of fifty, keenly aware of our own mortality. Through it all, the familiar, ever-present uncertainty of having a financially successful exhibition only added to our weariness. We were looking forward to a restful night's sleep before the opening reception the next evening.

Since 1974, we had lived and worked in a converted barn in Averill Park, New York—a quiet upstate town where our neighbors are hardworking and respectful of one another. Our summer exhibition in Saratoga gave us our only glimpse, from our rural location, of an art market capable of supporting a contemporary artist.

All year, working under the professional name Jenness Cortez, Jenness painted images depicting the pageantry and excitement of horse racing at the prestigious Saratoga race-course. Then, each summer, we hung our exhibition in the ballroom of a major hotel hoping that the money we earned through the sale of paintings would keep us going for another season.

Over the years, Cortez paintings provided the public a poetic reflection of a world filled with fast horses and colorful people—horse owners, trainers, jockeys, breeders, show business personalities, race fans and politicians. Through Jenness's creations and my efforts to sell them, we were able to support ourselves, and the Daymon Runyon-like cast of characters and wanna-bes were able to see themselves as part of a time-honored tradition. Without exaggeration, by 1995 Jenness's paintings and the public perception of Saratoga had become virtually synonymous.

When we began to prepare for our first Saratoga show back in 1976, doors of opportunity were graciously opened to us. Public relations officials from the New York Racing Association (owners and operators of the racetrack) literally took us on guided tours of the facility to point out dozens of scenes they thought would make beautiful paintings.

Over the years, we happily granted the Racing Association (NYRA) permission to reproduce many of Jenness's paintings on their daily race program, Christmas card greetings, promotional calendars and newsletters—all without financial remuneration.

As the informal relationship developed and continued, the thought of charging NYRA money for the rights to reproduce Jenness's paintings never even occurred to us. This was simply a mutually beneficial relationship. NYRA was able to use the romantic Cortez images to promote its business and Jenness's art received an entree to a responsive audience.

The Lawsuit

By the early 1990s, however, the relationships began to change.

Technically, NYRA is a privately run, non-profit corporation—granted permission by the State of New York to own and operate a thoroughbred racetrack in Saratoga and to administer wagering for the state. However, because NYRA collects hundreds of millions of gambling dollars and its administrative operations fall under the legislative scrutiny of state government, the courts have determined that NYRA is legally a "quasi-governmental agency" of New York.

As the decade of the 1990s began, the thoroughbred racing industry was under intense financial pressure from an array of factors. These included an aging and dwindling fan base, the proliferation of numerous state lotteries and casino gambling operations, and the appearance of off-track betting parlors in virtually every neighborhood in the state.

In light of the competition, NYRA officials sought to

maximize profits. One novel idea they considered was to enter the burgeoning business of sports licensing. NYRA was aware of the lucrative trademark licensing programs already instituted by other sports. Major League Baseball, the National Football League and the National Basketball Association were already making millions of dollars by reproducing team logos on an array of products, and NYRA decided to explore the financial potential for its own sport.

Against this backdrop, NYRA filed a federal trademark for the word "Saratoga" in 1990—claiming it owned exclusive rights to the word "Saratoga" in connection with horse racing, as well as the right to all images of horse racing at the Saratoga Racecourse. For many residents of Saratoga County and the City of Saratoga Springs—the history of which dates to the American Revolution—this action was shocking.

Even though the law allows an individual or corporation the legal right to trademark any word, enforcing a trademark claim is a different issue altogether. Usually, in order to substantiate a contentious claim, a powerful corporation like NYRA—in this case, with the muscle and influence of the State of New York behind it—would first try to intimidate a smaller and weaker competitor into conceding its own legitimate rights under the threat of expensive legal proceedings. If that approach failed, the owner of a trademark would then have to rely on the courts. In other words, a non-acquiescing competitor would be sued in an attempt to convince a judge to enforce such a claim.

By the time our summer exhibition was hung in 1995, NYRA officials had already approached us about their trademark claims. They demanded that we pay them 15 percent of our income generated through the sale of Jenness's artwork containing the word "Saratoga" in the title or depicting images of Saratoga horse racing in its composition. With the sole exception of original paintings, NYRA demanded payment on original, hand-drawn lithographs and etchings, signed, open-edition prints, greeting cards and art shirts.

When pressed by our attorneys to explain their legal

justification for such demands, NYRA officials claimed they did not want to explain their rights because, in their own words, "We don't want to be limited by what we say. What if an artist comes up with a novel idea we hadn't considered? Would that mean NYRA didn't own the image?"

Our legal research, however, had concluded just the opposite—NYRA had no legal precedent to justify its claim. Counsel advised us that we had not broken any laws; that NYRA was merely trying to increase its own revenues by rewriting the intellectual property law. But this intimidating negotiation tactic ended abruptly.

When we arrived home from Saratoga on that July afternoon in 1995, we were informed that a reporter from the local NBC affiliate had telephoned. When Jenness returned the call, the question awaiting her was anything but usual. It was a bombshell! "What is your reaction," the reporter asked, "to the lawsuit filed against you in federal court by the New York Racing Association?"

We were in shock—filled with embarrassment, fear and then anger. We felt as if an intruder had broken into our home in the middle of the night and slammed us from behind with a two-by-four. Totally abandoning their negotiating strategy, NYRA had abruptly decided to litigate. We had become the legal test case for their trademark claims, and the events that followed would forever change our lives.

The next days, weeks and months were filled with meetings, affidavits, court appearances, emotional roller coaster rides, the slow deterioration of income, and the loss of many social and business associations because we were on the politically incorrect end of the lawsuit. And, of course, piles and piles of bills. Our attorneys had told us right from the first legal volley that our position was sound; that we had not broken the law, and that NYRA was merely exhibiting greed.

In moments of frustration and doubt, we would have preferred to run away or just accept NYRA as an undesirable partner. As we analyzed our situation, we understood how Arjuna must have felt on the eve of his great battle in the

Bhagavad Gita. Like Arjuna, we faced powerful emotions of fear, anger and despondency that were undermining our willingness to fight. Yet, despite the anguish, we knew intuitively that we were being asked by Divine Providence to fight this fight; to protect ourselves and to fulfill our duty (*dharma*) by defending every artist's constitutional right of free expression. After much deliberation, we decided to commit ourselves (and our limited resources) to what local newspaper columnists were already calling a real-life David and Goliath battle.

A Divine Alliance

Throughout this difficult ordeal, the philosophy and science of yoga gave us the insight and inner strength to face each decision and turn of fortune. We realized that we were being tested. We had been studying and assimilating the wisdom of yoga for many years. Now, in order to be true to that teaching, we were being asked to make difficult decisions that reflected our theoretical and intellectual understanding. And it was not easy.

The traditional definition of the word Islam is "trustful surrender to Divine Providence," and that essence of Islam is reflected in every spiritual tradition. Through our studies, we had learned (intellectually) that there is only One Absolute Reality and that each of us exists inseparable from a larger, conscious whole. When we are in harmony with that consciousness, we know that each individual manifestation supports every other expression. Our studies had taught us that everything we perceive has been manifested by the Divine Reality and that each relationship has the potential of leading us for our highest and greatest good—regardless of the protests and anguish of the limited ego.

For us, being sued by the New York Racing Association was a life-altering experience. Because NYRA represented an enormously powerful economic and social presence in our small upstate community, we knew that many relationships would change. If we chose to accept the financial demands of

NYRA, we would not be true to our conscience. If, on the other hand, we fought the legal fight—regardless of whether we won or lost—we ran the risk of being ostracized by the powerful political and economic interests behind the corporate facade of NYRA. And that's what happened.

Saratoga Springs, like other "company towns," still reflects aspects of feudal society. In feudal times, if the lord of a manor wrongfully discriminated against one of his vassals, the other vassals would likely distance themselves from the spurned party in order to maintain their good standing with the lord.

In fact, when the powerful New York Racing Association sued us, we immediately lost the support and friendship of other artists exhibiting in Saratoga, prominent banking, business and political leaders who had previously been our patrons, the Saratoga and Rensselaer County arts councils, the local Saratoga newspaper and the very hotel where we had been exhibiting Jenness's paintings for fifteen consecutive years.

We were not, however, totally abandoned. The regional print and television press corps understood the constitutional issues and were very supportive, as were the Albany-Schenectady League of Arts, the American Civil Liberties Union, SUNY Empire State College, the many Cortez art collectors who cheered us on, and our immediate families and friends. Of course, our greatest source of comfort and support was our *sadhana* and the teachings of yoga science.

Through the pain, fear and anger of the ordeal, our philosophy of life and the skills learned through the practice of yoga science gave us the strength, insight, discrimination and will power to make the moment-by-moment, thought-by-thought decisions that ultimately helped us experience the liberating truth of the knowledge we had assimilated.

Throughout our ordeal, the Old Testament story of Joseph gave us strength and inspiration. His jealous brothers, as you might remember, sold Joseph into slavery. Years later, after Joseph had become governor of Egypt, the brothers came petitioning for grain during a time of widespread famine.

Upon discovering that the governor of Egypt was actually their long-lost brother, they began to cry and beg for Joseph's forgiveness. Joseph's response was not vengeful. Rather, it reflected a profound understanding of the yogic philosophy of trustful surrender to Divine Providence. In modern vernacular, Joseph told them, "There is no need to forgive you, my brothers, for it was not you who sold me into slavery. It was the Lord who sold me into slavery—using you as instruments—so that I could be here today to feed you and all who are hungry."

After NYRA sued us, the rapid succession of changes we experienced meant the death of many comfortable habits and relationships. Our everyday expectations about earning a living and relating to our local community were being taken away from us.

Yet, in the midst of this upheaval, we found ourselves aware of a calm, contented center. Our study and practice of yoga science was providing us the freedom and insight to grasp the positive value of circumstances even when they were accompanied by pain.

The philosophy of life we embraced enabled us to transform debilitating *preya* thoughts and emotions and to become fearless in the face of fear. Our *sadhana* helped us recognize that it wasn't really the New York Racing Association foisting this unjust lawsuit upon us. Rather, we trusted that NYRA, like Joseph's brothers, was merely serving as an instrument of Divine Providence bringing revolutionary change into our lives for some as yet unknown higher and greater good. By centering ourselves in the peace of that understanding—the same still-point we experienced in meditation—we witnessed the transformation of our fear, anger and self-willed desires.

The seed must be split in order for a plant to sprout, and the decomposing hull of the seed fertilizes the new growth. In addition to signaling the end of an era, this lawsuit also served as a catalyst for the dawning of a new life for us. By relying on the philosophy of yoga science in all our choices, we were able to employ a practical and powerful mechanism for turning painful and potentially devastating experiences into growth and creativity. Our ordeal had spawned in us an immense gratitude to our teachers, and led to a growing desire to pass this knowledge on to others.

Against this backdrop, in July 1996—almost one year to the day after we had been sued—two pivotal events occurred.

First, Federal District Court Judge Frederick J. Scullin, Jr. rendered a courageous First Amendment decision in our case, completely supporting the artist's constitutional right to free expression. For all intents and purposes, the lawsuit was over, and we were legally free to continue creating and selling Jenness's artwork depicting horse racing at the historic Saratoga racecourse.

Secondly, we received a letter from Swami Rama, our spiritual teacher who was living in India. Although we knew he was ill at the time, we had no idea he would live for only another four months. The letter itself was unusual. It marked the first and only occasion in our relationship when Swami Rama gave us such a direct and unequivocal order. The entire message read: "Start teaching now."

While succinct and emphatic, the letter did not instruct what, where or how we were to teach—only to begin *now*! Yet, even in the face of this seeming vagueness, the instruction left us no room for misunderstanding.

By using the word "now" in his instruction, the universal *light of guru*, through the personage of Swami Rama, was clearly reminding us of how that same word is used in the opening verse of the *Yoga Sutras*. In that ancient text, the Sanskrit verse states: *Atha yoganushasanam*: "Now begins instruction in the discipline of yoga."

As Swami Rama himself had previously taught us, the word "now" in the *Yoga Sutras* is used to note an auspicious moment of transition. The sages of yoga science carefully chose to use the word "now" to indicate that satisfactory preparation had been completed, and that the student was ready to undertake a new aspect of his or her spiritual practice. By using the phrase "start teaching now," Swami Rama was disclosing to us that we were adequately prepared in our studies and that *now*, at this auspicious moment, we were ready to become teachers in the tradition of yoga science.

CHAPTER 42

Birth of AMI

The wood does not change the fire into itself, but fire changes the wood into itself. So we are changed into God, that we shall know Him as He is.

GEORGE BERNARD SHAW

As we read and reread Swami Rama's written instructions to "start teaching now," two important memories came to mind.

Our first meeting with Swami Rama took place in May 1991. Although Jenness and I had been studying yoga science and philosophy as serious students since 1976, it was not our habit to attend lectures or retreats. Our personalities seemed better suited to reading the classical and contemporary writings of both East and West, and to fashioning our own spiritual practice based on what felt right in our hearts, minds and bodies.

However, our *sadhana* had accelerated and expanded to such an extent that we were curtailing social and business relationships in order to give more attention to our studies and practice. As we simplified our lives, we felt healthier and more content, but grew uneasy about the many and profound changes we were making. Although the alterations were benefiting us, no one in our immediate family, social or business community had any interest in, nor understanding of, our spiritual practice. Feeling a bit as if we were out on a limb, we decided to seek advice from someone who had walked this path before—someone we respected.

Although we had never met Swami Rama, by 1991 we had been studying his books for thirteen years. Since both of us acknowledged him as our primary teacher, we decided to write to ask if he would see us. Two days after we mailed our letter, Swami Rama's secretary, Kamal, telephoned us from his teaching facility in Pennsylvania to say Swami Rama wanted to initiate us into the Himalayan tradition as soon as possible. We subsequently learned that Swami Rama had already begun to retire from his worldly activities at that time, and was only rarely initiating students. We now cherish that experience as an auspicious gift.

The night before our initiation, we met informally with Swami Rama for the first time. He asked if I were a teacher. "No," I replied, "I'm an art dealer." His response was swift and precise: "You are a teacher, and many people will come to you. And I will help you."

The second memory that came to mind as we read the instructions to "start teaching now" was of an August day in 1992. Swami Rama had accepted our invitation to visit our annual painting exhibition in Saratoga Springs. We were very proud and excited as Swami Rama, dressed in his burgundy robe, strolled regally into our gallery with three of his disciples trailing behind him. The August show represented a year's labor and, as we had discussed with him before, it was our only opportunity to sell Jenness's paintings so close to home.

After respectfully greeting the Swami, we slowly escorted him around the exhibition, stopping at each painting as Jenness presented personal and artistic insights. The entire tour took about twenty minutes and, when it concluded, we and his entourage stood at his side, eagerly anticipating the master's comments.

A few suspenseful seconds of silence passed. Then, Swami Rama's lips began to move and his words became audible. "This should not be here!" he decreed.

What could he mean?! We were both in shock. We knew

from studying his writings and through our own experience of him, that Swami Rama measured his words very carefully. He was known as a "seer," one who sees things as they are rather than as they appear. His spare sentences were often like riddles to be studied and deciphered. But, "This should not be here!" Why would he say such a thing? Did he think we could have found a better location for the exhibition?

In the interlude of silence that followed, both of us independently decided we could make no immediate reply, although we knew we'd have to contemplate his words very seriously. Under the circumstances, however, "Anyone for lunch?" seemed the easiest response.

Later, as we became embroiled in litigation with the Racing Association, the meaning of Swami Rama's pronouncement that "This should not be here" began to make sense. It became clear that attachments to the status quo had been clouding our vision at the time Swami Rama visited us in Saratoga, but the subsequent pain of the NYRA lawsuit helped us to sacrifice many of our limitations and re-order our priorities.

We came to realize that yoga science was our strongest and most reliable ally. Nothing else could make sense of our predicament. The difficult circumstances motivated us to intensify our *sadhana* and earnestly align our thoughts, words and deeds with the intuitive wisdom of the *buddhi*.

By making every choice a means for our spiritual unfoldment, we came to see, in retrospect, that the beneficent force of *guru* had been subtly advising us that our creative energies had been misdirected for quite some time. At long last we knew the time had come to move on, and that the suffering we were experiencing by defending the artist's constitutional right of free expression was only a reflection of our resistance to that transformation.

Challenging and painful as the battle was, it provided a catalyst for seeing many issues in clearer perspective. NYRA's incomprehensible legal actions were instrumental in our decision to follow the intuition of our hearts, and not to continue business as usual.

In fact, we could find only one real motivation for maintaining the status quo, and that was fear—fear that we wouldn't be able to find another creative outlet for our energies and talents while still making a living. Ultimately, however, our fear, powerful as it was, was not enough to keep us from exploring other possibilities the universe was presenting to us.

In retrospect, we recognized that we had spent twenty years creating and selling horse racing paintings of Saratoga. At the half-century mark of our lives we had to ask ourselves realistically, "How many twenty-year periods do we have remaining to give to any worthwhile project?" The answer was sobering, and although we found it difficult to admit, our course now seemed obvious.

As part of our *sadhana*, we decided to renounce attachment to our fear. Jenness would no longer paint images of Saratoga horse racing. As an act of faith in yoga philosophy, we sacrificed the sporting art market that had supported us for most of our adult years, opening ourselves up to whatever Divine Providence would bring into our lives. From that moment on, we agreed, Jenness would apply her artistic talents to other subjects, and together, we would offer to students a practical teaching we understood through our own personal experience.

Having received direct instructions in the summer of 1996 to "start teaching now," we began to discuss the form, content and location of that teaching. At first we assumed that we should teach at Swami Rama's *ashram* in Pennsylvania where we had been initiated. To our surprise, however, the new director of that organization refused our numerous attempts to discuss the matter.

After that rejection and a great deal of soul searching, I finally understood the meaning of Swami Rama's first words to me in May of 1991: "You are a teacher, and many people will come to you. And I will help you." Had Swami Rama known immediately that students would seek me out where I lived? Suddenly, my path was clear: I was to teach where I lived, and through our earnestness Providence would sustain that effort.

We also gained clarity on the issue of what to teach. We

decided that the only subjects we could offer with honesty and authority were those we practiced. We knew their merits well. Throughout the emotional onslaught of the legal battle, the dissolution of our livelihood and the loss of friends and business associates, our spiritual practice had kept us balanced, upright and creative.

If the practical application of yoga science and philosophy worked so well for us in such demanding circumstances, we concluded, it could work for others as well—assuming they were interested and earnest. So, we started outlining a curriculum of the practices that formed our own daily *sadhana*.

What evolved was the birth of a growing number of classes and an association of students that we eventually named the American Meditation Institute for Yoga Science and Philosophy. We did not choose this name casually. In addition to honoring the lineage of teachers who preceded us, we wanted our teaching to reflect our own American roots. After all, we were part of the post-World War II American baby boom. We were the first generation influenced by television and such personalities as Davey Crockett, Roy Rogers, Eleanor Roosevelt, Elvis Presley, John F. Kennedy, Martin Luther King, Jr., Bob Dylan and the Beatles. Our early lives had been shaped by experiences of the Cold War, the Peace Corps and Vietnam; by liberalized sexual mores, the increasing availability and reliance on drugs and by a rampant materialism embraced as a remedy for our persistent mental and emotional pain.

Although we were Western by birth and experience, our earnest desire to diminish our own dis-ease had led us to investigate the messages of the East as well as the West. In that search, we discovered that the essence of Eastern thought is present in Western philosophy and science. Through our study and practice, a rich tapestry of Eastern and Western wisdom began to reveal itself.

Again and again the same message appeared to us in the context of many different traditions. The scriptures of the Old Testament, New Testament, Quran, *Bhagavad Gita, Upanishads, Dhammapada*, Talmud and Kabbala supported and enriched one another. The philosophies enunciated by Jesus in the Sermon on the Mount, St. Francis of Assisi, Shakespeare, Meister Eckhart, Teihard de Chardin, Rumi, Kabir, Black Elk, Emerson, Thoreau and Whitman all began to echo and reinforce one another. Our study and practice helped us realize that on the highest level of consciousness, only one truth exists. Names and forms, places of origin, personalities, historical and cultural contexts may differ, but truth remains the same.

For us, the science and philosophy of yoga represents a practical, common sense methodology for experimenting with truth—a profound process for transforming the energy of the mind into meaningful, creative and joyful life experiences.

But please, don't believe us. If you are at all interested, take the knowledge we offer and experiment with it every day in your life like a real yoga scientist, because your own experience is the only mechanism by which you will come to know the truth of this knowledge. Then, experience by experience, take what resonates as truth and consciously discard that which does not. On your journey, never be guided by the suggestions of others—unless those suggestions are endorsed by your own common sense, your own discrimination, your own heart, your own inner *guru*.

CHAPTER 43

Uncomplicating Modern American Life

> *Manifest plainness.*
> *Embrace simplicity.*
> *Reduce selfishness.*
> *Have few desires.*
>
> LAO TZU

> *Be ye therefore perfect,*
> *Even as your Father which is in heaven is perfect.*
>
> JESUS THE CHRIST

Without question, modern American life is fast-paced and hectic. When you stop to think about all your duties and responsibilities, you may sometimes feel overwhelmed and under-equipped to handle them.

If you have a spouse and children, they require a great deal of time and loving attention. You may also be facing challenging situations with aging parents, siblings, work and your ability to pay all the bills. Simply maintaining your own good health can become a major issue.

As if that weren't enough, there are concerns about the economy, your dwindling retirement nest egg and the persistent threat of terrorism—all of which underscore the unspoken fear of your own mortality. Being human is a challenging assignment.

Like the proverbial rat in a maze, most of us attempt to cope with stress by treating ourselves to more and more of what we see as the world's pleasures. Diversions like television, movies, vacations, exercise, consumerism and alcohol can all provide temporary relief from our dis-ease, but eventually the weight of the world reappears. When we are enslaved to the matrix, it is impossible to explore new possibilities that might free us from our bondage.

Everyday life does not have to remain as stressful, worrisome and unfulfilling as it currently appears to be. According to the sages of all traditions, we can gain access to a Divine intelligence greater than the human mind, and if relied upon, Its wisdom can uncomplicate modern American life. Many books have been written about this knowledge and teachers willingly share their experiences, but this wisdom can transform our lives only when we implement Its inherent power.

Toward the end of the Sermon on the Mount, Jesus the Christ shares this practical understanding with his apostles when He explains, "Whosoever heareth these sayings of mine, and doeth them, I will liken him unto a wise man, which built his house upon a rock: And the rain descended, and the floods came, and the winds blew, and beat upon that house; and it fell not: for it was founded upon a rock." Then Jesus makes it very clear that the rock upon which to base our lives is not mere belief in Him. Belief, Jesus the Christ insists, must manifest in actions that acknowledge and serve Divine will. "Not every one that saith unto Me, 'Lord, Lord,' shall enter into the kingdom of heaven; but he that doeth the will of my Father who is in heaven."

The science of yoga teaches that *buddhi*, the discriminating power of the human mind, is the mirrored reflection of the will of the Divine Reality, and is the rock upon which Jesus the Christ teaches us to base our lives. In the ancient Christian tradition, *buddhi* is spoken of as the Holy Spirit, and Western culture acknowledges it as the conscience.

Most of us sense that we are citizens of two worlds: the

manifest world that is known and seen, and the unmanifest world of consciousness that is unseen and usually unknown. Still, we don't fully understand how to access the power of the unmanifest world for our unbounded Happiness—here and now, in this lifetime.

If we live predominantly in the outer world of names and forms, and if the inner world of thoughts, desires and emotions is not in harmony with the intuitive discrimination of *buddhi*, we separate ourselves from the truth and blessings of the Absolute Reality. Under such circumstances, our alienation from Divine wisdom leaves us no other option than to base our actions on habit, the lure of the senses and the suggestions of others.

Yoga science and meditation create the bridge between the inner and outer worlds. In the *Ashtavakra Gita*, King Janaka is enlightened upon hearing the teachings of the great sage Ashtavakra. As soon as King Janaka awakens to the realization of his true Self and receives instruction on how knowledge of the subtle world leads to success in the material world, the illusion of separateness—the cause of his suffering and bondage—disappears.

At that moment, King Janaka exclaims the joy of Self-realization: "O, wonder that I am! I salute Myself who knows no decay and survives even the destruction of the entire universe. O, wonder that I am! I salute Myself who, though with a body, am one who neither goes anywhere nor comes from anywhere but ever abides pervading the universe. O, wonder that I am! I salute Myself, none more capable, who is bearing the burden of the entire universe without even touching it with my body."[1]

When you are able to skillfully walk the bridge between the inner and outer worlds, your life becomes Divinely directed. As the intuitive power of *buddhi* guides you, the stress you once experienced from everyday circumstances will begin to vanish.

[1] *Duet of One*, by Ramesh S. Balsekar, ©1989 Advaita Press, PO Box 3479, Redondo Beach, California 90277.

On that day, no matter what calamities befall you, every relationship that requires an action is seen as a means to spiritual unfoldment and liberation. What was once complicated becomes uncomplicated. What was once overwhelming becomes energizing. What was once infuriating becomes instructive, and the one who was once fearful becomes fearless.

When there is no longer any distinction between you and the Absolute Reality, you move through the world free from both attachment and aversion alike, and you abide in a peace in which all sorrows end.

Recognizing the Power of Desire

Several years ago our young friend fell in love with a wonderful girl, and, as the relationship developed, they talked of marriage. Eventually he wanted to buy her an engagement ring. As he thought more about the ring, he spoke to friends who advised him that the best place to buy a ring was the diamond district in New York City.

Now, this was a fellow who was so nervous about travel that he avoided visiting the next town twelve miles away, but as his desire for the engagement ring grew, he considered taking an unusual action to fulfill a powerful desire. One morning he woke up early, took $1,800 in cash from his savings, taped it to his ankle, pulled his sock over the money, gathered all his courage, copied down the address of a recommended jeweler in the diamond district, and took a train 143 miles south into what he truly believed to be the bowels of hell. When he arrived at Grand Central Station, he took a cab to the jeweler's, bought the ring, and then headed back home.

This story clearly provides scientific evidence of the power of desire. It was the power of desire that propelled this apprehensive, two hundred-pound human being a distance of 143 miles. Without the desire, such an undertaking would have been absolutely impossible.

In the language of the physical sciences, energy is the

capacity to move an object a certain distance through space. In the practice of yoga science, desire is energy, and attention is the mechanism that transforms potential energy into kinetic energy and unusable energy into usable energy—all for the purpose of realizing the goals we most cherish in life.

Unifying the Power of Desires

In every facet of life the supreme human desire for unbounded Life, Liberty and Happiness is expressed through one of four basic categories of desire. In yoga science these desires are known as:

Artha — material comfort and security.

Kama — emotional, intellectual or physical pleasure (the desire that, when thwarted, gives rise to anger; when fulfilled, it may give rise to selfishness, attachment, jealousy or pride).

Dharma — the eternal law that maintains individual and social order. Duty; right action.

Moksha — realization of unbounded Life, Liberty and Happiness; liberation from the pain, misery and bondage experienced in human life.

The fulfillment of each of these four categories of desire is considered essential to living a rewarding human life. No one can be truly happy or fully content unless the desires for *artha*, *kama*, *dharma* and *moksha* are recognized, honored, explored and balanced. These four are listed in order from the most gross (*artha*) to the most subtle (*moksha*), for this is the sequence in which they motivate most of us.

The more we rely on the intuitive wisdom of the *buddhi* to consciously transform the energy of desires for *artha* and *kama*, the greater will be our personal fulfillment. Conversely, the more we remain attached to fulfilling selfish desires, the greater will be our physical, mental, emotional and spiritual dis-ease. The choice is ours.

In order to consciously shape our destiny, we need to know what we want most in life, and adopt a philosophy that helps us reach our goal. This means working toward the fulfillment of our higher desires for *dharma* and *moksha*—even during our pursuit of *artha* and *kama*. The Divine wisdom of *buddhi* equips us to fulfill all these desires in a creative and gratifying way.

When we unify the energy of our many smaller desires to serve the one deep, driving desire for *moksha* (liberation), all our thoughts, words and actions will manifest what we need: health, security, happiness, creative work, and loving relationships. By choosing the *shreya* over the *preya* in fulfilling our desires for *artha* (security) and *kama* (pleasure), we automatically achieve fulfillment in our *dharma*. These three desires, rightly expressed, result in *moksha* (the realization of unbounded Life, Liberty and Happiness, and liberation from all pain, misery and bondage).

As we examine and prioritize all the little desires we previously thought would make us happy, we move toward acknowledging life's true goal through our consistent choice of the *shreya*. Remember the instruction of the ancient *Upanishads*: "You are your deepest driving desire. As your deepest driving desire is, so is your will. As your will is, so is your deed. As your deed is, so is your destiny."

By recognizing *moksha* as our deepest driving desire, we effectively define the standard of *shreya* against which all our physical, mental, emotional, spiritual, vocational, social, familial and financial desires will be measured. Then, every relationship becomes a means for our spiritual unfoldment.

When we harmonize every thought, word and action with *buddhi*'s discrimination by surrendering our many, small desires for the *preya*, we will no longer be bound.

The process of sacrifice and *renunciation* of *preya* is transformation, not repression, and must always be guided by *ahimsa* (non-injury), yoga's first and highest principle. This means that we should never give up too much too soon. Remember, we cannot unify our desires by merely renouncing the worldly objects we possess. Rather, it is by joyful surrender of our attachments to lesser desires that we are led to the freedom we truly seek.

We develop *shraddha* (trust and faith) in direct proportion to the amelioration of the physical, mental and emotional pain we once experienced. It's simple physics: when we clear and purify the mind, our innate and profound Happiness will have room to unfold effortlessly in our lives. By harnessing the energy of all our desires, we gain access to our hidden power and create a destiny that reflects our highest aspirations.

CHAPTER 44

Living Free from Worry

I am an old man and have had many troubles,
most of which never happened.

MARK TWAIN

On a basic level, fear can be a healthy expression of our desire for self-preservation. Obviously, it's prudent to want to protect ourselves, but yoga science reminds us of two important points: first, when the body is truly in danger, animal instinct for self-preservation reliably comes forward to guide our actions against any real or imminent threat; and second, when we become aware of "what-if" situations, it's quite possible to consider these while remaining secure, confident and creative.

If we are courageous enough to examine our fears, we discover them to be based on a false premise. We worry when we forget our true Self. If we believe, "I am the limited body or I am the fallible mind (*jiva*)," we will constantly worry about not getting what we want or losing what we have.

Antidote for Worry

In 1989 we traveled to California to visit one of our dearest teachers, Eknath Easwaran. While with him, we explained that yoga science had become the guiding force in our lives, but we still worried about money. It seemed to us, we told him, that this philosophy would work best for people certain of receiving a paycheck every week. We, on the other hand, were self-employed. The fact that Jenness was a painter and I was an art dealer meant that we never knew from one day to the next if we would have enough money to pay our bills. So we asked for some advice.

Without hesitation, and with a loving twinkle in his eye that I still recall to this day, Easwaran responded, "Your problem is this: you consider yourself self-employed. I am employed by the Self." Hearing that one turn of phrase, we recognized that the antidote for all our worries could be found by earnestly practicing yoga science.

Easwaran's reply taught us that the mental and emotional pain we suffered by worrying was a direct consequence of being enslaved to the limited perspective of the *jiva*. To end our dis-ease, we'd have to expand our sense of "I-ness." We'd have to willingly surrender our small, separate sense of self by relying exclusively on the Divine wisdom of the *buddhi* for every decision—including those about whether or not to worry.

Easwaran's insight made sense to us, so we decided to experiment. Through our own personal experience, we discovered that yoga science is not just a scholarly pursuit. It is a moment-by-moment and thought-by-thought practical guide for living. Our path became clear. In order to end our worries and mental anguish, we simply had to become loyal employees—of the Self. This meant not repressing our worries, but welcoming, witnessing and honoring them without being controlled by them. This detached perspective on circumstances (*vairagya*) helped calm our minds and allowed us to hear and to serve the *buddhi*.

As we consistently were able to surrender the alluring *preya* of worrisome thoughts, the material and spiritual support we needed began to naturally flow into our lives. Trustful surrender to Divine Providence effectively freed us from debilitating *samskaras* while increasing our reserves of energy, will and creativity.

It's Not Ten O'clock Yet

During her recent visit to the American Meditation Institute, our colleague, Ginger Cunes, told an inspiring story that speaks to this very point. In 1994, Ginger and her daughter Jill were planning to visit Swami Rama in India. Because of some frustrating difficulties with the Indian Consulate, however, they had still not received their passports the night before their flight. Yet, on the morning of their departure, Ginger awakened Jill well before sunrise and told her to get dressed and prepare for their 10 A.M. ride to the airport. Jill's reaction was predictable. Why should they be rushing to the airport if they had no passports? But Ginger was persistent: "To get to the airport on time, we must leave the house by 10 A.M. Until ten o'clock, we have no problem. Just get ready." Jill, despite her protests, finished packing.

At precisely 9:55 A.M., the postman rang the doorbell. "I have a special delivery package," he announced. "Of course you do," Ginger exclaimed. "It's our passports!" And it was. The moral of the story is this: no matter how bleak things may appear, if it's not ten o'clock yet, there's no problem and no need to worry.

Swami Rama often reminded his students that "whatever is going to happen is going to happen, and whatever is not going to happen is not going to happen." In any given situation, if we are secure in the Self and our actions reflect the wisdom of *buddhi*, we can free ourselves from worries simply by resting our consciousness in the fullness of the present moment.

When we learn this skill, we recognize that there is, in fact, no actual connection between one moment and the next or between one thought and the next. Every moment and every thought is fresh and unique. When we abide in the present, not overly concerned with our own self-will, we allow a great creative force to shine forth through our words and deeds. The fruits of those actions will not only transform our limiting personality, but also the world.

CHAPTER 45
Epilogue

If you did not desire your present position, You would not be doing everything possible to maintain it.

LEO TOLSTOY

You are in pain because you don't want what you have and you don't have what you want. The solution is so simple: Just want what you have and don't want what you don't have.

NISARGADATTA MAHARAJ

Become the change you seek in the world.

MAHATMA GANDHI

Whether we consciously acknowledge it or not, each of us is on a journey. We have come from somewhere, and we are headed somewhere. Throughout this brief interlude called life, we have unwittingly created bundles of habit patterns for ourselves; deep *samskaras* of fear, anger and greed that cause us to view life through the lens of our own ignorance—the habit of ignoring our own Divinity. We are like the man of perfect proportion who goes on a crash diet after seeing himself in a distorting mirror that makes him look as if he weighs three hundred pounds.

The practices of yoga science provide opportunities to unburden ourselves of those habits that have kept us enslaved to the pain of our own ignorance. We have the great gift of a human birth. We now have a body. We have a mind. We have five senses and the unique faculty of *buddhi*. Thanks to our humanity, we have all the necessary tools to leave behind the suffering brought about by indulging our animal nature and to reclaim the Divine treasure hidden deep within our consciousness. But to accomplish this goal, we must learn to be present in each moment to make discriminating, conscious choices.

In 1962, President Kennedy announced that the United States would place a man on the moon before the end of that decade. "We choose to go to the moon," Kennedy said, "not because it is easy, but because it is hard; because that goal will serve to organize and measure the best of our energies and skills; because that challenge is one that we are willing to accept, one we are unwilling to postpone."

At first, meditation and yoga science may seem difficult, but most of us have already tried the easy path, skimming along the surface of consciousness, led by our fears, anger and selfish desires. When students claim that changing old habits is too hard, we simply ask, for whom is it too hard? Who is the *real* you? The truth is that you are the Supreme Reality having a limited human experience. Is there anything too difficult for the Lord of the Universe or the Divine Mother? Certainly not. As part of your *sadhana*, simply refuse to identify with your small self.

For the earnest seeker, the initially required discipline soon yields to love, because *sadhana* makes one feel better physically, mentally, emotionally and spiritually. Meditators may appear to be disciplinarians, but are not. Meditators are pleasure seekers of the highest order.

Beware the "Yeah, But" *Mantra*

The transition from discipline to love, however, can sometimes be quite challenging. For that reason it's essential that you remain on guard for one of mankind's most debilitating *mantras*: "Yeah, but." Trying to maintain its power, the ego will surreptitiously undercut your resolve by first acknowledging the value of the teaching, and then by denying its appropriateness for you. "Yeah," the ego agrees, "this knowledge is very profound—*but* it's just not right for us at this time." As part of your *sadhana*, whenever you hear this kind of seductive argument, confront it immediately and let the *buddhi* expose the ego's nefarious attempt to play one of its trump cards.

The truth is, there's no greater adventure awaiting any of us. Taking to the spiritual life is like continually surfing the big wave. Being consistently present in each moment transforms an ordinary life into a perpetually thrilling sequence of relationships. You never know from one moment to the next what action will be required of you—until the *buddhi* reflects intuitive wisdom from the Center of Consciousness and discriminates between the *preya* and *shreya*. Then, as a yoga scientist, you choose your response and employ it, with the skill and grace that are your birthright.

Every time we think, speak or act, we use some of our vital *prana*. That might not have concerned us in our teens or twenties, but for those living into their forties, fifties, sixties and beyond, a technology for renewing that creative force is invaluable. Regardless of age, everyone wants to be happy, healthy, creative, productive, loving and nurtured. Merely professing to be the architects of our lives does not assure a destiny free from the debilitating strictures of stress and disease. To attain the unbounded Life, Liberty and Happiness we seek, we need a practical framework that helps us transform every thought, word and deed into energy, will power and creativity. In our experience, yoga science is such a framework.

A Bird in the Hand

We conclude by sharing the story of a young man who was the student of a renowned sage. Like most intelligent young people, the student enjoyed impressing his celebrated teacher.

One day he devised a scheme to prove his intelligence and also to impress his fellow classmates.

The student decided to bring a songbird to class, hold the bird in his closed hand, and ask the teacher if the bird were alive or dead. If the teacher said the bird were alive, the boy planned to crush and kill the bird, open his hand and show the teacher that the bird was dead. This, of course, would prove the teacher wrong.

If, however, the teacher said the bird were dead, the child planned to open his hand carefully, allowing the bird to fly away. And again the teacher would be proven wrong. The student believed that regardless of how the teacher answered his question, it would be the wrong answer.

The day finally arrived and the boy came to class with the bird. When called on by the teacher, the young man rose from his seat and in front of all the students asked, "Sir," in my hand I have a bird. Is the bird alive or is the bird dead?"

The teacher thought for a moment and looked at the lad. Then he replied, "My son, the life or death of the bird lies in your hand."

The same is true for yoga science and meditation. We have been richly blessed by wonderful teachers over the past thirty years. Now, with enormous gratitude in our hearts, we lovingly pass this knowledge on to you. To the best of our ability, we have offered you our experiences and practical understanding.

However, even if we have been one hundred percent successful in sharing what we have gained through our own *sadhana*, that would equal only fifty percent of the equation—for the "life or death of this bird" (the bird of *Peace, Happiness and Freedom from Fear*) "lies in your hand."

Be That which You Are

The practice of yoga science is not a pill you swallow to eliminate pain or instantly gain something you want. The extent to which you work with this teaching is entirely up to you. If you are sincerely interested in becoming free from pain and bondage, and are willing to transform your own fear, anger and self-centered desires into a loving, creative and uplifting force, your life will become the magnificent symphony the world is waiting to hear.

The Bible says, "Ask, and it shall be given you; seek, and ye shall find; knock, and it shall be opened unto you." But nowhere in the scriptures is there an instruction to knock only once. "Keep knocking; keep practicing," the sages would urge, "and the gates of heaven will open to you."

Students often ask if there is a higher level to this teaching, or some advanced course they should take. The answer is yes. The higher level and advanced course lies in your next thought. Who are you, and what are you going to do with that thought?

If you are curious and motivated to experiment with the practices presented in this book, always remember that you are indeed the architect of your life. Your thoughts determine your destiny. But each thought that comes into your awareness is only a suggestion of what to give your attention to. It is not an imperial command.

Every thought is a manifestation of your most powerful and abundant natural resource. Every thought has the potential to transform your life from its present limited condition into poetry and song. Developing the skills to steward this natural resource, therefore, is the most important task in life. The practices presented here are proven catalysts for that transformation—if you are earnest and sincere. Ultimately, everything yields to your earnestness.

The sages of all traditions teach that joy and fearlessness are the birthrights of every human being, and our own personal studies have taught us that yoga science and meditation are powerful and practical mechanisms for reclaiming this misplaced inheritance.

By relying exclusively on the Divine wisdom of the *buddhi* to determine which thoughts are served and which are not—in your mind, action and speech—you will experience a peace and creativity beyond your imagination.

Consciously and willingly control, conserve and transform

the energy of your mind, and claim your abundant human potential—as it was recognized by America's founding fathers. Remember: unbounded Life, Liberty and Happiness are your own unalienable rights because they *are* your Divine Self. The limitations of worry and fear have no valid place in your life. Be That which you are and live your life in freedom and joy.

May God bless you.
Om.
Shanti. Shanti. Shanti.
Peace. Peace. Peace.

Peace within you.
Peace within your immediate personal relationships.
Peace throughout the universe.

In service—with love,
your own Self in the forms of
Leonard Perlmutter and Jenness Cortez Perlmutter.

We pray to the Divinity in you.

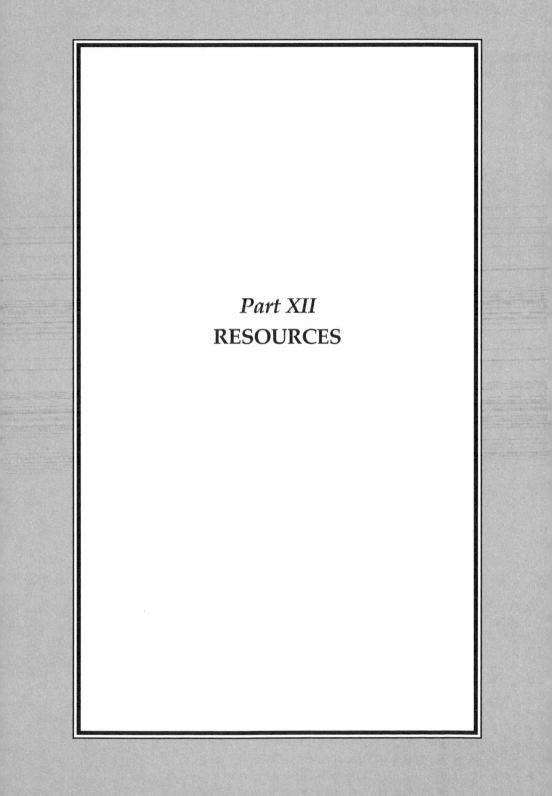

Part XII
RESOURCES

Glossary of Terms

ABHYASA – Constant spiritual practice.

ABHYANGA – In *Ayurveda*, a warm sesame oil massage.

ADONAI – A Hebrew name for the Divine Reality.

AGNI – The Sanskrit name for the fire element.

AHAMKARA – Ego or I-maker (one of the four major modifications or functions of the mind). See also *manas, chitta* and *buddhi*.

AHIMSA – The highest precept of yoga science and the first of Patanjali's *yamas* and *niyamas*. It means non-injury or non-harming. Since there is but one true reality (*Sat-Chit-Ananda*) from which all subtle and gross objects are manifest, if we think, speak or act in a harmful manner, somewhere in space and time that injury will come back on us. "As you sow, so shall you reap." It is equally true that if we think, speak or act in a selfless manner toward another, somewhere in space and time some benefit will be added unto us. "Blessed are the merciful, for they shall obtain mercy."

AJNA CHAKRA – The sixth *chakra*, located at the space between the two eyebrows.

ANAHATA CHAKRA – The fourth, or heart *chakra*, located at the midpoint between the two breasts. It is considered to be the demarcation between the lower animal consciousness primarily concerned with self-preservation, and the higher *chakras* that lead to an expansion of the self and union with the Divine.

ANANDA (ANAND) – Bliss or fullness; an aspect of our Essential Divine Identity. The other two aspects are *Sat* (eternal) and *Chit* (conscious).

ANNAMAYA KOSHA – The physical body; sheath of food and water.

APARIGRAHA – Non-possessiveness; the fifth yogic virtue presented in the *yamas*.

ARTHA – Material and social security (one of the fourfold goals of achievement for a successful human life). See also *dharma, kama* and *moksha*.

ASANA – Physical posture; the third rung of classical yoga science.

ASHRAM – A place where yoga scientists gather to study and to practice *sadhana* in a protected setting.

ASHTANGA YOGA – Literally, "eight-limbed" yoga. Also known as *raja yoga*, it is the basis of yoga science as codified around 200 A.D. by the sage Patanjali in the Yoga Sutras. It consists of spiritual practices of internal purification for the purpose of Self-realization. See *yama, niyama, asana, pranayama, pratyahara, dharana, dhyana* and *samadhi*.

ASTEYA – Non-stealing; the third yogic virtue presented in the *yamas*.

ATMAN – The pure Self; the Divine Reality (*Sat-Chit-Ananda*) that resides within the individual *jiva* (body-mind-sense complex). Just as the space of one room in a house is the same as the space in every other room, the *Atman* is identical in every being. Differing walls and furnishings make two rooms appear dissimilar, but the space in one does not differ from the space in the other. Different bodies and habits make human beings appear to be separate, but the Essential Nature of all is one and the same *Atman*. The collective *Atman* is called *Brahman*.

AUM – The sacred *mantra* or vibration of creation (*OM*). The A, U, M and the silence that follows represent the four states of consciousness: waking, dreaming, deep sleep and *turiya* (the transcendent state existing beyond the limitations of mind). *AUM* is considered to be the "mother of all *mantras*" because it contains all past, present and future manifestations.

AYURVEDA – Science of Life. A medical system intuited by meditators approximately five thousands years ago. *Ayurveda* is based on the concept that within the parameters of our genetic make-up, optimal health is achieved by maintaining the unique balance of the five basic elements with which we were born. These elements are ether (space), air, fire, water and earth. See *vata*, *pitta* and *kapha*.

BINDU – Point of concentrated attention.

BRAHMACHARYA – Moderation of energy, commonly translated as chastity; the fourth yogic virtue presented in the *yamas*.

BRAHMA – God as the creator; one aspect of the Hindu trinity.

BRAHMAN – The absolute, undifferentiated Divine Reality. See *Atman*.

BUDDHI – That function of the mind that has the power to discriminate, determine, judge and decide (conscience, Holy Spirit). *Buddhi* discriminates between the *preya* and *shreya*. It reflects intuitive wisdom from the Center of Consciousness (*Chit*), unerringly advising us which action will lead us for our highest and greatest good. Dis-ease occurs when our thoughts, words and deeds are not in harmony with the *buddhi*.

CAVE OF THE HEART – A space in the subtle body, located at the level of the heart, between the two breasts.

CHAKRA – Literally, wheel or circle. In yoga science, it refers to a psychoenergetic center of consciousness. The seven primary *chakras* are situated between the base of the spine and the crown of the head. The lower *chakras* represent our animal consciousness, dealing with self-preservation and reproduction. The higher *chakras* represent our expanding consciousness and identification with the Divine unity of all life. See also *muladhara*, *svadhishthana*, *manipura*, *anahata*, *vishuddha*, *ajna* and *sahasrara chakras*.

CHIT – Consciousness; awareness and wisdom—an aspect of our true Divine identity. See also *Sat* and *Ananda*.

CHITTA – Unconscious mind; the function of the mind that serves as the storehouse of consciousness (merits and demerits). It consists of information related to self-preservation, attachments and our learned mental processes for dealing with emotions, desires, memories and imaginings.

CHRIST – From the Greek word meaning "the anointed one."

In yoga science the *Christ* represents the wisdom of Divine light within each human being.

CONTEMPLATION – A daily review of all our actions (thoughts, words and deeds), assessing which opportunities were successfully acted upon for our highest good and which were not.

CORPSE POSE – The yoga posture known as *shavasana* in which the student lies motionless on the back with arms away from the torso, legs apart, and the palms of the hands facing upward.

CROCODILE POSE – A yoga posture in which the correct movement of diaphragmatic breathing is easily experienced while lying on the floor.

DESIRE – The fuel of action. Every desire is composed of energy, will power and consciousness. See *kama*.

DHARANA – One-pointed attention. This is the sixth rung of classical yoga science.

DHYANA – Meditation. This is the seventh rung of classical yoga science. .

DHARMA – The eternal law that upholds and maintains individual and social order. Also, the spiritual and ethical disciplines that, if practiced, guide humanity toward its highest destiny. Duty; right action. One of the fourfold goals of achievement for a successful human life. See *artha, kama* and *moksha*.

DIS-EASE – Pain is the shadow of the outstretched hand of Divine Providence. Physical, mental or emotional dis-ease, therefore, is usually an indication that our thoughts, words and/or actions are not completely aligned with the wisdom of the *buddhi*; not in harmony with *ahimsa*.

DOSHA – In *Ayurveda*, any of the three basic constitutions or body types: *vata, pitta* and *kapha*.

DVESHA – An aversion to the unpleasant (dislike); the opposite of *raga*, an attraction to the pleasant (that which is liked).

EGO – *Ahamkara* or I-Maker. In yoga science, ego is the psychological conditioning by which a person experiences himself or herself as an individual—apart from other animate and inanimate manifestations. Identification with the ego is said to be the root cause of pain and is a major stumbling block on the spiritual path.

ERETZ YISRAEL – Land of Israel (land of milk and honey) refers to the Inner Witness in the cave of the heart. *Eretz Yisrael* has nothing to do with geography or statehood. As Jesus the Christ taught, "The kingdom of heaven is within."

GUNAS – The three forces active in all physical, mental and emotional aspects of the phenomenal world (*prakriti*). See *tamas, rajas* and *sattva*.

GURU – The force of Divine light and wisdom that dispels the darkness of ignorance.

HATHA YOGA – The first four limbs (*yamas, niyamas, asana* and *pranayama*) of *raja yoga* that combine to prepare a student for higher meditation practices.

HEART CHAKRA – See *anahata chakra*.

I AMNESS – The first human differentiation in the One Absolute Reality; individual consciousness. By contemplating the *I-amness*, we become aware of the Eternal Witness within and are led to a direct experience of Divine Reality. See *Sat, Chit* and *Ananda*.

IDA – A primary *nadi* located along the left side of *sushumna* channel. It represents passive and intuitive feminine energy. The *ida* stimulates the brain's right hemisphere, controls mental processes and exemplifies the coolness of the moon.

ISHVARA PRANIDHANA – Surrender to the Ultimate truth; the fifth yogic virtue presented in the *niyamas*.

JAPA – Continuous attention to the silent repetition of the *mantra*. In Christianity, *japa* is known as prayer without ceasing.

JIVA – A living human being; the entity comprised of the soul (*Atman*) plus the physical body-mind-sense complex.

KAMA – Pleasure in fulfilling desires. One of the four-fold goals of achievement for a successful human life. See also *dharma, artha* and *moksha*.

KAPHA – In *Ayurveda*, the body type (*dosha*) in which the elements of water and earth predominate.

KARMA – Action; especially past actions that will lead to certain results in a cause and effect relationship. According to yoga traditions, a *karma* performed with selfish motivation results in bondage, while the same *karma,* if performed selflessly—in the service of *dharma*—brings freedom.

KARMA YOGA – Action performed for the welfare of another and in fulfillment of one's *dharma.* Giving away the fruit of one's action.

KRODHA – Anger.

KUNDALINI – The feminine creative energy, *shakti*; the power of consciousness.

MALA – A rosary-like string of beads used in the meditational practice of *japa.*

MANAS – That modification of the mind that organizes information received from the senses, ego and the unconscious, and presents alternatives and their probable consequences to our awareness. *Manas* is constantly asking the question, "Should I do it, or should I not do it?"

MANIPURA CHAKRA – The third, or navel, *chakra.*

MANTRA – A compact prayer, examples of which are found in all spiritual traditions. *Mantras* usually contain the name of the Divine Reality. Repetition of the *mantra* generates love, fearlessness and strength. Through its earnest repetition, the *mantra* leads to Self-realization. See *japa.*

MAYA – The illusory force (an aspect of the One Reality) that produces the appearance of the external world, the deception of bondage and the delusion that there is something to be liberated from.

MOKSHA – Liberation; freedom from all pain and bondage. One of the fourfold goals of achievement for a successful human life. See *artha, kama* and *dharma.*

MULADHARA CHAKRA – The first, or root, *chakra,* located at the base of the spine.

NADI – A channel, or river, of moving energy (*prana*) in the subtle body. The complex network composed of thousands of *nadis* sustains human life. See *ida, pingala, sushumna* and *pranamaya kosha.*

NADI SHODHANA – A *pranayama* practice that focuses and quiets the mind and oxygenates the blood, thereby increasing physical and mental energy.

NAMASTE – The traditional greeting of India and yoga scientists, "I pray to the Divinity in you."

NETI POT – The small vessel from which warm saline water is passed through the nasal passages to rinse away mucus, allergens and airborne particles.

NIRVANA – Literally, "blow out" or "extinguish." In Buddhism, the illuminated state of consciousness in which all pain and suffering subsides; freedom from desire. An approximate equivalent of *samadhi*, the eighth rung of classical yoga science.

NIYAMAS – Restraints; disciplinary guidelines for self-transformation. This is the second rung of classical yoga science, consisting of purity (*saucha*), contentment (*santosha*), austerity (*tapas*), self-study (*svadhyaya*) and surrender to the Ultimate truth (*Ishvara pranidhana*).

OM – See *AUM*.

PINGALA – A primary *nadi* located along the right side of the *sushumna* channel. It represents active male energy. The *pingala* stimulates the brain's left hemisphere, controls the body's vital processes and exemplifies the heat of the sun.

PITTA – In *Ayurveda*, the body type (*dosha*) in which the elements of fire and water predominate.

PRAKRITI – The basic unconscious principle or substance of the phenomenal world, composed of the three *gunas*. See also *Purusha*.

PRANA – The first unit of life; life force. In breathing, air is the vehicle for vital *prana* to enter and animate the city of life (body-mind-sense complex).

PRANAMAYA KOSHA – The energy body; the subtle sheath of *nadis* and *prana*.

PRANAYAMA – Literally, control of the life force; yogic breathing exercises. This is the third rung of classical yoga science.

PRATYAHARA – Control of the senses. This is the fifth rung of classical yoga science.

PRAYER – An essential element in the practice of yoga science and philosophy. God-centered prayer develops a positive relationship with the Divine Inner Dweller.

PREYA – Short-term ego or sense gratification.

PURUSHA – The conscious principle; the eternal Divine Self (*Sat-Chit-Ananda*). Through the conscious power of *Purusha*, *prakriti* (the individual *jiva*) becomes the enjoyer of pleasure and the sufferer of pain.

RAGA – That which is liked (pleasant); the opposite of *dvesha*, that which is disliked (unpleasant).

RAJA YOGA – Literally, the royal path. See *ashtanga* yoga.

RAJAS – One of the three attributes (*gunas*) of *prakriti*. The qualities of activity and restlessness. See also *tamas* and *sattva*.

RENUNCIATION – Surrender or sacrifice. In order to attain freedom from pain, misery and bondage, every thought, word and action that serves the *preya* (as suggested by *buddhi*) is to be renounced in favor of the *shreya*. See *buddhi*, desire.

REPENTANCE – A pledge to the Divine Self that the next time a particular *preya* presents itself, the seeker will choose the *shreya* and surrender the *preya*—in mind, action and speech.

SADHANA – Commitment to spiritual practices associated with meditation and the science of yoga. See yoga, *abhyasa*.

SADHAKA – A practicing spiritual seeker; a yoga scientist.

SAHASRARA CHAKRA – The seventh and highest *chakra*, located at the crown of the head; the thousand-petaled lotus.

SAMADHI – The merging of individual consciousness with the Absolute Reality. This is the eighth rung of classical yoga science.

SAMSKARA – A deep-seated inclination to think or behave in a certain way; a habit pattern created in the unconscious mind (*chitta*) and sustained by our attention and attachment.

SANKALPA – Resolve, will; the power of determination.

SANTOSHA – Contentment; the second yogic virtue embodied in the *niyamas*.

SAT – That aspect of our essential Divine Identity that is eternal—subject neither to birth nor death. *Sat* is self-existent—

dependent on nothing else for its creation or sustenance. See *Chit* and *Ananda*.

SATSANG – Company of the wise. Often refers to a gathering of like-minded spiritual seekers for the purpose of enhancing their *sadhana*.

SATTVA – One of the three attributes (*gunas*) of *prakriti*. The qualities of tranquility, equanimity, lightness and illumination. See also *rajas* and *tamas*.

SATYA – Truthfulness; the second yogic virtue presented in the *yamas*.

SAUCHA – Purity; the first yogic virtue presented in the *niyamas*.

SHANTI – Peace.

SHAVASANA – See corpse posture.

SHAKTI – The dynamic, manifesting power of consciousness; the source of the phenomenal world; *kundalini*.

SHIVA – God as the destroyer; one aspect of the Hindu trinity. Also, pure, unmanifested consciousness, existence, bliss. For the yoga scientist, *Shiva* is the aspect of the Divine that dissolves our limitations.

SHRADDHA – A firm faith born of personal experience; trust. This is not blind faith, but the calm conviction that yoga science and philosophy can always be relied upon to remedy any dis-ease in one's life. This growing confidence grants the *sadhaka* an ease of being, in every circumstance.

SHREYA – That which may be initially neither attractive nor pleasant, but that leads us for our highest and greatest good. See *buddhi, preya*.

SUSHUMNA – The central *nadi* or channel; the conduit for the feminine energy of consciousness (*kundalini*). It runs from the base of the spine (*muladhara chakra*) to the crown of the head (*sahasrara chakra*). When both *ida* and *pingala* are flowing equally, the central channel is opened and the mind enters a meditative state. See *ida, pingala* and *nadi*.

SVADHISHTHANA CHAKRA – The second *chakra*, located at the level of the pubic bone. *Shakti's* true abode.

SVADHYAYA – Self-study; the fourth yogic virtue presented in the *niyamas*.

TAMAS – One of the three attributes (*gunas*) of *prakriti*. The qualities of lethargy, inertia, heaviness and darkness. See also *rajas* and *sattva*.

TAPAS – Austerities, self-discipline; the third yogic virtue presented in the *niyamas*.

TATTVA – Any of the five basic elements of the manifest world: space (ether), air, fire, water and earth.

TURIYA – The fourth, transcendent state of consciousness beyond the waking, dreaming and deep sleep states.

UPANISHAD – Literally to sit down devotedly at the foot of a teacher. Any one of several philosophical Indian scriptures which form the foundation of yoga science.

VAIRAGYA – Detachment, non-attachment, dispassion; an invaluable aid in making reliable decisions. Love in action.

VASANA – A latent tendency that gives rise to the formation of a *samskara*.

VATA – In *Ayurveda*, the body type (*dosha*) in which the elements of ether (space) and air predominate.

VICHARA – Inquiry into the nature of the Self. For instance, contemplation of the question, "Who am I?"

VISHNU – God as the sustainer of the universe; an aspect of the Hindu trinity. See also *Brahma* and *Shiva*.

VISHUDDHA CHAKRA – The fifth *chakra*, located at the pit of the throat.

VIVEKA – The power of discrimination; the employment of the *buddhi*—that which reflects the wisdom of the supercon-scious mind.

YAJNA (YAGNA) – Offering or sacrifice—the very nature of the universe; the act or attitude that helps create and maintain harmony in our personal, social and cosmic lives.

YAMAS – Controls or observances. This is the first rung of classical yoga science consisting of non-violence (*ahimsa*), truthfulness (*satya*), non-stealing (*asteya*), moderation of energy (*brahmacharya*), non-possessiveness (*aparigraha*).

YOGA – An ancient philosophy and science codified by Patanjali. Yoga, which literally means "yoke" or union, is a system of physical and mental practices that manage and purify the energy and internal processes of the *jiva* to facilitate conscious union with *Brahman*.

YOGA SUTRAS – Text written by Patanjali around 200 A.D. codifying the ancient oral teachings of yoga science. The *yoga sutras* delineate the science and philosophy known as *ashtanga* or *raja yoga*.

The Illumined Man

Bhagavad Gita, Chapter 2, Verses 54-72

ARJUNA:

Tell me of the man
Who lives in wisdom,
Ever aware of the Self, O Krishna;
How does he talk, how sit,
How move about?

SRI KRISHNA:

He lives in wisdom
Who sees himself in all and all in him,
Whose love for the Lord of Love
Has consumed every selfish desire
And sense-craving tormenting the heart.
Not agitated by grief
Nor hankering after pleasure,
He lives free from lust and fear and anger.
Fettered no more
By selfish attachments,
He is not elated by good fortune
Nor depressed by bad.
Such is the seer.

Even as a tortoise draws in its limbs
The sage can draw in his senses at will.
An aspirant abstains from sense-pleasures,
But he still craves for them.
These cravings all disappear
When he sees the Lord of love.
For even of one who treads the path
The stormy senses can sweep off the mind.
But he lives in wisdom who subdues them,
And keeps his mind ever absorbed in Me.

When you keep thinking
About sense-objects,
Attachment comes.
Attachment breeds desire,
The lust of possession which, when thwarted,
Burns to anger.
Anger clouds the judgment
And robs you of the power
To learn from past mistakes.
Lost is the discriminative faculty,
And your life is utter waste.

But when you move
Amidst the world of sense
From both attachment
And aversion freed,
There comes the peace
In which all sorrows end,
And you live in the wisdom
Of the Self.

The disunited mind is far from wise;
How can it meditate?
How be at peace?
When you know no peace,
How can you know joy?
When you let your mind

Follow the siren call of the senses,
They carry away your better judgment
As a typhoon drives a boat
Off the charted course to its doom.

Use your mighty arms
To free the senses
From attachment and aversion alike,
And live in the full wisdom of the Self.
Such a sage
Awakes to light in the night
Of all creatures.
Wherein they are awake
Is the night of ignorance to the sage.

As the rivers flow into the ocean
But cannot make
The vast ocean o'erflow,
So flow the magic streams
Of the sense-world
Into the sea of peace that is the sage.

He is forever free
Who has broken out
Of the ego-cage of *I* and *mine*
To be united with the Lord of love.
This is the supreme state.
Attain thou this
And pass from death to immortality.

ॐ

Translated by Eknath Easwaran, from *God Makes the Rivers to Flow*. Copyright ©1982, 1991 by the Blue Mountain Center of Meditation. Reprinted by permission of Nilgiri Press, P. O. Box 256, Tomales, California 94971. www.nilgiri.org.

Recommended Reading

Swami Rama of the Himalayas: *Art of Joyful Living, Life Here and Hereafter, Living With The Himalayan Masters, Love and Family Life, Path of Fire and Light (Vols. I and II), Perennial Psychology of the Bhagavad Gita, Sacred Journey, Sadhana, Science of Breath.*

Eknath Easwaran: *End of Sorrow, Like A Thousand Suns, To Love Is to Know Me, Conquest of Mind, Dhammapada, Dialogue With Death, Gandhi the Man, God Makes the Rivers to Flow, Original Goodness, Upanishads, Words to Live By.*

Swami Veda Bharati: *Light of Ten Thousand Suns, Philosophy of Hatha Yoga.*

Leonard Perlmutter: *Life, Liberty and Happiness* CD.

Ramesh Balsekar: *Duet of One, Final Truth.*

Various Authors: *Anatomy of Hatha Yoga*, Dr. David Coulter; *Autobiography of a Yogi*, Paramahansa Yogananda; *The Ayurvedic Cookbook*, Amadea Morningstar; *I Am That*, Nisargadatta Maharaj; *Perfect Health*, Deepak Chopra; *Sermon on the Mount According to Vedanta*, Swami Prabhavananda.

Healthful Items:
Neti Pot, Breath Pillow.

Each book and healthful item has been personally chosen by Leonard and Jenness Perlmutter to aid your understanding and experience of the heart and science of yoga. All are available through the American Meditation Institute bookstore.

www.americanmeditation.org **Tel. (800) 234-5115**

Practices and Important Principles

About the Authors

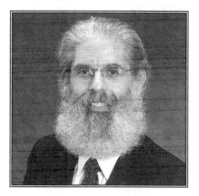

Leonard Perlmutter
Founder and Co-Director, American Meditation Institute

Leonard Perlmutter has been a student of yoga science since 1975 and has served on the faculties of the New England Institute of Ayurvedic Medicine in Boston, Massachusetts and the International Himalayan Yoga Teachers Association in Calgary, Canada. Leonard is currently an adjunct professor at the College of St. Rose in Albany, New York where he teaches yoga and meditation. He has studied in Rishikesh, India and is a direct disciple of Sri Swami Rama of the Himalayas. Leonard graduated from the American University with degrees in Political Science and International Relations and attended the George Washington University School of Law. From 1971 to 1975 he was the editor and publisher of the *Washington Park*

Spirit newspaper in Albany, New York. In 1976 he produced a bi-centennial film history of Troy, New York entitled, *The Collar City Song*, and from 1977 to the present, has been president of Classic Gallery. In 1996 he founded the American Meditation Institute for Yoga Science and Philosophy in Averill Park, New York. He currently serves as the director of the Institute.

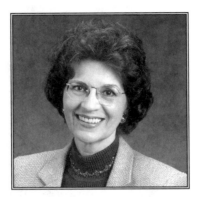

Jenness Cortez Perlmutter
Founder and Co-Director, American Meditation Institute

Jenness Cortez Perlmutter also has been a student of yoga science since 1975. Like her husband, Leonard, she has studied in Rishikesh, India and is a direct disciple of Sri Swami Rama of the Himalayas. Jenness graduated from the Herron School of Art with a five-year degree in Fine Arts and attended the Art Students League in New York. She is an internationally renowned artist.

American Meditation Institute
For Yoga Science and Philosophy

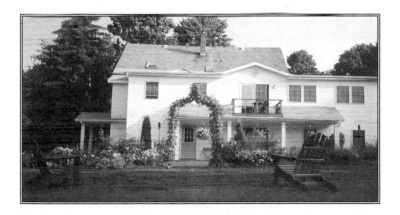

The American Meditation Institute was established in 1996 for the teaching and practice of authentic yoga science and philosophy. Located in the picturesque foothills of the Berkshire Mountains, *AMI* provides a peaceful, healthy setting to learn practical, holistic skills that improve physical, mental, emotional and spiritual well being.

Drawing upon all major meditation traditions, *AMI* offers a variety of classes and retreats that:

1. Empower students by awakening them to their individual potentials, freedom of choice and a vision of their own true spiritual nature.

2. Help students build confidence in their discriminative

capacity through daily exercise of conscious attention to the thought process and contemplation of their personal experiences.

3. Help students embrace those values which have the power to protect, uphold and transform the individual and society.

4. Help students understand and implement these values through the regular, systematic practice of meditation and yoga science in their daily lives.

5. Help students recognize and appreciate that these same values are also found within their own spiritual traditions.

Classes, Retreats, Newsletter and Home-Study

Weekly classes, special retreats, a home-study course and an inspiring *Transformation* newsletter are offered throughout the year. Call, or visit our website for specific details.

Membership

The American Meditation Institute is a 501(c)3 non-profit educational organization. Please call, write or visit our website for information on how you can support this teaching.

Teachers' Training Program

If you would like to become a teacher of yoga science under the personal direction of Leonard Perlmutter, please inquire about our program for certification.

Speaker's Bureau

If you or your school, church, temple, yoga center, government, business, or civic organization is interested in hosting a workshop by Leonard Perlmutter, please contact the American Meditation Institute to make arrangements.

How to Contact AMI

For information about our programs, please contact us at 60 Garner Road, Averill Park, NY 12018, Tel. (800) 234-5115, www.americanmeditation.org.

Index

Acknowledgements on this page constitute an extension of the copyright page.

Grateful acknowledgement is made to the following
for the use of new and previously published material:

Cover photograph: *"Lotus—Purity,"* © 2002, Gerry Gantt, GerryGantt@att.net, Fairfax, Virginia.

Illustrations on pages 246, 247, 261 and 263 Copyright © 2004, William B. Westwood, Westwood Medical Communications, Albany, New York.

Photographs on pages 146, 147, 252, 254, 255, 264, 370-390, 393-400 Copyright © 2004, Michael Dzamen Photography, Troy, New York. Photographs on pages 489 and 490 by Joseph Mulone, The Photographers & Co., Schenectady, New York.

All excerpts from the *Bhagavad Gita* on pages 55, 61, 408 and 481 and the *Katha Upanishad* on pages 38 and 283 are from *"God Makes the Rivers to Flow,"* by Eknath Easwaran, founder of the Blue Mountain Center of Meditation. Copyright 1982, 1991 by the Blue Mountain Center of Meditation. These passages are reprinted by permission of Nilgiri Press, P. O. Box 256, Tomales, California 94971. www.nilgiri.org.

Excerpts on pages 46, 222, 293, 299 and 408 are from *"Dialogue With Death"* by Eknath Easwaran. Copyright ©1981 by the Blue Mountain Center of Meditation. Reprinted by permission of Nilgiri Press, P. O. Box 256, Tomales, California 94971. www.nilgiri.org.

Excerpts on pages 21, 90, 189, and 194-195 from *"I Am That: Talks with Shri Nisargadatta Maharaj"* translated from the Marathi tape recordings by Maurice Frydman." (1999) Copyright © 1973, Nisargadatta Maharaj. Used by permission of The Acorn Press, PO Box 3279, Durham, NC 27715.

The poem *Pillar of Light* by Swami Veda Bharati is reprinted from *"The Light of Ten Thousand Suns,"* © 1998, Published by Yes International Publishers, St. Paul, MN, www.yespublishers.com.

Notes